Future Opportunities and Tools for Emerging Challenges for HIV/AIDS Control

Edited by Samuel Okware

Published in London, United Kingdom

Future Opportunities and Tools for Emerging Challenges for HIV/AIDS Control
http://dx.doi.org/10.5772/intechopen.100820
Edited by Samuel Okware

Contributors
Rima Bazzi, Kayla Aleshire, Ramakrishna Prakash, Mysore Krishnamurthy Yashaswini, Ricardo Roberto De Souza Fonseca, Luiz Fernando Machado, Silvio Menezes, Aldemir Branco Oliveira-Filho, Carlos Gomes, Rogério Valois Laurentino, Tatiany Oliveira de Alencar Menezes, Tábata Resque Beckmann Carvalho, Paula Gabriela Faciola Pessoa de Oliveira, Erich Brito Tanaka, Jorge Sá Elias Nogueira, Marcelo Newton Carneiro, Paula Mendes Acatauassú Carneiro, Oscar Faciola Pessoa, Patricia de Almeida Rodrigues, Aluísio Ferreira Celestino Junior, Douglas Magno Guimarães, John Rubaihayo, Nazarius Mbona Tumwesigye, Josephine Birungi, Daniel Mesafint Belete, Manjaiah D. Huchaiah, Gordon Ogweno, Seggane Musisi, Noeline Nakasujja, Adenike O. Soogun, Ayesha B.M. Kharsany, Temesgen Zewotir, Delia North, Jacqueline Carol Matthews-Mthembu, Gadija Khan, Nirmala Pillay, Samuel Okware

First published in London, United Kingdom, 2023 by IntechOpen
IntechOpen is the global imprint of INTECHOPEN LIMITED, registered in England and Wales, registration number: 11086078, 5 Princes Gate Court, London, SW7 2QJ, United Kingdom
Printed in Croatia

British Library Cataloguing-in-Publication Data
A catalogue record for this book is available from the British Library

Additional hard and PDF copies can be obtained from orders@intechopen.com

Future Opportunities and Tools for Emerging Challenges for HIV/AIDS Control
Edited by Samuel Okware
p. cm.

This title is part of the Infectious Diseases Book Series, Volume 16
Topic: Viral Infectious Diseases
Series Editor: Alfonso J. Rodriguez-Morales
Topic Editor: Shailendra K. Saxena

Print ISBN 978-1-80356-176-9
Online ISBN 978-1-80356-177-6
eBook (PDF) ISBN 978-1-80356-178-3
ISSN 2631-6188

For EU product safety concerns:
IN TECH d.o.o., Prolaz Marije Krucifikse Kozulić 3, 51000 Rijeka, Croatia,
info@intechopen.com or visit our website at intechopen.com.

IntechOpen Book Series

Infectious Diseases

Volume 16

Aims and Scope of the Series

This series will provide a comprehensive overview of recent research trends in various Infectious Diseases (as per the most recent Baltimore classification). Topics will include general overviews of infections, immunopathology, diagnosis, treatment, epidemiology, etiology, and current clinical recommendations for managing infectious diseases. Ongoing issues, recent advances, and future diagnostic approaches and therapeutic strategies will also be discussed. This book series will focus on various aspects and properties of infectious diseases whose deep understanding is essential for safeguarding the human race from losing resources and economies due to pathogens.

Meet the Series Editor

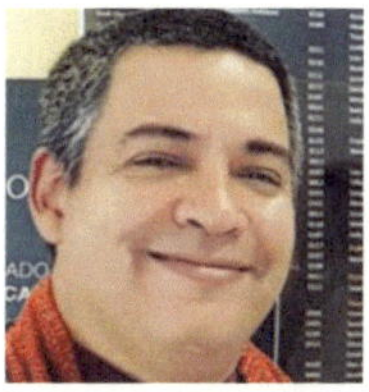

Dr. Rodriguez-Morales is an expert in tropical and emerging diseases, particularly zoonotic and vector-borne diseases (especially arboviral diseases). He is the president of the Travel Medicine Committee of the Pan-American Infectious Diseases Association (API), as well as the president of the Colombian Association of Infectious Diseases (ACIN). He is a member of the Committee on Tropical Medicine, Zoonoses, and Travel Medicine of ACIN. He is a vice-president of the Latin American Society for Travel Medicine (SLAMVI) and a Member of the Council of the International Society for Infectious Diseases (ISID). Since 2014, he has been recognized as a Senior Researcher, at the Ministry of Science of Colombia. He is a professor at the Faculty of Medicine of the Fundacion Universitaria Autonoma de las Americas, in Pereira, Risaralda, Colombia. He is an External Professor, Master in Research on Tropical Medicine and International Health, Universitat de Barcelona, Spain. He is also a professor at the Master in Clinical Epidemiology and Biostatistics, Universidad Científica del Sur, Lima, Peru. In 2021 he has been awarded the "Raul Isturiz Award" Medal of the API. Also, in 2021, he was awarded with the "Jose Felix Patiño" Asclepius Staff Medal of the Colombian Medical College, due to his scientific contributions to COVID-19 during the pandemic. He is currently the Editor in Chief of the journal Travel Medicine and Infectious Diseases. His Scopus H index is 47 (Google Scholar H index, 68).

Meet the Volume Editor

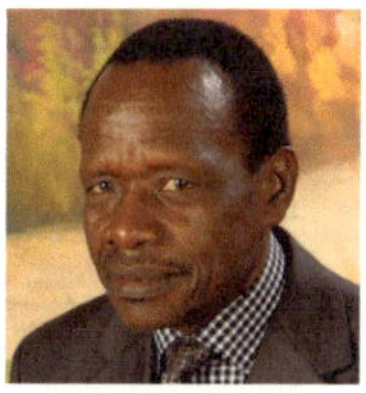

Samuel Okware is a public health specialist with a Ph.D. in Emerging Infections. He pioneered early studies that contributed to major declines in HIV infections in Uganda. He held several national public health appointments coordinating disease control, maternal and child health, and outbreak emergency response. He was a member of the WHO Expert Committee on Research and Development. He is the director general of the Uganda National Health Research Organization, which coordinates health research. He has published and edited several books on HIV and emerging infections. Dr. Okware is also an Associate Professor of Public Health and Epidemiology at Busitema University, Uganda, and the Uganda Christian University. He has received several national and international awards in recognition of his contributions to public health.

Contents

Preface

This book reviews and discusses future opportunities and tools for emerging challenges in HIV/AIDS control. The introductory section provides background on the progress and achievements made in the prevention and control of HIV/AIDS. Over time, new behavioral and societal challenges have emerged. For instance, prevention messages on risk reduction are being undermined by the successes in effective antiretroviral treatment. Complacency among the public, especially the youth, is gradually increasing. There are also emerging challenges on stagnating uptake of testing. The introduction briefly discusses these challenges and suggests future opportunities and tools for enhanced response.

Section 2 discusses challenges in surveillance and prevention. Behavior change is key to safe sexual practices and abstinence, and fidelity and condom use are key to prevention. However, surveillance systems for both case reporting and behavioral surveillance are poor in low-resource countries. Chapter 2 presents a systematic review of literature from thirteen countries, highlighting the obstacles that impact outcomes. The discussion concludes that deterioration of physical health, HIV-associated stigma, and costs, among other shortcomings, are major reasons for reduced uptake and access to services. The challenges undermining surveillance are also discussed. For instance, the chapter analyzes the risk factors associated with non-suppression of HIV viral load. The methodology used involves two sequential cross-sectional surveys conducted in 2014 and 2015 of viral load measurements in South Africa. The analysis is based on data from the HIV Incidence Provincial Surveillance System (HIPSS), which monitors HIV-related measures of HIV prevalence and incidence. According to the results, nearly half of the women surveyed had a non-suppressed viral load. Factors associated with non-suppression among women include a lack of knowledge of their HIV status, having a moderate-to-low perception of contracting HIV, and being unable to access antiretroviral therapy. Another study in Chapter 3 assesses spatial and temporal risk factors associated with the prevalence of opportunistic infections. With antiretroviral therapy, the frequency of such infections has been declining steadily, but with variations by region. The trends of these infections by region show that the commonest comorbidity by region is tuberculosis, whereas cancers are very rare. These findings are contrasted with those from the developed world.

Deep learning is a recent approach to predicting HIV test results and supporting testing services. The model in Chapter 4 analyzes demographic and sero-survey datasets from population surveys, following which the deep learning tool identifies people with HIV and estimates the prevalence of infection in the community. The model was used to construct an HIV status prediction system and results show that it has predictive accuracy of 85.3%. Such an approach based on demographic and survey data may be used to predict and forecast the HIV status of individuals. The modeling in the study supports planning and strategy development.

Section 3 discusses some emerging challenges in laboratory testing and the need for rapid, reliable, and relevant testing. Chapter 5 examines current HIV diagnostic tests and explains and provides a rationale for the use of these tests. It also discusses the various indications and criteria for HIV testing, and detection by stages and phases. It examines the difficulties encountered during the early window period of infection and suggests appropriate detection tools. It also describes the classifications of tests from first generation to fourth generation and makes recommendations for their appropriate and rational usage. Suggestions are also made for ideal screening and confirmatory tests for each stage of the disease.

There is also growing attention on platelet functions in people living with HIV/AIDS because of the high reported incidence of cardiovascular adverse effects, including thrombosis, in these individuals. Furthermore, the effects of antiretroviral therapy on platelet functions are not well understood. Chapter 6 reviews HIV-associated thrombocytopenia and discusses the immune complexes' environment including the cytokines and inflammatory markers in cytokine elaboration. The value of tests based on platelet aggregation is discussed by region, race, and ethnicity. The concept of "platelet exhaustion" where activated platelets continued to circulate in HIV infection but with decreased aggregation is also examined.

Section 4 discusses challenges in care. It includes specific systematic reviews of challenges in the care and management of perinatal HIV/AIDS. The prevention and management of perinatal HIV infections involves the administration of antiretroviral therapy to both the pregnant person and their child after delivery, in combination with regular HIV tests. The recommendations for ART medication in pregnant persons and neonates are often modeled after data obtained from non-pregnant adults or older children thus impacting efficacy and safety. Maternal physiology also changes throughout the gestational period and the pharmacodynamic parameters of a drug may be altered as the pregnancy progresses. In neonates, physiologic considerations are important when selecting safe and effective medications. Due to the underdeveloped immune system of the infant, an antigen test is not as sensitive as virologic testing. Chapter 7 examines subsequent implications, identifies barriers, and suggests options for treatment success. The study proposes revised treatment guidelines for the perinatal period for the mother and neonate. Chapter 8 discusses oral lesions common in people infected with HIV. Periodontal disease can be categorized simply as gingivitis and periodontitis and necrotizing periodontitis. It is an infectious and inflammatory disease with multifactorial etiology. This chapter provides an update on periodontal disease, discussing risk factors for oral lesions and their mechanisms.

Section 4 also addresses mental health. Effective lifelong treatment for HIV/AIDS requires a sound mind to ensure compliance and adherence. Mental disorders are often neglected, yet they undermine treatment and prevention. Chapter 9 discusses disorders such as antisocial personality disorders and borderline personality disorders. It presents a detailed examination of the various acute psychological reactions following HIV diagnosis and makes recommendations for how to manage such problems as an integrated component of HIV/AIDS. The analysis demonstrates that mental illnesses compromise treatment outcomes and undermine HIV care and prevention. The chapter concludes by recommending the integration of mental health care into HIV prevention and prevention programs.

Section 5 discusses the implications of social stigma on the health outcomes of marginalized groups. Chapter 10 focuses on the stigma associated with HIV, mental health, and sexual orientation and gender identities. Public education to regulate sexual behavior is often associated with stigma. These forms of stigma often lead to discrimination and lowered self-esteem as well as social devaluation in society. The chapter presents a systematic review of experiences in South Africa, a country with a history of complex socially structured norms based on stereotypes. The discussion suggests that the multi-layered nature of stigma and its interconnectivity makes it difficult to implement robust interventions. The chapter discusses policy implications and makes key recommendations for promoting social inclusion and improving access to care.

Social frameworks are needed to promote social inclusion and gainful social integration. These additional social issues require action as the elimination of HIV is targeted.

Section 6 reviews the health and human rights associated with HIV/AIDS. The epidemiological, and clinical approaches to HIV/AIDS are inextricably intertwined with the protection of health and human rights. Chapter 11 examines the legal human rights and health rights aspects and discusses the extent to which HIV/AIDS litigation has advanced the prevention, control, and treatment of HIV/AIDS and related issues on health and human rights. Advancing health rights through the courts highlights the limitations of law as a human rights tool in holding government service providers more accountable. The chapter examines several successful examples in which courts not only upheld the rights of individuals but also forced governments to address the holistic management of people living with HIV. The chapter recommends that the full realization of health rights to achieve health equity requires that rights-based approaches be mainstreamed into national public and private health service strategic plans and research.

I thank the chapter authors for their contributions. I also thank Author Service Managers Josip Knapić and Marica Novakovic at IntechOpen for their invaluable support and assistance.

Samuel Okware, Ph.D.
Associate Professor Public Health,
Busitema University,
Busitema, Uganda

Section 1

Introduction

Chapter 1

Introductory Chapter: Future Opportunities and Tools for Emerging Challenges for HIV/AIDS Control

Samuel Okware

1. Introduction

It is almost 40 years since the first cases of HIV/AIDS were identified. The disease was a tragedy of monumental dimensions. Millions have died leaving families helpless especially in developing countries. Experiences of unprecedented suffering and social disruption prevailed in the early part of the pandemic. Orphans became heads of households and carried the family burden as the disease killed both parents. Gradually over time, some feelings of hope emerged following the launch of the UN Global Strategy for Prevention and Control of HIV/AIDS. Steady progress was made in prevention and management of persons living with HIIV/AIDS. Anti-retroviral treatment offered the best hope for the patients. The quality of life for people living with HIV/AIDS steadily improved on with anti-retroviral treatment. Mortality has reduced and AIDS is no longer a death sentence, but a chronic disease. Longevity too for them has improved significantly since the introduction of Anti-Retroviral Therapy in 2003. Opportunistic Infections, the major causes of death too have declined. New infections and HIV-related mortally is declining worldwide [1, 2]. The UNAIDS global HIV/AIDS program [3] based on combination strategy for risk reduction targeting sexual behavior has successfully reversed trends in new infections. The current UNAIDS Global Strategy targets elimination of infection by 2030 by focusing more on reducing inequities hindering progress, enhancing people-centered services, and removing legal and social constraints that hamper human rights. The overall goal of the strategy is based on human rights, gender equity free of discrimination. The strategy prioritizes the elimination of HIV infection particularly among children. The new strategy priorities the interventions for the prevention of mother to child transmission with a target of elimination of mother-to-child transmission. Reviews on the evolution of the disease are helpful in realizing missed opportunities to help in the future outbreaks.

2. Challenges in behavior change

Behavior change for safe sexual practices is essential in mitigation of spread of infection. The key components of the these safe sexual practices include abstinence, fidelity, and condom use and have been vital to HIV prevention [4]. Messages need

IntechOpen

to be targeted using more accurate, rational, and evidence-based interventions. However, poor surveillance systems for both case reporting and behavioral surveillance remains weak especially where HIV burden is greatest. Furthermore, stigma and societal issues persist, which are barriers that have partly promoted perceived low risk among the communities [5]. There are instances where intensified implementation of the combination interventions on key populations within the context of the highest-risk scenarios and targeting local HIV epidemiology has yielded good results. Such outstanding examples ought to be shared as we approach the last mile in our containment efforts. Targeting of appropriate packaged messages has worked in some communities, the experience of which could be benchmarked toward the elimination of infection.

Other new behavioral and societal challenges have emerged in some instances. For instance, prevention messages on risk reduction are being undermined by the successes following effective and successful anti-retroviral treatment. Complacency among the general public especially the youth is gradually growing. The youth do not see the disease as a threat encouraged by the absence of the earliest typical clinical features of extreme body wasting associated with high fever and diarrhea [6]. Special interventions including condoms are to be scaled up for key populations. The high prevalence of discordancy of infection among couples in committed relationships needs to be addressed. Instead of focusing on individuals, programs should aim at couples as an entity since the risks are similar so as to maintain the discordancy in stable relationships.

Behavior and mental health are often linked. However, this relationship is often missed when planning for prevention strategies and behavior change. Sexual compulsivity and hyperactivity, for instance, are rarely considered yet it is a mental behavioral deficit that needs attention in some communities. This trait may be associated with high risk and addressing it could have some impact in reduction of HIV transmission. Mental health should be integrated into the next programs for the elimination of infection.

3. The test and treat policy

The test and treat policy is regarded as an effective way to reduce infections because undetectable viral load translates into no transmission in most circumstances. This approach should significantly support the elimination of infection. The UNAIDS global 90–90–90 strategy for the elimination of the scourge by 2030 is being implemented worldwide, but with varying levels of success. This strategy is based on test and treat policy and the sustenance of quality undetectable viral loads. For such intervention to be effective, the tests need to be accessible. Equally important for the client is that access is user-friendly. While the classifications of tests from first generation to fourth generation is well described for appropriate usage, the limited financial environment presents challenges for optimal work and calls for rational more appropriate tools. For instance, the challenges of screening and detection during the acute and the window period post infection should be examined to enhance accuracy and appropriateness. The tests should be rapid and of high quality. Such tests are most appropriate in low resource settings where costs and convenience remain a major consideration. This challenge is most pronounced in low-income countries. While early testing and diagnosis are key to achieving zero new infections, universal access to testing and treatment remains a herculean task. In Sub-Saharan Africa, for instance, testing is not optimal due to weak health systems and costs. Other impediments may include deterioration of clinical status or death of a partner. In local settings this can significantly impact on uptake [5]. Some countries have coped with this by the expansion of primary health care through community engagements strategy and effort.

4. Challenges in perinatal diagnosis and care

Perinatal care and management of mother and baby need clear guidelines. Perinatal diagnosis preceding management in particular remains a challenge. For instance, the guidelines for the management of perinatal transmission in neonates remain unclear. This is primarily due to the administration of Anti-retroviral Therapy to pregnant mothers and her child after delivery. Thus, the identification and management of HIV infection among neonates during the perinatal period are yet to be made clearer. Thus, there is a paucity of evidence for the rationale management of HIV-infected neonates. The discussion should be made on the implications and barriers for treatment guidelines for successful outcomes for neonates and should be examined for the better management of these cases.

Overall some laboratory functions and parameters functions are yet to be clarified. For instance, the role of platelet parameters and pathophysiology is not fully understood in the managing people living with HIV/AIDS. There should therefore be increasing attention on platelet functions among this group because of reported cardiovascular severe adverse effects and thrombosis and related conditions [7]. More studies and evidence are required to improve care and social well-being.

5. Responding to challenges for the elderly

The elderly living with HIV/AIDS will increase with improved anti-retroviral treatment. A resurgence of noncommunicable diseases is bound to grow. Diabetes and hypertension usually associated with obesity will present special challenges during this life extension. Additional social programs will be needed to provide amenities for the elderly. They will need support to promote social inclusion and gainful integration in order to participate in community and societal agendas. Frameworks for housing, jobs, and direct financial support are challenges to consider during the HIV/AIDS long-term recovery.

The book chapters in the proposed updates will examine and discuss arguments on these crucial issues, the consideration of which could be the recipe for the improvement of strategies for the elimination of HIV/AIDS by 2030 and wellness for all.

Author details

Samuel Okware
Uganda National Health Research Organization, Uganda

*Address all correspondence to: okwares@gmail.com

References

[1] Kambugu A, Rhein J, O'Brien M, Janoff EN, Ronald AR, et al. Outcomes of cryptococcal meningitis in Uganda before and after the availability of HAART. Clinical Infectious Diseases. 2008;**46**(11):1694-1701

[2] Morgan D, Mayanja B, Whitworth JA. Progression to symptomatic disease in people infected with HIV-1 in rural Uganda: Prospective cohort study. BMJ (Online). 2002;**324**:193-196

[3] Global AIDS Strategy 2021-2026 — End Inequalities. End AIDS. Available from: 21 March 2021

[4] Okware S et al. Fighting HIV/AIDS: Is success possible? Bulletin of the World Health Organization. 2001;**79**(12):1113-1120

[5] Musheke M, Ntalasha H, Gari S, et al. A systematic review of qualitative findings on factors enabling and deterring uptake of HIV testing in Sub-Saharan Africa. BMC Public Health. 2013;**13**:220. DOI: 10.1186/1471-2458-13-220

[6] Okware SI. Towards a national AIDS-control program in Uganda. The Western Journal of Medicine. 1987;**147**(6):726-729

[7] Ahonkhai AA, Gebo KA, Steiff MB, Moore RD, Segal JB. Venous thromboembolism in patients with HIV/AIDS. A case-control study. Journal of Acquired Immune Deficiency Syndromes. 2008;**48**(3):310-314

Section 2

Surveillance and Prevention

Chapter 2

Spatial Variation and Factors Associated with Unsuppressed HIV Viral Load among Women in An HIV Hyperendemic Area of KwaZulu-Natal, South Africa

Adenike O. Soogun, Ayesha B.M. Kharsany,
Temesgen Zewotir and Delia North

Abstract

New HIV infections among young women remains exceptionally high and to prevent onward transmission, UNAIDS set ambitious treatment targets. This study aimed to determine the prevalence, spatial variation and factors associated with unsuppressed HIV viral load at ≥400 copies per mL. This study analysed data from women aged 15–49 years from the HIV Incidence Provincial Surveillance System (HIPSS) enrolled in two sequential cross-sectional studies undertaken in 2014 and 2015 in rural and peri-urban KwaZulu-Natal, South Africa. Bayesian geoadditive model with spatial effect for a small enumeration area was adopted using Integrated Nested Laplace Approximation (INLA) function to analyze the findings. The overall prevalence of unsuppressed HIV viral load was 45.2% in 2014 and 38.1% in 2015. Factors associated with unsuppressed viral load were no prior knowledge of HIV status, had a moderate-to-low perception of acquiring HIV, not on antiretroviral therapy (ART), and having a low CD4 cell count. In 2014, women who ever consumed alcohol and in 2015, ever ran out of money, had two or more lifetime sexual partners, ever tested for tuberculosis, and ever diagnosed with sexually transmitted infection were at higher risk of being virally unsuppressed. The nonlinear effect showed that women aged 15 to 29 years, from smaller households and had fewer number of lifetime HIV tests, were more likely to be virally unsuppressed. High viral load risk areas were the north-east and south-west in 2014, with north and west in 2015. The findings provide guidance on identifying key populations and areas for targeted interventions.

Keywords: Bayesian, spatial effect, geoadditive model, integrated nested Laplace approximation, unsuppressed viral load, women, UNAIDS 95–95-95 target, South Africa

1. Introduction

In 2014, the Joint United Nations Programme on HIV/AIDS (UNAIDS) set ambitious 90–90-90 HIV testing and treatment target to achieve the 73%

composite viral suppression target by the year 2020 towards ending the epidemic by year 2030 [1]. While few countries like Australia and Botswana achieved this target [2, 3], the global public health community failed to achieve this target [4]. Therefore, in 2021 the UNAIDS Global AIDS strategy raised the targets to 95–95-95 with an overall viral suppression of 86% to be met by 2025 including prioritising sexual reproductive health and rights for women living with HIV (WLHIV), with the aim of controlling the epidemic by the year 2030 [5]. The "first 95" represents 95% of people living with HIV knowing their HIV status; the "second 95" represents 95% of people who know their HIV-positive status and are on antiretroviral therapy (ART); and the "third 95" represents 95% of HIV positive people who know their HIV status are on ART and are virally suppressed [1, 4]. At the country and global level, commitment, and resources to meet these indicators has been prioritised as the strategy was expected to prevent onward transmission of HIV and reduce HIV incidence [5–7].

In 2020, globally, 36 million adults over the age of 15 were living with HIV [4]. Out of these, 84% knew their status, 73% were accessing treatment and 66% were virally suppressed [4]. South Africa contributes approximately 22% of the global HIV burden [4, 8], and KwaZulu-Natal province is the epicentre [9, 10], where the UNAIDS targets has not been met [11, 12]. Whilst South Africa has substantially scaled-up ART provision, having the largest HIV treatment programme globally, has resulted in reducing number of HIV related death [8]. However, country level HIV prevalence of 14.0%, with an estimated 231,000 new infections remains persistently high [13], and almost a fourth of women in their reproductive ages (15–49) were HIV positive at the end of 2020 [8]. KwaZulu-Natal has the highest HIV burden with prevalence of 18.1% compared to Western Cape with a prevalence of 6.8% [14]. Heterosexual sex is the key path to HIV transmission and acquisition in this region [15], where women of reproductive age are disproportionately affected [16, 17], thus increasing the potential of mother to child transmission (MTCT) of HIV during pregnancy, childbirth, or breastfeeding [13, 18]. Thus, viral suppression is critically important among this key population for the prevention of mother-to-child transmission (PMTCT) of HIV [18, 19] and transmission to sexual partners.

Small area location-based approaches have been recommended for targeted interventions, scale up of treatment and identify spatially distributed structural and behavioural risk factors towards achieving the UNAIDS targets and to help to reduce the overall HIV burden [20]. Evidently, their exist geographic variation in the complexity of HIV epidemiological measures [21]. Therefore, spatial analysis and modelling accounting for the presence of spatial autocorrelation between observation and residual must be considered [20, 21]. Failure to account for spatial heterogeneity and possible causes could result in misleading epidemiologist, public health institutions, and policy makers. The national HIV prevalence survey among pregnant women that also examined socioeconomic factors associated with unsuppressed viral load did not account for the nonlinear effect of continuous covariates or mapped the spatial effect [22]. Therefore, the aim of this study was to determine factors associated with unsuppressed HIV viral load among women living with HIV while accounting for nonlinear effects of some continuous covariates and mapping spatial risk effect using Bayesian inference. Furthermore, the study assessed progress towards UNAIDS indicators, examined the prevalence and hotspots of unsuppressed HIV viral load among women in an HIV hyperendemic area of KwaZulu-Natal, South Africa. This study applied the Bayesian hierarchical Geoadditive model technique to identify risk factors associated with unsuppressed HIV viral load and mapping the spatial areas in KwaZulu-Natal, South Africa.

2. Methods

2.1 Sources of data, design, and procedures

This analysis was based on data from HIV Incidence Provincial Surveillance System (HIPSS) that monitored HIV related measures of HIV prevalence and incidence in association with the programmatic scale of HIV prevention and treatment efforts in a "real world" non-trial setting. The study undertook two sequential cross-sectional surveys with the first survey from June 2014 to 18 June 2015 (2014 Survey) and the second survey from 8 July 2015 to 7 June 2016 (2015 Survey). All study participants provided written informed consent and or assent, completed a face-to-face questionnaire to obtain socio-demographic, behavioural, knowledge of HIV testing, sexually transmitted infections (STI) and tuberculosis (TB) history and biological information. From a total of 600 Enumeration Areas (EAs), 591 EAs with more than 50 households were systematically selected at random, of which 221 were drawn for the 2014 Survey and 203 were drawn for the 2015 Survey. Households were randomly selected using multi-stage random sampling, were geo-referenced and one individual per household, within the age range 15–49 years old was randomly selected and invited to participate in the study. In the 2014 Survey a total of 9812 participants were enrolled, of whom 6265 were women, whilst in the 2015 Survey a total of 10,236 participants were enrolled, of whom 6341 were women. All enrolled participants had HIV antibody and viral load testing undertaken. In the 2014 Survey, 2955 were HIV positive and 2946 had viral load measurement, whilst 9 participants had missing viral load measurement. In the 2015 Survey, 2947 women were HIV positive and 2946 had viral load measurements, whilst 1 participant had missing viral load measurement.

HIPSS study was conducted in accordance with the approval by the Biomedical Research Ethics Committee of the University of KwaZulu-Natal (Reference number BF269/13), the KwaZulu-Natal Provincial Department of Health (HRKM 08/14), and the Associate Director of Science of the Centre for Global Health (CGH) at the United States Centre for Disease Control and Prevention (CDC) in Atlanta, United States of America (CGH 2014–080). Details about HIPSS study design, objectives and study and data collection procedures have been described elsewhere [10, 11].

2.2 Study population and geographic area

HIPSS was conducted in a geographically defined region of rural Vulindlela and peri urban Greater Edendale areas in the Msunduzi municipality, uMgungundlovu district of KwaZulu-Natal province in South Africa. Whilst this community has basic access to water, electricity and free health facilities, the area is characterised by high rates of unemployment, poverty, and HIV. The EAs are located between 29°39' South and 30°17 East of KZN, covers a total of 33 wards in the Msunduzi and a part of uMngeni municipalities, in uMgungundlovu district.

2.3 Study variables

2.3.1 Dependent variable

The primary outcome variable was HIV viral load status among women living with HIV (WLHIV) in this community, which was categorised as binary outcome:

$$\pi_{ij} = \begin{cases} 1 \text{ viral load} \geq 400 \text{ copies/mL (unsuppressed)} \\ 0 \text{ viral load} < 400 \text{ copies/mL (suppressed)} \end{cases} \quad (1)$$

This threshold was used in accordance with the country revised ART treatment guideline [23, 24] as well as evidence from several studies on transmission potential at this cut off [25, 26]. Unsuppressed viral load calculation and definition was based on the composite viral suppression of all WLHIV irrespective of being on ART or not.

2.3.2 Explanatory variables

Initial data exploration to identify potential factors associated with unsuppressed viral load was established using multiple correspondence analysis and random forest analysis [27]. The explanatory variables considered in the study comprised of socio-demographic, behavioural, knowledge of HIV status and HIV testing, medical history, and biological variables. These included age, marital status, education level, community duration, migration history, monthly income, accessing health care, meal cut, income loss, place of residence, number of household members, had sex in the last 12 months, number of sexual partners in the last 12 months, number of total lifetime sex partners, forced first time sex, ever consumed alcohol, ever tested for HIV, number of lifetime HIV test, knowledge of HIV status, perceived risk of contracting HIV, exposed to TB last 12 months, ever diagnosed of TB, had any STI symptoms, ever diagnosed of STI, ever pregnant, currently on antiretrovirals (ARV) and current CD4 cell count. The variance inflation factors (VIF) was used to check for collinearity among continuous independent variables and all variables with VIF < 4 was assumed that multicollinearity was not significantly present. Also, non-linear effect of all continuous variables was also examined, of which only age, household size, number of lifetime HIV test and total number of children ever born displayed a significant nonlinear effect and were considered in the fitted model while the remaining independent variables were included as linear fixed effect.

2.4 Statistical data analysis

To account for the complex multilevel sampling design, weighted percentage and frequency were used to describe and summarise the study characteristics across both surveys. Progress towards each of the 95-95-95 indicators and composite viral suppression was estimated. Comparisons of weighted proportion of viral load status was estimated with associated 95% confidence intervals (CIs) and p values using Taylor series methods. Initial non-spatial bivariate survey logistic regression was used to test association between each background characteristics and the dependent variable using Rao-Scott chi-square test. Statistical analyses were performed using SAS (SAS Institute, Cary, North Carolina) version 9.4. Covariates with significant association at 5% significant level for each study year was included in the multivariate model.

Suppose γ_{ijkl} denote the viral load status of women and $P\left(\gamma_{ijkl}=1\right)=\theta_{ijkl}$ is the probability that woman l in household k within cluster j and district i is unsuppressed and $P\left(\gamma_{ijkl}=0\right)=1-\theta_{ijkl}$ is the probability that the woman is suppressed. This assumes that the response variable γ_{ijkl} is Bernoulli distributed. Thus, the hierarchical Geoadditive model is given as:

$$logit\left(\theta_{ijkl}\right)=X_{ijkl}\,\beta+d_1Y_{ijkl1}+d_2Y_{ijkl2}+d_nY_{ijkln}+d_{spatial}\left(g_h\right) \qquad (2)$$

Eq. 2 is a semi-parametrical model, where $logit\left(\theta_{ijkl}\right)$ is the logit link function, and $X_{ijkl}\,\beta+d_1Y_{ijkl1}+d_2Y_{ijkl2}+d_nY_{ijkln}+d_{spatial}\left(g_h\right)$ is the Geoadditive predictor. Parameter β is the vector of the linear fixed effects which we modelled parametrically. The unknown smooth function of the non-linear effect is denoted as $d_a(.), a=1, \dots .n$, which was modelled non-parametrically. $d_{spatial}\left(g_h\right)$ is the spatial effect covariate of district g_h in which a woman resides, which symbolises the unaccounted and unobserved effect that are not included in the model [28–30]. Thus, resulting in the partitioning of this spatial effect into a spatially correlated (structured) and uncorrelated (unstructured) effect, given as:

$$d_{spatial}\left(g_h\right)=d_{struct}\left(g_h\right)+d_{unstruc}\left(g_h\right) \qquad (3)$$

The argument is that spatial effect is the proxy of most unobserved influence, under which spatial structure assumption must be followed. The structured spatial effect accounts for the assumption that location close in proximity are more likely to be correlated in respect of their outcome. While the unstructured spatial effect accounts for the spatial variation because of the effects of interminable district-level factors that are not related spatially [31–33].

The study utilised a fully Bayesian inference, hence all parameters and functions were considered as random variables and thus assigned with appropriate prior. Parameter β was assigned vague Gaussian priors N (0, 1000). The Bayesian penalised spline (P-splines, second-order random walk smoothness prior and third-degree spline) was adopted for the unknown smooth function $d_a(.)$ [34, 35]. Borrowing strength from neighbouring locations, the intrinsic Gaussian Markov random field (IGMRF) prior as specified by Besag et al. [34] was used for the structured spatial effect $d_{struct}\left(g_h\right)(.)$ [36, 37]. Two regions $\left(g_h\right)$ *and* $\left(g_i\right)$ are referred to as neighbours if they share common boundary, thus the spatial extension of random walk model was modelled by assuming the Besag-York-Mollie Conditional Autoregressive (CAR) prior given as:

$$d_{struct}\left(g_h\right)|d_{struct}\left(g_i\right), h\neq 1\sim N\left(\frac{1}{w_{g_h}}\sum\nolimits_{g_i\in g_h}d_{struct}\left(g_i\right), \frac{1}{w_{g_h}\tau^2{}_{struct}}\right) \qquad (4)$$

Where w_{g_h} is the number of neighbours in district g_h, and $g_i\in g_h$ represents that g_i is a neighbour of district g_i. Thus, the conditional mean of $d_{struct}\left(g_i\right)$ is the average function of $d_{struct}\left(g_h\right)$ of neighbouring districts.

Independent and identically distributed random variable (i.i.d) Gaussian priors were assigned to the unstructured spatial effect to account for the unobserved covariates that are inherent within the districts, denoted as:

$$d_{unstruc}(g_h) \sim \mathrm{N}\left(0, \frac{1}{\tau^2{}_{struct}}\right) \tag{5}$$

where the variance $\tau^2{}_{struct}$ is the unknown parameter to be estimated. Hyperpriors defined as log-gamma m, n distribution, where $m, n = 1$ *and* $n = 0.001$ were assigned at the second stage of the hierarchy. Non-linear and spatial effect were imposed with a sum-to-zero limit in order to distinguish between the effects and intercepts.

Lastly, the posterior distributions of all the parameters $\pi(\theta)$ and the likelihood function $L(x|\theta)$ was estimated. The study then assumes that θ denotes vectors of the unknown parameters in the model and likelihood $L(.)$ is the product of individual likelihood. Thus, the posterior distribution is written as:

$$\pi(\theta|x)\ \alpha\ L(y|\beta_1, d_1, \ldots.., \beta_n d_n, \varphi) \prod\nolimits_{h=1}^{p} \pi\ (\beta_h|d^2)\ d_h^2 \tag{6}$$

This is a high dimensional model and analysis which sometimes require good knowledge of advance mathematical and statistical computation. So, Markov chain Monte Carlo (MCMC) algorithm is required to generate samples from this distribution which comes with much computational difficulties. To circumvent this problem and difficulties, the Integrated Nested Laplace Approximation (INLA) was used to obtain the estimate [38, 39]. The outmost goal is to estimate marginal posterior distribution for the latent Gaussian model which was used to compute the summary statistics of interest like posterior mean, standard deviation, and 95% credible interval.

Three models were considered for comparison namely:

Model 1: Generalised Additive model (GAM): All categorical and some continuous variables were modelled as linear fixed effect, and nonlinear effects of covariates age, household size, total number of children ever born and number of lifetime HIV test.

Model 2: Structured Additive model (SAM), extension of GAM with the inclusion of CAR prior.

Model 3: Unstructured Geoadditive model (UGM), Model 2 with the inclusion of the spatial effect and modelled using i.i.d.

Deviance information criterion (DIC) of each model were compared. The final Geoadditive model was selected based on smallest DIC which was considered as good predictive performance and best fit model [40, 41]. The summary results give the posterior mean estimates with associated credible interval as well as the spatial effect map. The enumeration area shapefile was created in ArcGIS using the geographic attributes. Bayesian inference was analysed using INLA package in R software [37, 42].

3. Findings

3.1 Study characteristics

Table 1 shows the sample size and characteristics of HIV positive women in rural and peri urban areas of KwaZulu-Natal, South Africa. Almost half (45.2%) of the women had unsuppressed viral load in 2014 and about one third (38.1%) in 2015. Majority of WLHIV were aged between 20 and 44 years; 86.9% in 2014 and 85% in 2015 with median age and interquartile range (IQR) of 31(25–39) in 2014 and and 32 (26-40) years in 2015. Majority of the women were never married; 84.6% in 2014 and

Characteristics	2014 Survey[α]	2015 Survey[β]
Total	2955	2948
Age median (IQR)	31 [25–37]	32 [26–39]
Socio-demographic characteristics		
	n (%)	**n (%)**
Age groups (in Years)		
15–19	131 (4.6)	133 (4.9)
20–24	436 (14.3)	337 (11.2)
25–29	578 (20.3)	606 (20)
30–34	561 (20.7)	674 (21.1)
35–39	517 (18.4)	510 (18.8)
40–44	426(13.2)	431 (13.9)
45–49	306 (8.5)	257 (10.2)
Marital Status		
Never married	2468 (84.6)	2364 (81)
Ever married	478 (15.4)	584 (19)
Level of Education		
No Schooling	137 (2.9)	37 (1.4)
Incomplete High School	1525 (53.5)	1688 (57.3)
Complete high school	1293 (43.7)	1223 (41.2)
Duration in Community		
Always	2290 (76.7)	1504 (54.8)
Moved here less than 1 year ago	88 (2.3)	122 (3.8)
Moved here more than 1 year ago	577 (21.0)	1322 (41.4)
Away from home last 12 months		
Yes	311 (10.2)	217 (7.3)
No	2644 (89.9)	2731 (92.7)
Monthly Income[a]		
No income	602 (17)	50 (1.3)
≤ R2500	2177 (75.5)	1657 (53.0)
> R2500	169 (7.5)	1241 (45.8)
Run out of money[b]		
Yes	682 (24.5)	1477 (50.8)
No	2273 (75.5)	1469 (49.2)
Meal cut[c]		
Yes	606 (22.1)	1330 (46.2)
No	2342 (77.9)	1616 (53.8)
Accessing health care[d]		
Yes	1216 (44.9)	2168 (73.3)

Characteristics	2014 Survey[α]	2015 Survey[β]
No	1732 (55.1)	778 (26.7)
Place of Residence		
Rural	1009 (57.6)	954 (36.2)
Urban	1946 (42.4)	1994 (63.8)
Behavioural characteristics		
Had sex in the last 12 months		
Yes	2218 (77.2)	2501 (83.5)
No	737 (22.8)	447 (16.5)
Number of sex partner in the last 12 months		
1 partner	1178 (53.3)	1824 (72.9)
2 or more partners	1034 (46.7)	677 (27.1)
Number of lifetime sex partner		
1 partner	533 (22.2)	455 (15.7)
2 or more partners	1844 (77.8)	2429 (84.3)
Forced first time sex		
Yes	72 (2.5)	100 (3.3)
No	2831 (95.9)	2833 (96.1)
Do not remember	52 (1.6)	15 (0.5)
Ever consumed alcohol		
Yes	390 (11.5)	536 (18.5)
Never	2564 (88.5)	2412 (81.5)
HIV knowledge and risk perception		
Ever tested for HIV		
Yes	2513 (88.9)	2868 (96.9)
No	442 (11.1)	80 (3.1)
Number of lifetime HIV test		
Never	442 (11.1)	81 (3.1)
1 time	769 (26.2)	765 (27.1)
2 or more times	1744 (62.7)	2102 (69.8)
Knowledge of HIV status		
Yes	1870 (65.6)	2219 (73.7)
No	1085 (34.4)	729 (25.3)
Perceived risk of contracting HIV		
Likely to acquire HIV	573 (19.3)	461 (16)
Not likely to acquire HIV	686 (21.5)	405 (14.1)
I am already infected	1696 (59.2)	2082 (70)
TB/STI history		

Characteristics	2014 Survey[α]	2015 Survey[β]
Exposed to TB last 12 months		
Yes	103 (3.6)	162 (5.9)
No	2853 (96.6)	2786 (94.1)
Ever diagnosed with TB		
Yes	251 (9.6)	363 (12.7)
No	2704 (90.4)	2585 (87.3)
On medication to prevent TB		
Yes	219 (9.0)	449 (14.9)
No	2736 (91.0)	2499 (85.1)
Tested for TB		
Yes	1245 (47.1)	1689 (57.4)
No	1710 (52.9)	1259 (42.6)
Ever had any STI symptoms		
Yes	163(4.5)	80(2.9)
No	2792(95.5)	2868(97.1)
Ever diagnosed with STI		
Yes	213 (9.1)	320 (11.3)
No	2742 (90.9)	2628 (88.7)
Clinical characteristics		
Ever pregnant		
Yes	2346 (79.6)	2595 (88.1)
No	600 (20.4)	353 (11.9)
On ARV		
Yes	1346 (48.8)	1775 (59.8)
No	1600(51.2)	1172 (40.2)
ART dosage		
Single/fixed	1079 (86.3)	1580 (88.5)
Multiple	172 (13.7)	196 (11.5)
Current CD4 cell count[f]		
<350 cells per μL	696 (23.1)	634 (21.7)
350–499 cells per μL	639 (21.1)	576 (19.7)
≥500 cells per μL	1593 (55.8)	1729 (58.6)

Participants missing for: a = 7, and f = 27 in 2014; b, c and d = 2, f = 9 in 2015. No response: e: = 879(64) for 2014(2015). Missing data were excluded from percentage calculation. ZAR = South African Rand (ZAR15 ~ US$1).
TB = tuberculosis, STI = sexually transmitted infections, ARV = antiretroviral drugs, ART = antiretroviral therapy, Ever had any STI symptoms = any symptoms of abnormal vaginal discharge, burning or pain when passing urine or presence of any genital warts/ulcers.

Table 1.
Characteristics of HIV positive women in Vulindlela and Greater Edendale, KwaZulu-Natal, South Africa, 2014–2015.

81% in 2015. More than half had incomplete high school education 53.5% in 2014 and 57.3% in 2015. Most women had always lived in the community; 76.5% in 2014 and 54.8% in 2015 whilst never being away from home in the last 12 months was 89.8% in 2014 and 92.7% in 2015. In 2014 75.5% and in 2015, 53.0% of women reported a monthly income of ≤R2500 More than half of women sampled (57.6%) in 2014 were from rural area whilst the majority (63.8%) in 2015 were from urban areas. Overall 77.2% in 2014 and 83.5% in 2015 had engaged in sex in the last 12 months, whilst 46.7% in 2014 and 22.1% in 2015 reported having had two or more number of sex partners in the last 12 months. Overall, the majority; 77.8% in 2014 and 84.3% in 2015 reported having had two or more lifetime sex partners. Almost all the women were not forced to have sex at their first-time sex encounter. Regarding their HIV testing knowledge and perception, 88.9% of women in 2014 and 98.9% in 2015 reported having had an HIV test with 62.7% in 2014 and 69.8% had HIV test more than twice in their lifetime. In 2014, 21.5% had a perception of not likely to contract HIV, while only 14.1% in 2015. Overall, 79.6% of women in 2014 and 88.2% in 2015 had reported having been pregnant in their lifetime. Less than half, 48.8% in 2014 reported to be on ART, though this increased to 59.8% in 2015. More than half of the women 55.8% in 2014 and 58.6% in 2015 had a current CD4 cell counts of ≥500 cells per μL and 23.1% in 2014 and 21.6% in 2015 had CD4 cell counts of <350 per μL.

3.2 Progress towards UNAIDS 95-95-95 indicators

Figure 1 provides the status on the UNAIDS 95–95-95 indicators. Of the 2955 women in 2014 and 2948 in 2015 who tested positive for HIV, 9 and 1 participants respectively had no viral load measurement. Thus, 2946 women in 2014 and 2947 women in 2015 had viral load measurements. In 2014, to meet the "first 95", 65.5% (95% CI, 62.9–68.2) (n = 1890/2955) were aware of their HIV positive status and for the "second 95", 74.2% (95% CI, 71.6–76.8 (n = 1348/1870) had initiated ART and for the "third 95", 82.9% (95% CI, 80.4–85.4) (n = 1105/1346) had achieved viral suppression, and overall viral suppression among all HIV positive women was 54.8% (95% CI, 52.0–57.5) (n = 1574/2946). While in 2015, progress towards 95–95-95 targets were: 74.7% (95% CI, 72.7–76.6) (n = 2219/2948) were aware of their HIV status; 80.0% (95% CI, 78.1–82.0) (n = 1777/2219) of these had initiated ART and 88.2% (95% CI, 86.6–89.9) (n = 1551/1777) of those on ART had achieved HIV viral suppression, resulting in the overall viral suppression among all HIV positives to be 61.9% (95% CI, 59.7–64.1) (n = 1828/2947).

Disaggregated by age groups, **Figure 1a** shows the progress towards the "first 95" Knowledge of HIV status increased from 65.6% in 2014 to 74.7% in 2015, and across age groups, with highest achieved among 35–39 (86.5%), 40–44 (82.4%) and 45–49 (82.4%) in 2015. Highest increase in the knowledge of HIV positive status was in the age group 15–29, increasing from 25.8% in 2014 to 46.7% in 2015. **Figure 1b** shows the progress towards the "second 95". Overall proportion of women who knew their HIV positive status and were on ART increased from 74.2% in 2014 to 80.0% in 2015. The uptake of ART varied across age groups, uptake was high in the 15–19 years age group at 74.8% in 2014 and 75.9% in 2015; in ages 30–34 uptake was 77.2% in 2014 and 80.5 in 2015; in ages 35–39 years uptake was 77.8% in 2014 and 85.6% in 2015; in ages 40–44 years uptake was 77.1% in 2014 and 84.6% in 2015 and in age 45–49 uptake was 79.1% in 2014 and 84.2% in 2015. However, ART uptake in the age group 20–24 years was lowest at 62.4% in 2014 and 62.8% in 2015. **Figure 1c** shows the progress towards the "third 95", that is the proportion of HIV positive women who knew their HIV

DOI: http://dx.doi.org/10.5772/intechopen.105547

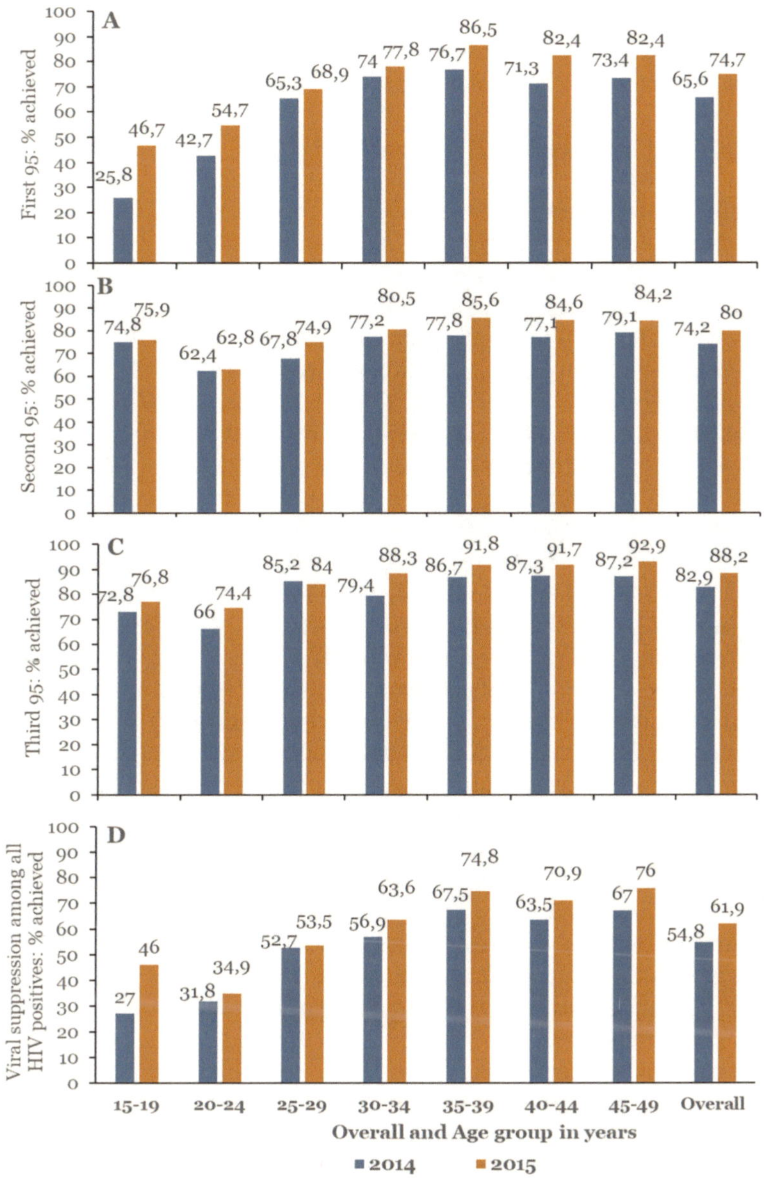

Figure 1.

Progress of the UNAIDS 95–95-95 indicators by age group and overall, among HIV positive women (2014–2015). (A). First 95: Women living with HIV who knew they were HIV positive. (B). Second 95: Women who knew they were HIV positive and were taking ART. (C). Third 95: Women who knew they were HIV positive, were on ART and had achieved HIV viral suppression at HIV viral load <400 copies/ml. (D). UNAIDS composite measure towards achieving HIV viral suppression among all HIV positive women.

positive status, were on sustained ART and who had achieved viral suppression of <400 copies per mL. Proportion varied across ages group; HIV viral suppression was lowest at 66% among 20–24 years old in 2014 and increased to 74.4% in 2015. Viral suppression of 92.9% was achieved among 45–49 years old and 91.7% among 40–44 years old and 91.8% among 35–39 years old in 2015. **Figure 1d** shows the overall UNAIDS 95–95-95 composite measure of achieving viral suppression of 86% among all HIV positive women. Overall, 54.8% of women in 2014 and 61.9% in 2015 had achieved HIV viral suppression of <400 copies per mL. Substantial variation existed across the age groups, with 27% among 15–19 years in 2014 and increased to 46% in 2015. Highest achievement was observed with 76% among 45–49 years old.

3.3 Prevalence of unsuppressed HIV viral load

Table 2 shows that overall prevalence of unsuppressed HIV viral load was 45.2% (95 CI, 42.5–48.0), (n/N = 1372/2946) in 2014 and 38.1% (95% CI, 35.9–40.3), (n/N = 1119/2947) in 2015. Viral suppression increased by 7.1% over the study period. Unsuppressed viral load prevalence decreased as age increased and it was 72.9% (95% CI, 62.7–83.2), (n = 95/130) in 15–19 years age group, 68.2% (95% CI, 62.4–73.9), (n = 290/433) in the 20–24 years age group, 47.3% (95% CI, 41.9–52.7), (n = 299/577) in 25–29 years age group, 43.1% (95% CI, 37.9–48.3), (n = 248/561) in 30–34 years age group, 32.5% (95% CI, 26.6–38.4), (n = 185/513) in 35–39 years age group, 36.5% (95% CI, 30.6–42.4), (n = 153/426) in 40–44 years age group, 33.0% (95% CI, 26.6–39.3), (n = 102/306) in 45–49 years age group. In 2015, prevalence also decreased by age and it was 56.0% (95% CI, 43.8–64.1), (n = 74/133); 65.1 [59.5–70.7], (n = 210/337); 46.5 [41.4–51.5], (n = 279/606); 36.4% (95% CI, 32.1–40.8), (n = 244/674); 25.2% (95% CI, 20.9–29.4), (n = 125/509); 29.1% (95% CI, 24.0–34.2), (n = 120/431); 24.0% (95% CI, 18.3–29.8), (n = 67/257) in the 15–19, 20–24, 25–29, 30–34, 35–39, 40–44, and 45–49 years age categories (X^2 trend $P < 0.001$).

Whilst unsuppressed viral load prevalence was similar across most variables, decrease in the trends over the study years was observed. In 2014 unsuppressed viral load prevalence was 50.1%, (n = 152/311) and declined to 20.2%, n = 113/217) in 2015, among women that were away from home in the last 12 months (compared to those that were never away from home; 44.7%, (n = 1220/2635) in 2014 and 37.2%, n = 1006/2730) in 2015. Among those that ever-consumed alcohol 58.8%, (n = 229/390) in 2014 and declined to 44.4%, n = 249/536) in 2015 compared to those that never consumed alcohol and 43.9%, (n = 1143/2556) (36.6%, n = 870/2411) also among those that never had HIV test 68.1%, (n = 286/441) (63.4%, n = 53/80). Among those that ever had an HIV test 42.4%, (n = 1086/2505) in 2014 and 37.3%, n = 1066/2867) in 2015 had unsuppressed viral load. Similarly, among women who did not know their HIV status 72.0%, (n = 753/1081) in 2014 and 74.3%, (n = 528/729) in 2015 compared to those who knew their status 31.2%, (n = 619/1875) in 2014 and 25.8%, n = 591/2218) in 2015 had unsuppressed viral load. Women who perceived they are not likely to contact HIV 70.7%, (n = 478/682) in 2014 and 70.2% (n = 281/405) in 2015 compared to those who already perceived they had been infected 28.9%, (n = 530/1692) (24.6%, n = 529/2081), also women who have ever been diagnosed of STI 43.7%, (n = 98/213) (47.7%, n = 155/320), among women who had never been pregnant 59.4%, (n = 343/600) (49.3%, n = 169/352) compared to those that has ever been pregnant 42.5%, (n = 1029/2346) (36.6%, n = 947/2595), likewise among WLHIV and not on ART 72.1% (n = 1131/1600) (77.3%, n = 899/1172) in comparison with those on ART 17.1% (n = 241/1346) (11.8%, n = 220/1775). Prevalence was higher among women whose current CD4 cell count were < 350 count per μ/L, 69.3%, (n = 493/695) (68.5%, n = 430/633), and those with CD4 cell count of between 350 and 499 count per μ/L 49.1%, (n = 315/638) (42.0%, n = 247/576) compared to those 500 count per μ/L 33.2%, (n = 546/1591) (25.6%, n = 437/1729) in 2014(2015) respectively.

Figure 2 shows the observed prevalence map of unsuppressed viral load. Highest prevalence was observed in the north and south of Vulindlela and east part of Greater

Characteristics	2014 Survey			2015 Survey		
	n/N	**% [95 CI]**	**P-value**	**n/N**	**% [95 CI]**	**P-value**
Overall						
≥400 copies per mL	1372/2946	45.2 [42.5–48.0]		1119/2947	38.1 [35.9–40.3]	
<400 copies per mL	1574/2946	54.8 [52.0–57.5]		1828/2927	61.9 [59.7–64.1]	
Age median (IQR)	31 [26–39]			32 [26–39]		
Socio-demographic characteristics						
Age groups (years)						
15–19	95/131	72.9 [62.7–83.2]	<0.0001	74/133	56.0[43.8–64.1]	<0.0001
20–24	290/433	68.2 [62.4–73.9]		210/337	65.1 [59.5–70.7]	
25–29	299/577	47.3 [41.9–52.7]		279/606	46.5 [41.4–51.5]	
30–34	248/561	43.1 [37.9–48.3]		244/674	36.4 [32.1–40.8]	
35–39	185/513	32.5 [26.6–38.4]		125/509	25.2 [20.9–29.4]	
40–44	153/426	36.5 [30.6–42.4]		120/431	29.1 [24.0–34.2]	
45–49	102/306	33.0 [26.6–39.3]		67/257	24.0 [18.3–29.8]	
Marital status						
Never married	1188/2468	46.4 [43.6–49.2]	0.03	948/2364	40.6 [38.1–43.2]	<0.0001
Ever married	184/478	39.0 [32.3–45.6]		171/583	27.4 [23.4–31.4]	
Level of Education						
No schooling	63/137	44.1 [34.8–53.4]	0.09	10/37	30.2 [12.8–47.6]	0.03
Incomplete High School	672/1521	43.2 [39.3–47.0]		605/1688	35.7 [32.8–38.6]	
Complete High School	637/1288	47.9 [44.4–51.4]		504/1222	41.7 [38.0–45.3]	
Duration in community						
Always	1078/2282	45.5 [42.7–48.4]	0.53	585/1504	39.0 [35.8–42.1]	0.04
Moved here less than 1 year ago	44/88	48.4 [34.3–62.4]		60/122	48.4 [38.1–58.7]	
Moved here more than 1 year ago	250/576	43.9 [38.3–49.5]		474/1321	36.0 [33.1–39.0]	
Away from home last 12 months						
Yes	152/311	50.1 [41.9–58.3]	0.21	113/217	50.2 [42.6–57.7]	0.01
No	1220/2635	44.7 [41.9–47.5]		1006/2730	37.2 [34.9–39.4]	
Monthly Income [a]						
No income	285/601	46.4 [41.0–51.7]	0.29	17/50	34.4 [19.8–49.0]	0.89
≤R2500	1017/2170	45.6 [42.4–48.8]		627/1656	38.0 [35.3–40.7]	
> R2500	67/168	38.8 [30.2–47.4]		475/1241	38.3 [34.9–41.7]	

Characteristics	2014 Survey			2015 Survey		
Run out of money[b]						
Yes	318/682	47.0 [41.2–52.7]	0.04	549/1477	37.7 [34.7–40.8]	0.02
No	1051/2257	44.7 [41.8–47.5]		569/1468	38.5 [35.4–41.6]	
Meal cut[d]						
Yes	285/606	47.4 [41.5–53.3]	0.38	499/1330	37.3 [34.0–40.5]	0.45
No	1084/2333	44.6 [41.8–47.5]		619/1615	38.8 [35.9–41.7]	
Accessing heath care[d]						
Yes	488/1212	41.7 [37.4–46.0]	0.03	769/2167	35.5 [33.0–38.1]	<0.0001
No	881/1727	48.1 [44.4–51.8]		349/778	45.2 [41.2–49.2]	
Place of residence						
Rural	457/1006	44.5 [40.3–48.7]	0.51	340/954	36.3[32.1–40.4]	0.25
Urban	915/1940	46.2 [43.4–49.1]		779/1993	39.1 [36.7–41.7]	
Behavioural characteristics						
Had sex last 12 months						
Yes	1052/2212	45.8 [42.8–48.8]	0.29	965/2501	38.8[36.4–41.3]	0.14
No	320/734	43.3 [38.9–47.7]		154/446	34.4[28.9–39.8]	
Number of sex partner last 12 months						
1 partner	908/1178	46.1 [43.0–49.2]	0.02	860/1824	38.2[35.6–40.7]	0.03
2 or more partners	464/1034	43.6 [39.1–47.4]		259/677	37.9[33.6–42.3]	
Total number of lifetime sex partners						
1 partner	265/532	48.3 [42.0–54.6]	0.01	185/455	39.4[34.7–44.1]	0.05
2 or more partners	828/1839	43.7 [40.7–46.8]		910/2428	37.9[354–40.2]	
Forced first time sex						
Yes	31/72	38.8 [26.1–51.5]	0.28	33/100	34.7[23.7–45.7]	0.74
No	1314/2822	45.2 [42.4–48.0]		1082/2832	38.3[36.0–40.6]	
Do not remember	27/52	56.1 [39.4–72.9]		04/15	30.4[1.1–59.7]	
Ever consumed alcohol						
Yes	229/390	58.8 [51.7–65.9]	<0.0001	249/536	44.4[39.4–49.5]	<0.0001
No	1143/2556	43.9 [40.6–46.3]		870/2411	36.6[34.2–39.1]	
HIV knowledge and risk perception						
Ever tested for HIV						
Yes	1086/2505	42.4 [39.5–45.3]	<0.0001	1066/2867	37.3[35.1–39.5]	<0.0001
No	286/441	68.1 [63.2–73.0]		53/80	63.4[51.4–75.4]	
Knowledge of HIV status						
Yes	619/1865	31.2 [28.1–34.3]	<0.0001	591/2218	25.8[23.6–28.0]	<0.0001
No	753/1081	72.0 [68.5–75.6]		528/729	74.3[70.7–77.8]	

Characteristics	2014 Survey			2015 Survey		
Perceived risk of contracting HIV						
Likely to Acquire HIV	364/572	67.4 [62.1–72.6]	<0.0001	309/461	69.0[64.0–74.0]	<0.0001
Not likely to Acquire HIV	478/682	70.7 [66.1–74.7]		281/405	70.2 [64.8–75.5]	
I am already infected	530/1692	28.9 [25.8–31.9]		529/2081	24.6[22.3–26.9]	
Number of lifetime HIV tests						
Never	286/441	68.1 [63.2–73.0]	<0.0001	54/81	63.7[51.8–75.6]	<0.0001
1 time	330/764	41.6 [37.1–46.2]		225/765	29.1[25.2–33.1]	
2 or more times	756/1741	42.7 [39.1–46.3]		840/2101	40.4[37.7–43.2]	
TB/STI history						
Exposed to TB in the last 12 months						
Yes	41/102	41.2 [27.8–54.6]	0.56	44/159	22.4[14.9–29.9]	<0.0001
No	1331/2844	45.4 [42.6–48.2]		1075/2786	39.0[36.8–41.3]	
Ever diagnosed with TB						
Yes	77/251	30.9 [23.2–38.6]	<0.0001	82/362	19.7[15.6–23.9]	<0.0001
No	1295/1295	46.8 [44.0–49.5]		1037/2585	40.8[38.4–43.2]	
On medication to prevent TB						
Yes	48/217	20.6 [13.6–27.6]	<0.0001	84/449	16.7[12.7–20.7]	<0.0001
No	1324/2729	47.6 [45.0–50.3]		1035/2498	41.8[39.4–44.3]	
Tested for TB						
Yes	417/1242	32.6 [28.8–36.4]	<0.0001	463/1688	27.1[24.7–29.5]	<0.0001
No	955/1704	56.5 [53.4–59.6]		656/1259	52.9[49.5–56.3]	
Had any STI symptoms						
Yes	65/162	37.3 [28.1–46.4]	0.08	30/80	37.4[23.0–51.9]	0.92
No	1307/2784	45.6 [42.9–48.4]		1089/2867	38.1[35.8–40.4]	
Ever diagnosed with STI						
Yes	98/213	43.7 [35.0–52.4]	0.71	155/320	47.7[41.5–53.9]	0.001
No	1274/2733	45.4 [42.5–48.3]		964/2627	36.9[34.5–39.3]	
Clinical characteristics						
Ever pregnant						
Yes	1029/2346	42.5 [39.6–45.5]	<0.0001	947/2595	36.6[34.3–38.9.5]	<0.0001
No	343/596	59.4 [53.7–65.1]		169/352	49.3[42.6–55.9]	
Currently on ARV						
Yes	241/1346	17.1 [14.6–19.6]	<0.0001	220/1775	11.8[10.2–13.5]	<0.0001
No	1131/1600	72.1 [68.9–75.3]		899/1172	77.3[74.4–80.2]	
ART dosage						
Single/fixed	127/1077	11.5 [8.9–14.0]	<0.0001	170/1579	24.4(17.1–31.7)	<0.0001

Characteristics	2014 Survey			2015 Survey		
Multiple	36/172	21.2 [12.3–30.1]		50/196	10.2(8.9–11.7)	
Current CD4 cell count [e]						
<350 per μL	493/695	69.3 [64.8–73.8]	<0.0001	430/633	68.5[64.4–72.5]	<0.0001
350–499 per μL	315/638	49.1 [43.2–55.0]		247/576	42.0[37.4–46.6]	
≥500 per μL	546/1591	33.2 [29.9–36.5]		437/1729	25.6[23.2–28.0]	

A total of nine women in 2014 survey and one woman in 2015 survey were missing viral load data. Participants missing for: a = 7, and e = 27 in 2014; b, c and d = 2, e = 9 in 2015.

Table 2.
Prevalence of unsuppressed viral load by study characteristics among women in Vulindlela and Greater Edendale, KwaZulu-Natal, South Africa, 2014–2015.

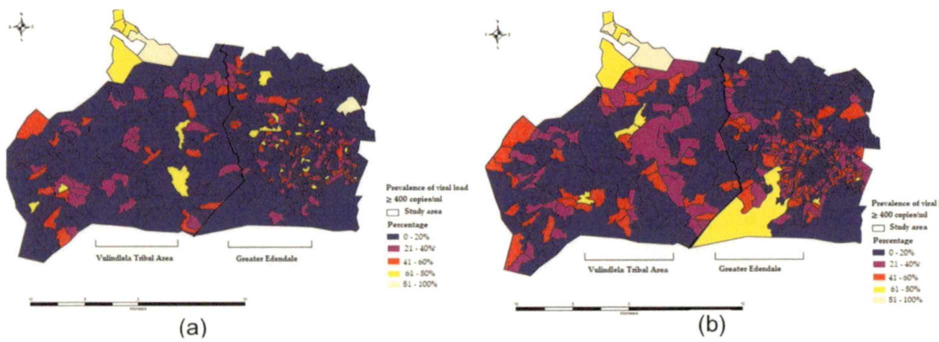

Figure 2.
Observed prevalence maps of unsuppressed viral load among women (a) 2014 and (b) 2015 in Vulindlela and Greater Edendale area in uMgungundlovu district, KwaZulu-Natal province, South Africa.

Edendale in 2014, while in the north part of Vulindlela and the south part of Greater Edendale in 2015. The north area (Mpophomeni) showed a consistently high prevalence across both surveys.

3.4 Model diagnostic measures

Table 3 shows values of the deviance information criterion (DIC) and effective numbers of parameters (pD) for each of the fitted model. Unstructured model has the minimum values (DIC = 2593.26 and 2087.70) for 2014 and 2015 respectively, thus attesting as the best fit model for the data sets, while GAM model offers the least fit. Besides, the unstructured model is of actual interest because it contains all the variables considered, and account for spatial autocorrelation and between clusters heterogeneity, failure to do so would have produced misleading and overfitting results. Thus, further results of this study are based on the unstructured model.

3.5 Non-linear effect of continuous covariates on women

Figure 3 shows the non-linear effect of continuous covariates after accounting for other variables. The results shows that current age, number of household members, total number of children ever born and total number of lifetime HIV test, had a non-

	2014 Survey			2015 Survey		
Parameters	**GAM**	**Structured**	**Unstructured**	**GAM**	**Structured**	**Unstructured**
DIC	2768.42	2597.64	2593.26	2097.27	2089.95	2087.70
DIC saturated	2998.34	2992.52	3004.69	2992.61	2987.95	2998.66
pD	44.92	48.88	49.23	46.53	46.50	47.55

DIC: Deviance Information Criteria. pD: effective numbers of parameters.

Table 3.
Model diagnostic.

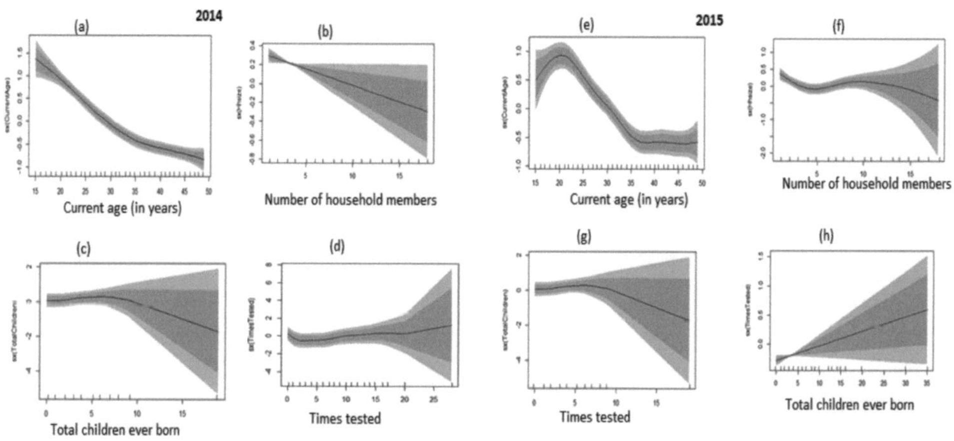

Figure 3.
Nonlinear effect of continuous covariate.

linear significant effect on women being virally unsuppressed in this study area. Furthermore, in **Figure 3a** and **e** shows a slight increase in effect among ages 15 to 20 in 2014 and sharp increase in 20 to 25 in 2015, after which the effect declined. Younger age 15 to 29 have higher risk of being virally unsuppressed compared to ages 30 above. **Figure 3b** and **f** shows that risk of unsuppressed viral load decreases with higher number of household members from 5 members. Also **Figure 3c** and **h** shows that the effect of total number of children ever born decreases the risk of being virally unsuppressed in 2014 but increases in 2015. Similarly, **Figure 3d** and **g** showed that the risk of unsuppressed viral load increased as the number of lifetime HIV tests increased in 2014, whilst in contrast unsuppressed viral load decreased as the number of lifetime HIV tests increased in 2015.

3.6 Fixed effect model

Table 4 displays the adjusted posterior mean estimates with their 95% credible intervals of the linear fixed effect from the multivariable model. If these intervals contain the number zero (0), then the parameter (estimate of the mean beta) is not significant; otherwise, it is significant. Factors associated with unsuppressed viral load across both years were knowledge of HIV status, low perceived risk of contracting HIV, ARV treatment and current CD4 cell counts. Women with no prior knowledge

	2014 Survey			2015 Survey		
Variables	**Posterior mean**	**Posterior SD**	**95 Credible intervals**	**Posterior mean**	**Posterior SD**	**95% credible intervals**
intercept	0.405**	0.075	(0.255, 0.551)	0.407**	0.076	(0.257, 0.557)
Marital status (ref: Ever married)						
Never married	0.032	0.017	(−0.002, 0.067)	0.005	0.021	(−0.035, 0.045)
Education status (ref: Complete high school)						
Incomplete high school	0.015	0.021	(−0.015, 0.045)	−0.005	0.014	(−0.032, 0.022)
Duration in community (ref: Always)						
Moved here less than 1 year ago	−0.016	0.042	(−0.099,0.068)	0.044	0.033	(−0.022, 0.109)
Moved here more than 1 year ago	0.002	0.019	(−0.034, 0.039)	0.002	0.014	(−0.025, 0.029)
Away from home last 12 month (ref: No)						
Yes	0.002	0.024	(−0.045, 0.048)	0.056 **	0.025	(0.007, 0.105)
Run out of money (ref: No)						
Yes	0.016	0.026	(−0.035, 0.067)	0.011 **	0.018	(0.024, 0.045)
Accessing healthcare (ref: Yes)						
No	0.018	0.016	(−0.013, 0.049)	0.014	0.015	(−0.016, 0.044)
Total number of sex partners last 12 months (ref: 1 partner)						
2 or more partners/no res	0.024	0.019	(−0.013, 0.061)	0.002	0.019	(−0.036, 0.039)
Total number of lifetime sex partners (ref: 1 partner)						
2 or more partners	0.037	0.027	(−0.016, 0.091)	0.049**	0.058	(0.102, 0.162)
Ever had alcohol (ref: No)						
Yes	0.058 **	0.022	(0.016, 0.101)	0.029	0.017	(−0.005, 0.063)
Ever tested for HIV (ref: Yes)						
No	−0.058	0.034	(−0.120, 0.014)	−0.022	0.045	(−0.110, 0.066)
Knowledge of HIV status (ref: Yes)						
No	−0.142 **	0.030	(−0.201, −0.084)	−0.200 **	0.030	(−0.259, −0.142)
Perceived risk of contracting HIV (ref: Already infected)						
Likely	0.095 **	0.025	(0.045, 0.144)	0.062**	0.028	(0.008, 0.116)
Not Likely	0.103 **	0.027	(0.050, 0.156)	0.074 **	0.029	(0.017, 0.131)
Ever tested for TB (ref: No)						
Yes	−0.034	0.018	(−0.069, 0.001)	−0.070**	0.015	(−0.099, −0.041)
Exposed to TB last 12 months (ref: No)						
Yes	0.061	0.041	(−0.019, 0.142)	−0.022	0.029	(−0.079, 0.035)

	2014 Survey			2015 Survey		
Variables	**Posterior mean**	**Posterior SD**	**95 Credible intervals**	**Posterior mean**	**Posterior SD**	**95% credible intervals**
Diagnosed of TB (ref: No)						
Yes	0.008	0.028	(−0.048, 0.064)	0.005	0.022	(−0.038, 0.048)
On medication to prevent TB (ref: No)						
Yes	−0.052	0.029	(−0.108, 0.004)	−0.027	0.019	(−0.064, 0.010)
Ever had any STI symptoms (ref: No)						
Yes	0.034	0.033	-(0.031, 0.100)	−0.077	0.039	(−0.084, 0.069)
Ever Diagnosed with STI (Ref: No)						
Yes	0.042	0.028	(−0.014, 0.097)	0.059**	0.021	(0.018, 0.099)
Ever Pregnant (ref: Yes)						
No	−0.065	0.019	(−0.103, 0.028)	0.001	0.018	(−0.156, 0.059)
on ART (ref: Yes)						
No	0.321**	0.030	(0.262, 0.379)	0.511**	0.031	(0.451, 0.571)
ARV dosage (ref: fixed/single)						
Multiple	0.251**	0.027	(0.199, 0.303)	0.242**	0.018	(−0.163, −0.093)
Current CD4 Cell count (cells per μl) (ref: < 350)						
350–499	−0.184 **	0.021	(−0.226, −0.143)	−0.157**	0.020	(−0.197, −0.118)
≥ 500	−0.319**	0.018	(−0.354, −0.285)	−0.287**	0.016	(−0.319, −0.254)

***Significant at 5% level of significance.*

Table 4.
Adjusted posterior means, standard deviation (SD) and 95% credible intervals for the best fitted model.

of their HIV status were more likely to be virally unsuppressed than those that knew their status. Women with either unlikely or likely perception of contracting HIV, not on ARV, and for those on ARV having multiple tablets of ARV had the highest risk of being virally unsuppressed compared to their reference categories. Additionally, in 2014 those that ever consumed alcohol were also at higher risk of having unsuppressed viral load. While in 2015, we also found that women that reported being away from home in the last 12 months, had a meal cut, being with two or more sexual partners in one's lifetime, ever tested with TB and ever diagnosed with STI had the highest risk of being virally unsuppressed compared to their counterparts.

3.7 Spatial effect map

Figure 4 shows the chloropleth spatial effect maps based on model 3, shows both positive and negative effects with predicted high and low risk areas of unsuppressed viral load. The colours on the chloropleth maps show the log-odds scale, indicating each area contribution to the odds of unsuppressed viral load in women. Predicted high risk areas are shaded in yellow and gold brown (0.00015 to 0.00020), in 2014, two distinct locations were in the north-east and south-west, while 2015 shows a clustered area in the south-east. Predicted lower risk areas are shaded in royal to dark

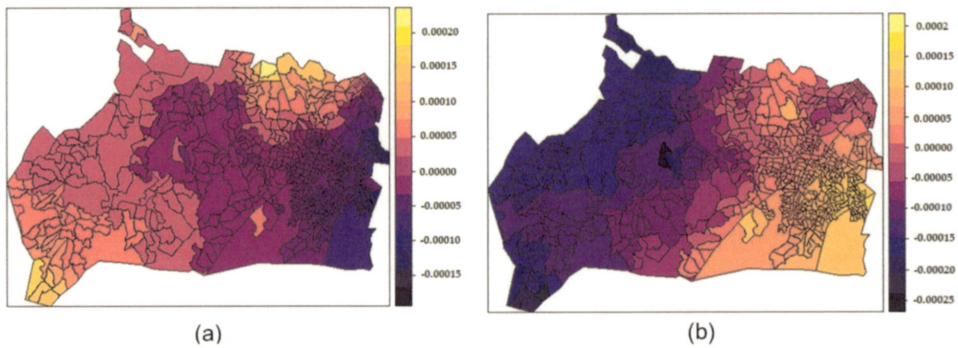

Figure 4.
Estimated posterior mean of the unstructured spatial effect map on the log-odds of unsuppressed viral load among women in uMgungundlovu district, KwaZulu-Natal province, South Africa (2014–2015). (a) 2014, (b) 2015.

blue (−0.00015 to −0.00025), the south-west in 2014, with both north and west in 2015. Evidently their exist spatial variation of unsuppressed viral load in this hyperendemic community.

4. Discussion

This analysis examined factors associated with unsuppressed viral load among women ages 15–49 years in peri-urban Greater Edendale and rural Vulindlela areas in the uMgungundlovu district, KwaZulu-Natal, South Africa between 2014 to 2015 while accounting for possible nonlinear effect of some continuous variables and mapping the unstructured spatial effects. We fitted hierarchical Bayesian Geoadditive multivariate model while controlling for the confounding effects of the explanatory variables. Bayesian spatial approach have numerous advantages over frequentist statistics, such as ability to account for and measure uncertainty in a model, minimise bias in complex data, ability to produce smoothed risk map, increased prediction accuracy, just to name a few [39, 43, 44]. Due to the strength of this approach many studies have emanated in investigating risk factors of anaemia in Sub Saharan Africa [33, 45], of HIV variation in Kenya [32], viral suppression [46] and other infectious disease globally [47]. Application of Bayesian spatial modelling therefore helped in identifying predictors and high-risk location of unsuppressed viral load among women in a small enumeration area. This enhancement of strategically identifying areas of key population is highly recommended as part of the global AIDS strategy to end inequality in resources allocation and provide localised HIV intervention in hyperendemic communities.

Our study found that knowledge of HIV status, perceived risk of contracting HIV, not on ART, and ART dosage were consistent significant factors associated with higher odds of being virally unsuppressed across both years. Having a CD4 cell count of >350 cells per μL was more likely to be associated with viral load <400 copies per mL Additionally, alcohol consumption was significant in 2014 while meal cut, total number of lifetime sex partner, ever tested for TB and ever diagnosed with STI were factors associated with unsuppressed viral load in 2015. These revealed the heterogeneity and need for continuous surveillance of HIV and its measures, as the predictors of this outcome are dynamic. Although fewer studies on women have been conducted in the country and other developing countries. Similar findings on the association of higher number of sexual partners were also reported among women in uMkhanyakude district of north KZN [48]. The use of ART and dosage of ARV was also found to be significant which is similar to past studies [49, 50]. Furthermore, similar studies have found higher CD4 cell count of >350 cells per μL to be predictive of being virally unsuppressed [51, 52]. We also found similar results on alcohol [53] from Western cape, South Africa and history of TB or STI in Kenya and Uganda [49, 54]. Alcohol use has been found to be associated with non-adherence to treatment in people living with HIV [55] and prevalence of which leads to high risk of transmission [56]. Several studies have shown relationship between TB and virological non-suppression [51, 57]. Similarly, concurrent ART and TB/STI treatment has been shown to increase the risk of virological non-suppression due to impaired treatment adherence and pharmacokinetics drug interaction [49].

The nonlinear effects of age, household size, total number of children ever born and total lifetime HIV test were considered. Across both years, risk of being virally unsuppressed decreases as age increases, with younger age 15–20 having a higher risk and being older associated with reduced risk of unsuppressed viral load. This is similar to past studies [48, 58]. Also risk of being virally unsuppressed decreases with increasing size of the family. Having 5 or lower number of family member showed a higher risk of being unsuppressed. This revealed that larger family members could bring more support to WLHIV. In contrast unsuppressed viral load decreases as number of children ever born increases in 2014 while the inverse was observed in 2015 (risk increases as number of birth increases). Recent study among pregnant women revealed significant association of currently breastfeeding with increase odd of viral load non-suppression [22, 59].

The unstructured spatial effect and observed prevalence map revealed the existence of localised positive spatial variation of unsuppressed viral load among women of reproductive age in this hyperendemic community. While higher prevalence was observed in the north area from both surveys and southern area in 2015. The predicted risk map revealed that in 2014 north-east and south-west as well as south-west in 2015 have an increase likelihood of being virally unsuppressed. This evidently shows that there are regional/district specific factors contributing to unsuppressed viral load with substantial spatial variation. Spatial variation in HIV and its measures has been reported by previous studies [16].

Among women in this community progress on 95–95-95 target was 65.5%, 74.2%, 82.9% in 2014 and 74.7%, 80.0%, 86.6% in 2015. The largest shortfall was in the first target, which is the entry point to health care system. None of the UNAIDS targets were met among this key population. Although, the country has made significant progress but has not achieved the UNAIDS 95–95-95 and 86% composite viral suppression target [14]. However, significant increase in viral suppression of 7.1% over a one year period was seen in this study, while ages 35 to 49 contributed to this increase, which could be attributed to the country commitment and effort in ART scaleup and intervention [27]. However, judging by the 90–90-90 indicator, our findings showed that the "third 90" target was met among age group 35–39, 40–44, 45–49 (91.8%, 91.7%, 92.9%) in 2015.

The key strengths of our study were the robustness of the study design, high participation rate, available of spatial variables and conducting the survey in a real time setting.

5. Limitation

This was a cross sectional population based study and not a randomised clinical trial with limited ART data available. Therefore, no causal effect could be established between unsuppressed viral load and women characteristics. The results are not generalisable to older individuals or children as study only accessed men and women aged 15–49 years.

6. Conclusion

Spatial effects in the model act as a representative of the unobserved predictors which strengthen the result. Identifying high risk areas could help policy maker, epidemiologist, and public health institutions to develop develop strategies and interventions that are suitable for women in the area, thus increasing the impact of allocated resources as well as effective monitoring to improve the health status of women in the community. Increase in progress of the 95–95-95 targets over time showed that the target is achievable in this community among this key population, with intensive HIV testing service, eradication of stigmatisation, ending inequality and increasing uptake of ART treatment. Knowledge of HIV status is a proxy and entry point to achieving the other indicators, generally women are more likely to test than men and receive optimum health care especially during pregnancy.

The likelihood of being virally unsuppressed was higher among younger age group, highlighting public health implication of sustained risk of HIV transmission. Aside clinical factors, family support cannot be underestimated as part of the factors that could help in achieving undetectable viral load among women of reproductive age. Right perception and knowledge of HIV positive status, being on ART and having a higher CD4 cell count contributed to achieving viral suppression. Thus, these remain multi-factorial and important public health priority to attain viral suppression towards the goal to end the epidemic by 2030.

Author details

Adenike O. Soogun[1,2*†], Ayesha B.M. Kharsany[2,3†], Temesgen Zewotir[1] and Delia North[1]

1 School of Mathematics, Statistics and Computer Science, College of Agriculture Engineering and Science, University of KwaZulu-Natal, Westville Campus, Durban, South Africa

2 Centre for the AIDS Programme of Research in South Africa (CAPRISA), University of KwaZulu-Natal, South Africa

3 School of Laboratory Medicine and Medical Science, Nelson R Mandela School of Medicine, University of KwaZulu-Natal, Durban, South Africa

*Address all correspondence to: nike.soogun@gmail.com; adenike.Soogun@caprisa.org

†Adenike O. Soogun and Ayesha B.M. Kharsany are Joint first authors

References

[1] UNAIDS. 90–90-90 an Ambitious Treatment Target to Help End the AIDS Epidemic. Geneva: UNAIDS; 2014. Available from: http://www.unaids/unaids.org/sites/default/files/media_asset/90-90-90_en.pdf

[2] Gaolathe T, Wirth KE, Holme MP, Makhema J, Moyo S, Chakalisa U, et al. Botswana's progress toward achieving the 2020 UNAIDS 90-90-90 antiretroviral therapy and virological suppression goals: A population-based survey. The Lancet HIV. 2016;**3**(5):e221-e230. DOI: 10.1016/S2352-3018(16)00037-0

[3] Marukutira T, Stoové M, Lockman S, Mills LA, Gaolathe T, Lebelonyane R, et al. A tale of two countries: Progress towards UNAIDS 90-90-90 targets in Botswana and Australia. Journal of the International AIDS Society. 2018;**21**(3):e25090. DOI: 10.1002/jia2.25090

[4] UNAIDS Global HIV & AIDS statistics: 2020 fact sheet. 2020. Available from: https://www.unaids.org/en/resources/fact-sheet [Accessed: November 30, 2021]

[5] UNAIDS. Global AIDS Strategy 2021–2026, End inequalities. End AIDS. 2021. Available from: https://www.unaids.org/sites/default/files/media_asset/global-AIDS-strategy-2021-2026_en.pdf [Accessed: November 30, 2021]

[6] Akullian A, Morrison M, Garnett GP, Mnisi Z, Lukhele N, Bridenbecker D, et al. The effect of 90-90-90 on HIV-1 incidence and mortality in eSwatini: A mathematical modelling study. Lancet HIV. 2020;7:E348-E358. DOI: 10.1016/S2352-3018(19)30436-9

[7] Pandey A, Galvani AP. The global burden of HIV and prospects for control. Lancet HIV. 2019;**6**(12):e809-e811. DOI: 10.1016/S2352-3018(19)30230-9

[8] Statistics South Africa (STATSA SA). Statistical release: Mid-Year population estimates. 2020. Available from: http://www.statssa.gov.za/publications/P0302/P03022020.pdf. [Accessed: November 30, 2021]

[9] Kharsany AB, Cawood C, Khanyile D, Lewis L, Grobler A, Puren A, et al. Community-based HIV prevalence in Kwa Zulu-Natal, South Africa: Results of a cross-sectional household survey. The Lancet HIV. 2018;**5**(8):e427-e437. DOI: 10.1016/S2352-3018(18)30104-8

[10] Kharsany AB, Cawood C, Lewis L, Yende-Zuma N, Khanyile D, Puren A, et al. Trends in HIV prevention, treatment, and incidence in a hyperendemic area of KwaZulu-Natal, South Africa. JAMA Network Open. 2019;**2**(11):e1914378. DOI: 10.1001/jamanetworkopen.2019.14378

[11] Grobler A, Cawood C, Khanyile D, Puren A, Kharsany ABM. Progress of UNAIDS 90-90-90 targets in a district in KwaZulu-Natal, South Africa, with high HIV burden, in the HIPSS study: A household-based complex multilevel community survey. Lancet HIV. 2017;**4**(11):e505-e513. DOI: 10.1016/S2352-3018(17)30122-4

[12] Huerga H, Van Cutsem G, Farhat JB, Puren A, Bouhenia M, Wiesner L, et al. Progress towards the UNAIDS 90–90-90 goals by age and gender in a rural area of KwaZulu-Natal, South Africa: A household-based community cross-sectional survey. BMC Public Health.

2018;**18**(1):303. DOI: 10.1198/1061860043010

[13] Simbayi LC, Zuma K, Zungu N, Moyo S, Marinda F, Jooste S, et al. South African National HIV Prevalence, Incidence, Behaviour and Communication Survey 2017 (SABSSM V): Towards Achieving the UNAIDS 90–90-90 Targets. Cape Town: HSRC Press; 2019

[14] Marinda E, Simbayi L, Zuma K, Zungu N, Moyo S, Kondlo L, et al. Towards achieving the 90–90–90 HIV targets: Results from the south African 2017 national HIV survey. BMC Public Health. 2020;**20**:1375. DOI: 10.1186/s12889-020-09457-z

[15] De Oliveira T, Kharsany AB, Graf T, Cawood C, Khanyile D, Grobler A, et al. Transmission networks and risk of HIV infection in KwaZulu-Natal, South Africa: A community-wide phylogenetic study. Lancet HIV. 2017;**4**:E41-E50. DOI: 10.1016/S2352-3018(16)30186-2

[16] Wand H, Dassaye R, Reddy T, Yssel J, Ramjee G. Geographical level contributions of risk factors for HIV infections using generalized additive models: Results from a cohort of south African women. AIDS Care. 2019;**31**: 714-722. DOI: 10.1080/09540121.2018.1556382

[17] Gibbs A, Reddy T, Dunkle K, Jewkes R. HIV-prevalence in South Africa by settlement type: A repeat population-based cross-sectional analysis of men and women. PLoS One. 2020; **15**(3):e0230105. DOI: 10.1371/journal.pone.0230105

[18] Wessels J, Sherman G, Bamford L, Makua M, Ntloana M, Nuttall J, et al. The updated south African national guideline for the prevention of mother to child transmission of communicable infections. South African Journal of HIV Medicine. 2020;**21**(1):1079. DOI: 10.4102/sajhivmed.v21i1.1079

[19] Horwood C, Vermaak K, Butler L, Haskins L, Phakathi S, Rollins N. Elimination of paediatric HIV in KwaZulu-Natal, South Africa: Large-scale assessment of interventions for the prevention of mother-to-child transmission. Bulletin of the World Health Organization. 2012;**90**(3):168-175. DOI: 10.2471/BLT.11.092056

[20] Manda S, Haushona N, Bergquist R. A scoping review of Spatial Analysis approaches using health survey data in sub-Saharan Africa. International Journal of Environmental Research and Public Health. 2020;**17**:3070. DOI: 10.3390/ijerph17093070

[21] Boyda DC, Holzman SB, Berman A, Grabowski MK, Chang LW. Geographic information systems, spatial analysis, and HIV in Africa: A scoping review. PLoS One. 2019;**14**(5):e0216388. DOI: 10.1371/journal.pone.0216388

[22] Woldesenbet SA, Kufa T, Barron P, Chirombo BC, Cheyip M, Ayalew K, et al. Viral suppression and factors associated with failure to achieve viral suppression among pregnant women in South Africa. AIDS. 2020;**34**(4): 589-597. DOI: 10.1097/QAD.0000000000002457

[23] SANAC. South Africa's National Strategic Plan for HIV, TB and STIs 2017–2022. 2016. Available from: https://sanac.org.za//wp-content/uploads/2017/06/NSP_FullDocument_FINAL.pdf

[24] South Africa National Department of Health (SANDoH). National Retention Adherence Policy: Policy and service delivery guidelines for linkage to care adherence to treatment and retention in care. 2016. Available from: https://www.

nacosa.org.za/wpcontent/uploas/2016/11/Integrated-Adherence-Guidelines-NDOH.pdf [Accessed: September 10, 2021]

[25] Quinn TC, Wawer MJ, Sewankambo N, Serwadda D, Li C, Wabwire-Mangen F, et al. Viral load and heterosexual transmission of human immunodeficiency virus type 1. The New England Journal of Medicine. 2000; **342**(13):921-929. DOI: 10.1056/NEJM200003303421303

[26] Ellman TM, Alemayehu B, Abrams EJ, Arpadi S, Howard AA, El-Sadr WM. Selecting a viral load threshold for routine monitoring in resource-limited settings: Optimizing individual health and population impact. Journal of the International AIDS Society. 2017;**20**:e25007. DOI: 10.1002/jia2.25007

[27] Soogun AO, Kharsany ABM, Zewotir T, North D, Ogunsakin RE. Identifying potential factors associated with high viral load in KwaZulu-Natal, South Africa using multiple correspondence analysis and random forest. BMC Research & Methods. 2022;**22**(174):1-16. DOI: 10.1186/s12874-022-01625-6

[28] Lawson AB. Statistical methods in spatial epidemiology. John Wiley & Sons; 8 Jul 2013

[29] Katarina V. Spatial autocorrelation of breast and prostate cancer in Slovakia. International Journal of Environmental Research and Public Health. 2020;**17**(12):4440. DOI: 10.3390/ijerph17124440

[30] Getis A. Spatial autocorrelation. Handbook of Applied Spatial Analysis. Springer; 2010. pp. 255-278. DOI: 10.1007/978-3-642-03647-7

[31] Lawson AB. Hierarchical Modelling in Spatial Epidemiology. Computational Statistics. 3rd Edition. CRC Press; 2014. DOI: 10.1002/wics.1315

[32] Ngesa O, Mwambi H, Achia T. Bayesian Spatial semi-parametric modelling of HIV variation in Kenya. PLoS One. 2014;**9**(7):e103299. DOI: 10.1371/journal.pone.0103299

[33] Roberts DJ, Matthews G, Snow RW, Zewotir T, Sartorius B. Investigating the spatial variation and risk factors of childhood anaemia in four sub-Saharan African countries. BMC Public Health. 2020;**20**:126. DOI: 10.1186/s12889-020-8189-8

[34] Besag J, York J, Mollié A. Bayesian image restoration, with two applications in spatial statistics. Annals of the Institute of Statistical Mathematics. 1991;**43**:120. DOI: 10.1007/BF00116466

[35] Greco F, Ventrucci M, Castelli EJ. P-spline smoothing for spatial data collected worldwide. Science Direct. 2018;**27**:1-17. DOI: 10.1016/j.spasta.2018.08.008

[36] Rue H, Held L. Gaussian Markov Random Fields: Theory and Applications. CRC Press; 2005. DOI: 10.1201/9780203492024

[37] Rue H, Riebler A, Sørbye SH, Illian JB, Simpson DP, Lindgren FK. Bayesian computing with INLA: A review. International Journal of Statistics and Applications. 2017;**4**:395-421. DOI: 10.1146/annurev-statistics-060116-054045

[38] Lindgren F, Rue H. Bayesian Spatial modelling with R-INLA. Journal of Statistical Software. 2015;**63**:1-25. DOI: 10.18637/jss.v063.i19

[39] Wang X, Yue Y, Faraway JJ. Bayesian Regression Modeling with

INLA. Chapman and Hall/CRC; 2018. DOI: 10.1201/9781351165761

[40] Spiegelhalter DJ, Best NG, Carlin BP, Van Der Linde AJ. Bayesian measures of model complexity and fit. Journal of the Royal Statistical Socirty Series B: Statistical Methodology. 2002; **64**:583-639. DOI: 10.1111/1467-9868.00353

[41] Shiffrin RM, Lee MD, Kim W, Wagenmakers EJ. A survey of model evaluation approaches with a tutorial on hierarchical Bayesian methods. Cognitive Science (Wiley online library). 2008;**32**:1248-1284. DOI: 10.1080/03640210802414826

[42] Rue H, Martino S, Chopin N. Approximate Bayesian inference for latent Gaussian models by using integrated nested Laplace approximations. Journal of the Royal Statistical Society Series B: Statistical Methodology. 2009;**71**:319-392. DOI: 10.1111/j.1467-9868.2008.00700.x

[43] Krainski E, Gómez-Rubio V, Bakka H, Lenzi A, Castro-Camilo D, Simpson D, et al. Advanced Spatial Modeling with Stochastic Partial Differential Equations Using R and INLA. Chapman and Hall/CRC; 2018. DOI: 10.1201/9780429031892

[44] Kang EL, Liu D, Cressie N, Analysis D. Statistical analysis of small-area data based on independence, spatial, non-hierarchical, and hierarchical models. Computational Statistics and Data Analysis. 2009;**53**: 3016-3032. DOI: 10.1016/j.csda.2008.07.033

[45] Ogunsakin RE, Akinyemi O, Babalola BT, Adetoro G. Spatial pattern and determinants of anemia among women of childbearing age in Nigeria. Spatial and Spatiotemporal Epidemiology. 2021;**36**:100396. DOI: 10.1016/j.sste.2020.100396

[46] Odhiambo C, Kareko MJ. An evaluation of frequentist and Bayesian approach to geo-Spatial Analysis of HIV viral load suppression data. International Journal of Statistics and Applications. 2019;**9**(6):171-179. DOI: 10.5923/j.statistics.20190906.01

[47] MacNab YC. Bayesian disease mapping: Past, present, and future. Spatial Statistics. 2022:2211-6753. DOI: 10.1016/j.spasta.2022.100593

[48] Tomita A, Vandormael A, Bärnighausen T, Phillips A, Pillay D, De Oliveira T, et al. Sociobehavioral and community predictors of unsuppressed HIV viral load: Multilevel results from a hyperendemic rural south African population. AIDS (London, England). 2019;**33**:559-569. DOI: 10.1097/QAD.0000000000002100

[49] Bulage L, Ssewanyana I, Nankabirwa V, Nsubuga F, Kihembo C, Pande G, et al. Factors associated with virological non-suppression among HIV-positive patients on antiretroviral therapy in Uganda, august 2014–July 2015. BMC Infectious Diseases. 2017;**17**:326. DOI: 10.1186/s12879-017-2428-3

[50] Desta AA, Woldearegay TW, Futwi N, Gebrehiwot GT, Gebru GG, Berhe AA, et al. HIV virological non-suppression and factors associated with non- suppression among adolescents and adults on antiretroviral therapy in northern Ethiopia: A retrospective study. BMC Infectious Diseases. 2020;**20**:4. DOI: 10.1186/s12879-019-4732-6

[51] Namale G, Kamacooko O, Bagiire D, Mayanja Y, Abaasa A, Kilembe W, et al. Sustained virological response and drug resistance among female sex workers

living with HIV on antiretroviral therapy in Kampala, Uganda: A cross-sectional study. Sexually Transmitted Infections. 2019;**95**:405-411. DOI: 10.1136/sextrans-2018-053854

[52] Abdullahi SB, Ibrahim O, Okeji A, Iliyasu Y, Bashir I, Haladu S, et al. Virological non-suppression among HIV-positive patients on antiretroviral therapy in Northwestern Nigeria: An eleven-year experience of a tertiary care Centre, January 2009–December 2019. BMC Infectious Diseases. 2021;**21**:1031. DOI: 10.21203/rs.3.rs-146794/v1

[53] Myers B, Lombard C, Joska J, Abdullah F, Naledi T, Lund C, et al. Associations between patterns of alcohol use and viral load suppression amongst women living with HIV in South Africa. AIDS and Behavior. 2021;**25**:3758-3769. DOI: 10.1007/s10461-021-03263-3

[54] Mwangi A, van Wyk B. Factors associated with viral suppression among adolescents on antiretroviral therapy in Homa Bay County, Kenya: A retrospective cross-sectional study. HIV/AIDS (Auckland, N.Z.). 2021;**13**: 1111-1118. DOI: 10.2147/HIV.S345731

[55] Lesko CR, Nance R. M, Lau B, Fojo AT, Hutton H. E, Delaney JA, et al. Changing patterns of alcohol use and probability of unsuppressed viral load among treated patients with HIV engaged in routine care in the United States. AIDS and Behavior 2021;**25**: 1072-1082. DOI: 10.1007/s10461-020-03065-z.

[56] Deiss RG, Mesner O, Agan BK, Ganesan A, Okulicz JF, Bavaro M, et al. Characterizing the association between alcohol and HIV virologic failure in a military cohort on antiretroviral therapy. Alcoholism: Clinical and Experimental Research. 2016;**40**:529-535. DOI: 10.1111/acer.12975

[57] Komati S, Shaw PA, Stubbs N, Mathibedi MJ, Malan L, Sangweni P, et al. Tuberculosis risk factors and mortality for HIV infected persons receiving antiretroviral therapy in South Africa. AIDS (London, England). 2010; **24**:1849-1855. DOI: 10.1097/QAD.0b013e32833a2507

[58] Atuhaire P, Hanley S, Yende-Zuma N, Aizire J, Stranix-Chibanda L, Makanani B, et al. Factors associated with unsuppressed viremia in women living with HIV on lifelong ART in the multi-country US-PEPFAR PROMOTE study: A cross-sectional analysis. PLoS One. 2019;**14**:e0219415. DOI: 10.1371/journal.pone.0219415

[59] Ngandu NK, Lombard CJ, Mbira TE, Puren A, Waitt C, Prendergast AJ, et al. HIV viral load non-suppression and associated factors among pregnant and postpartum women in rural Northeastern South Africa: Cross-sectional survey. BMJ Open. 2022;**12**(3): e058347. DOI: 10.1136/bmjopen-2021-058347

Chapter 3

Temporal and Spatial Distribution of Opportunistic Infections Associated with the Human Immunodeficiency Virus (HIV) in Uganda

John Rubaihayo, Nazarius Mbona Tumwesigye and Josephine Birungi

Abstract

The human immunodeficiency virus (HIV) remains one of the greatest challenges of the twenty-first century in the absence of an effective vaccine or cure. It is estimated globally that close to 38 million people are currently living with the HIV virus and more than 36 million have succumbed to this deadly virus from the time the first case was reported in early 1980s. The virus degrades the human body immunity and makes it more vulnerable to different kinds of opportunistic infections (OIs). However, with the introduction of highly active anti-retroviral therapy (HAART) in 2003, the pattern and frequency of OIs has been progressively changing though with variations in the different parts of the World. So this chapter discusses the temporal and spatial patterns of OIs in Uganda.

Keywords: HIV, opportunistic infections, temporal, spatial, distribution, Uganda

1. Introduction

Opportunistic infections (OIs) are the main cause of ill-health and mortality in persons living with HIV globally. OIs usually take advantage of a weakened immune system as found in persons infected with HIV to cause disease that may lead to death in the absence of effective treatment. Opportunistic infections can be viral, bacterial, fungal, or parasitic but their pattern of attack and frequency can vary in different individuals across the world [1–3]. Thus, while some HIV-infected individuals in developed countries rarely suffer from bacterial and protozoal infections, they are a major cause of morbidity and mortality in developing countries [2–4].

2. HIV and opportunistic infections

The human immunodeficiency virus (HIV) that causes acquired immunodeficiency syndrome (AIDS) remains one of the major global health challenges of the twenty-first century. According to the Joint United Nations Programme on HIV/AIDS (UNAIDS), 37.7 million people worldwide were estimated to be living with this deadly virus by the end of 2020 of which 25.3 million (67%) were in sub-Saharan Africa [5]. Since the outbreak of the HIV pandemic, an estimated 79.3 million cases have been recorded and 36. 3 million people worldwide have died and sub-Saharan Africa accounts for almost 70% of the total deaths [5].

HIV attacks and degrades the human body immune system rendering it defenseless against opportunistic infections normally checked by a competent immune system [6]. Opportunistic infections (OIs) remain the single main cause of ill-health and death among persons living with HIV. The natural history of HIV usually begins with an acute HIV syndromic phase, followed by an asymptomatic latency phase whose duration may vary from person to person (median duration ~10 years) to clinically apparent disease or symptomatic phase characterized by AIDS-defining opportunistic infections, and finally death from AIDS (**Figure 1**) [7].

During the asymptomatic phase, the T-cell-mediated immune system attempts to fight off the HIV infection but as the viral load increases, T-lymphocytes gets exhausted, CD4 cell count progressively falls down, and opportunistic infections start to appear in most cases when CD4 cell count has dropped below 200 cells/μl [7]. According to WHO, there are four clinical stages (WHO clinical stages) of HIV disease progression characterized by different opportunistic infections [8].

The first clinical stage is the asymptomatic phase in which the virus multiplies rapidly but is still hassling with the body immune system and no clinical signs are visible. The second clinical stage signals the end of the incubation period of the virus, and at this stage, its presumed viral load has significantly increased and CD4 cells significantly depleted allowing for the first opportunistic infections to appear, which may include herpes zoster, recurrent upper respiratory tract infections (bacterial sinusitis, tonsillitis, otitis media, and pharyngitis), fungal nail infections, recurrent oral or genital ulceration due to herpes simplex virus, extensive warts virus infection, or extensive molluscum

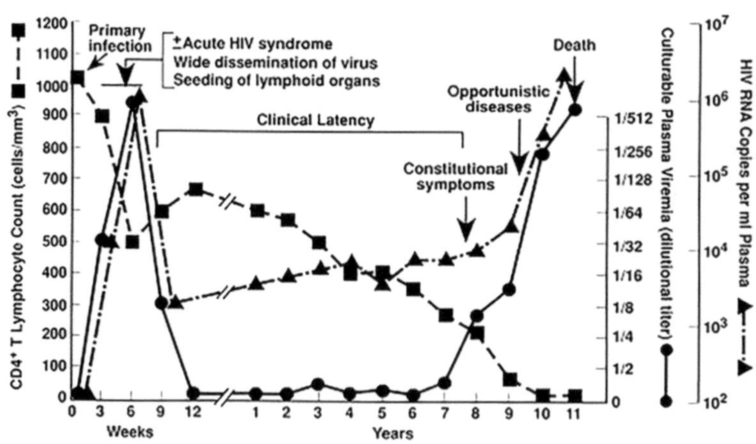

Figure 1.
The natural history of HIV infection (adopted from Pantaleo G, N Engl J Med 1993, 328:327–35).

contagiosum infection The third stage is the beginning of the AIDS (acquired immunodeficiency syndrome) stage in which the immune system is severely damaged and the persons becomes vulnerable to persistent diarrhea (>1 month), oral candidiasis, mycobacterium tuberculosis, oral hairy leukoplakia, and bacterial pneumonia.

The fourth and final stage is the climax of the AIDS stage characterized by multiple life-threatening opportunistic infections including pneumocystis jirovecii pneumonia, Kaposi's sarcoma, recurrent severe bacterial pneumonia, chronic herpes simplex viral infection, esophageal candidiasis, extra-pulmonary TB, cytomegalovirus infection, toxoplasmosis infection, cryptococcosis including meningitis, chronic cryptosporidiosis, chronic isosporiasis, extra-pulmonary histoplasmosis or coccidiomycosis, recurrent non-typhoid salmonella septicemia, and some may be hit by lymphomas (cerebral or B-cell non-Hodgkin).

3. The first opportunistic infection experience among HIV-positive individuals in Uganda

We conducted a study using clinical data obtained from the AIDS support organization database to assess the first opportunistic infection experience, and temporal and spatial distribution patterns of OIs in Uganda. TASO is one of the oldest and largest non-governmental organizations (NGO) providing HIV/AIDS care and treatment in Uganda and sub-Saharan Africa [9]. TASO was founded in 1987 and has 11 regional centers spread across Uganda which have been nationally recognized as centers of excellence (CoE) in HIV/AIDS care and treatment. Each center has four departments including administration, HIV counseling and psychosocial support, and medical (HIV clinic, pharmacy, medical laboratory, etc.) and data department. Additionally, TASO has 23 mini-TASO centers affiliated to public health facilities across the country. TASO serves predominantly HIV-positive patients of low socioeconomic status. All TASO centers offer free HIV testing and counseling, and comprehensive HIV treatment and care, including provision of free antiretroviral drugs and cotrimoxazole prophylaxis, home-based care, and psychosocial support [10].

National HAART rollout in Uganda started in 2004. Being one of the largest NGOs providing care and treatment to persons living with HIV, TASO has been instrumental in HAART rollout in Uganda. Initially, HAART access was based on the Ugandan Ministry of Health and WHO 2006 guidelines, that is, WHO stage 3 or 4 illness or a CD4 cell count <200 cells/μl for adults and adolescents and WHO stage III, advanced stage II or stage I with CD4 cell percentage less than 20% for those more than 18 months of age [11, 12]. However, following a policy review in HAART access, TASO adopted new HAART access guidelines in 2010 [13, 14] that raised the threshold for adults and adolescents to a CD4 cell count≤350 or WHO clinical stage 3 or 4 irrespective of CD4 cell count. In 2014, TASO started implementing the "test and treat" policy that recommends providing lifelong ART to all individuals who test HIV-positive irrespective of CD4 or WHO clinical stage. Initially, the target were HIV-positive pregnant or breast-feeding mothers, their children, HIV-positive individuals diagnosed with TB or hepatitis B co-infections, and HIV-positive individuals in sero-discordant relationships. Later in 2016, coverage was expanded to include everybody who test HIV positive to be eligible for HAART [15]. As part of comprehensive HIV care, TASO also implements universal cotrimoxazole prophylaxis as recommended by the Ministry of Health [16, 17].

The first opportunistic infection experience and the temporal and spatial distribution of each of the 17 selected OIs and Kaposi's sarcoma were assessed. Overall, opportunistic infections (OIs) accounted for 99% of all opportunistic events compared with 1% due to opportunistic cancers (Kaposi's sarcoma, malignant melanomas, Burkitt's lymphoma, and other lymphomas). This is also additional evidence that opportunistic infections are the primary cause of morbidity and mortality among HIV-positive individuals in sub-Saharan Africa.

We assessed data pre-HAART (2001–2003), early HAART (2004–2006), mid-HAART (2007–9), and late-HAART (2010–2013). During pre-HAART period, 84.7% (n = 6549) of the participants had cough with fever, which was later confirmed to be pulmonary TB as their first opportunistic infection and 15.3% had others (diarrhea, candida, herpes zoster, etc.) (**Figure 2**). In early HAART period, 48.4% (n = 7539) had pulmonary TB as their first opportunistic infection, 18.5% had upper respiratory tract infection, 13.5% had persistent diarrhea, 9.6% had herpes zoster, and 10.1% had others (candida, malaria, genital ulcer, etc.) as their first opportunistic infection

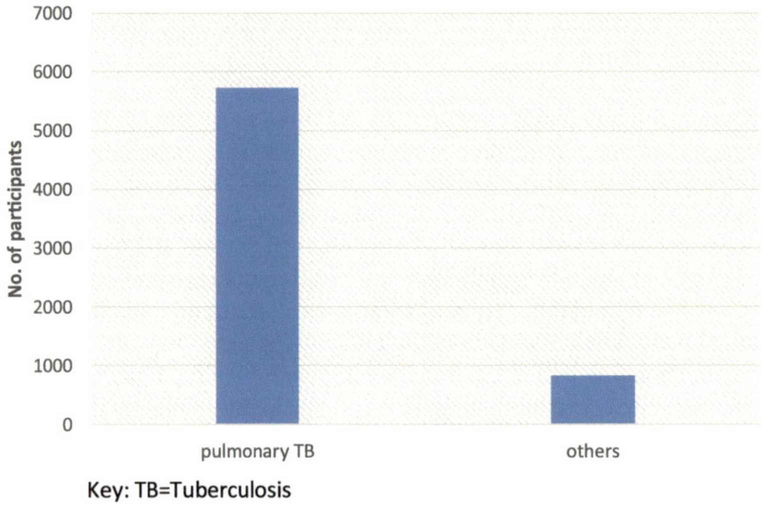

Figure 2.
First opportunistic infection to occur during pre-HAART (2001–2003). Key: TB = tuberculosis.

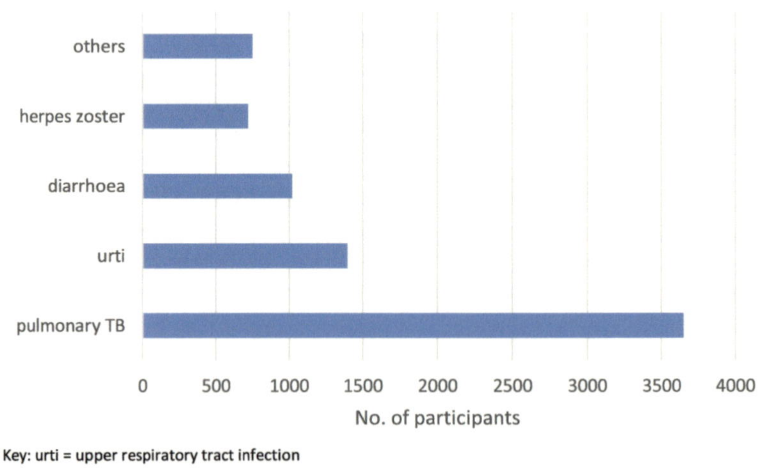

Figure 3.
First opportunistic infection to occur during early-HAART (2004–2006). Key: Urti = upper respiratory tract infection.

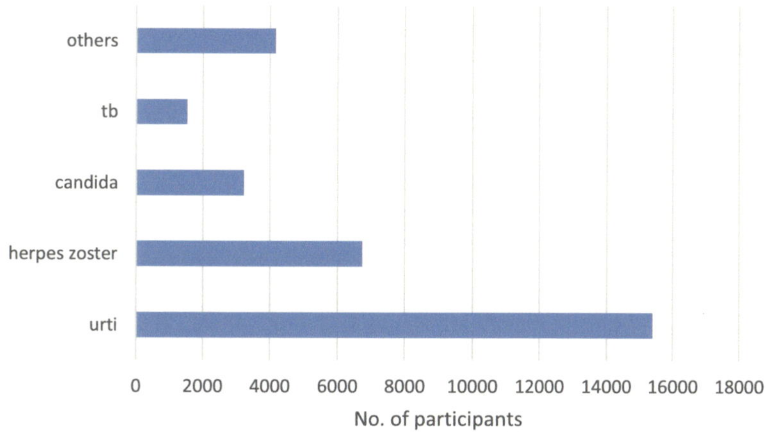

Figure 4.
First opportunistic infection to occur during mid-HAART (2007–2009).

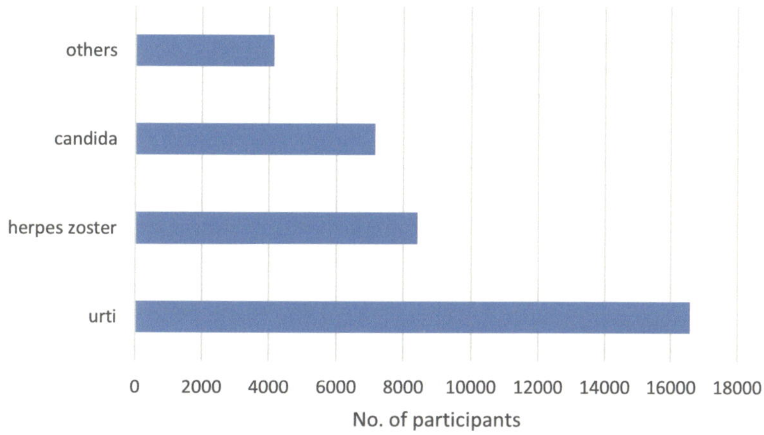

Figure 5.
First opportunistic infection to occur during late-HAART (2010–2013).

(**Figure 3**). In mid-HAART period, 49.6% (n = 31,032) had upper respiratory tract infection as their first opportunistic infection, 21.7% had herpes zoster, 10.4% had candida, 4.9% had pulmonary TB, 13.4% had others (diarrhea, toxoplasmosis, etc.) as their first opportunistic infection (**Figure 4**). In late-HAART period, 45.7% (n = 36,236) had recurrent upper respiratory tract infection as their first opportunistic infection, 23.2% had herpes zoster, 19.7% had candida, and 11.4% had others (pulmonary TB, diarrhea, etc.) as their first opportunistic infection (**Figure 5**).

4. Temporal and spatial distribution of opportunistic infections in Uganda

4.1 Fungal opportunistic infections

4.1.1 Candidiasis

Candidiasis caused by the fungus *Candida albicans* has been associated with HIV/AIDS from the very beginning of the HIV pandemic. Candidiasis can affect the

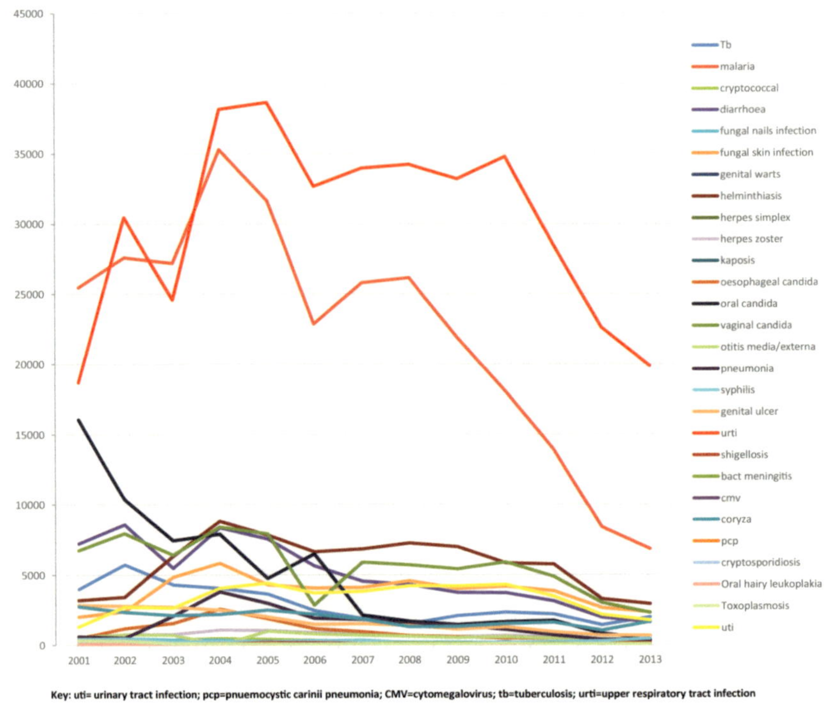

Figure 6.
Temporal distribution of OIs associated with HIV in Uganda.

skin, nails, and mucous membranes throughout the body. Most commonly associated with HIV are oral and esophageal candidiasis. Oral candidiasis is usually the first clinical manifestation of AIDS in most HIV-infected persons causing oral pain that can make eating of food very difficult resulting in malnutrition and HAART failure. Esophageal candidiasis appears later in advanced stages and can also cause a lot of pain in the chest making swallowing of food difficult and hence malnutrition and HAART failure. Studies in the developed countries show high prevalence of oral candidiasis (44.8%) and as high as 67% in sub-Saharan Africa before introduction of effective antiretroviral treatment [2, 18]. In Uganda, most studies before HAART reported high prevalence of both oral and esophageal candidiasis among HIV-infected persons [19–21].

In our recent study, prevalence of oral candida substantially reduced from 34.6% before HAART to 7.2% after HAART (**Figure 6**) [22].

Our recent study also shows that the frequency of oral candida varied by geographical area. HIV-positive patients in western Uganda had higher prevalence of oral candida compared with HIV-positive patients in other geographical areas. Geographical variation in prevalence of oral candidiasis could be an issue of genetic susceptibility and probably level of endemicity. In Netherlands, it was reported that compared with patients from Western Europe, Australia and New Zealand, patients of sub-Saharan African origin had a significantly lower risk for pneumocystis jiroveci pneumonia (PJP) and the authors suggested that differences in genetic susceptibility could be the reason for the lower PJP incidence in the African patients [23]. However, further research is required to gain more insight into the cause of this geographical variation in distribution pattern of oral candida in Uganda.

4.1.2 Pneumocystis carinii pneumonia (PCP) renamed pneumocystis jiroveci pneumonia (PJP)

PCP/PJP caused by *Pneumocystis carinii/jiroveci* used to be one of the most frequent OIs associated with advanced AIDS in the developed countries [24]. Previous studies show that over 80% of the AIDS patients develop PCP when their CD4 cell count drops below 200cell/μl [25]. Before the advent of HAART, it was the most prevalent opportunistic infection in both adults and children in the USA [2] and Western Europe [26, 27].

However following the introduction of HAART, PCP has virtually disappeared among HIV-positive patients in the developed countries [28]. Previous studies also show that PCP/PJP was very rare in sub-Saharan Africa [29–31].

In our recent study, PCP/PJP was very rare reinforcing previous evidence that this OI is not endemic in sub-Saharan Africa.

4.1.3 Cryptococcal meningititis

Cryptococcal meningitis caused by *Cryptococcus neoformans* is one of the most fatal fungal opportunistic infections associated with HIV/AIDS [6]. The disease spectrum includes pneumonia, cutaneous lesions, and meningitis [24]. Cryptococcal meningitis is the most common cause of mortality in adults with HIV [32]. It is the main single cause of death for 20–30% of persons with AIDS in sub-Saharan Africa [6, 33]. Cryptococcal meningitis is often the cause of poor prognosis on HAART [33].

Review of published literature on HIV-associated cryptococcal meningitis shows that its prevalence varies widely both within and between countries [34–37]. In the developed countries, the incidence of cryptococcal disease appears to have generally decreased during the era of HAART [34, 36, 38]. A review of studies on HIV/AIDS-related opportunistic infections in sub-Saharan Africa found 25% prevalence of cryptococcal meningitis among AIDS patients in Ethiopia [39] and 12–50% in South Africa accounting for 44% of the deaths [40]. In Uganda, a study at Mulago National referral hospital found out that the rate of cryptococcal infection among HIV-infected patients was more than double that reported in HIV patients in North America (40.4/1000 person-years vs. 17–20/1000 person-years) prior to the introduction of HAART [41]. In three separate cohort studies in Uganda, cryptococcal meningitis was the leading cause of death (20–40%) [37, 41, 42].

In our recent study findings, the frequency of cryptococcal meningitis substantially declined attributed to increased availability of highly potent systemic antifungal drugs such as fluconazole and HAART (**Figure 5**). Similar findings were also obtained in studied conducted elsewhere [43, 44]. Our recent findings also show that the prevalence was lower in western Uganda compared with the rest of the geographical areas studied probably because of variation in the endemicity of the causative agent. This is consistent with previous studies that show the prevalence of cryptococcosis varied widely both within and between countries [34, 36, 45].

4.1.4 Histoplasmosis

Histoplasmosis is a fungal infection caused by *Histoplasma capsulatum* considered diagnostic of AIDS in an HIV-infected person [24]. In about two-thirds of AIDS patients with histoplasmosis, it is the initial OI and over 90% of the cases have occurred in patients with CD4+ cell count <100 [46]. Though it is a major AIDS-defining illness in Central and South American countries [46], few studies about it have been published in Africa. In Uganda, a recent study confirmed its absence among HIV-infected individuals [22].

4.2 Viral opportunistic infections

4.2.1 Cytomegalovirus (CMV)

This virus causes HIV-associated retinitis resulting in eventual blindness [6]. Prior to the introduction of HAART, cytomegalovirus was commonly reported among HIV-infected patients in many developed countries [2, 26, 27]. A cross-sectional review of AIDS patients' medical records in France [27] found 37% of the patients suffered from cytomegalovirus infection. Another retrospective review of medical records in Italy [26] found 25.6% of the AIDS patients had cytomegalovirus infection. Cytomegalovirus was predominantly common at very low CD4 levels, with the majority of cases of CMV retinitis occurring at CD4 counts below 50 cells/mm^3. However, with the advent of HAART, there has been tremendous decline in the incidence of CMV in the developed countries.

The few studies that have reported on cytomegalovirus in sub-Saharan Africa show that it is very rare among HIV-positive patients. One study in Burundi reported cytomegalovirus retinitis diagnosed in only 1% of the AIDS patients [47] and also in only 1% of the AIDS patients in Malawi [48]. In our recent study in Uganda, it was found to be very rare (<1%) (**Figure 6**).

4.2.2 Herpes simplex virus types 1 and 2(HSV-1 and HSV-2)

Herpes infections are the most commonly diagnosed infections among HIV-positive patients both in developing and developed countries [49]. Both viruses cause severe and progressive rapture of the body mucus membranes. HSV-1 affects mainly the membranes of the nose and mouth leading to herpes-caused pneumonia, which can result into death in AIDS patients [49]. HSV-2 also affects the membranes of the anus and genitals causing severe peri-anal and genital ulcers, which can facilitate HIV transmission and is one of the most sexually transmitted co-infections with HIV [49–51]. Previous studies in Uganda found high prevalence of HSV-2 in HIV-positive patients with genital ulcer disease [52].

In our recent study, frequency of genital ulcers declined significantly attributed to increasing availability of HAART and effective treatment (**Figure 5**). Previous studies also showed that acyclovir significantly reduces both genital ulcers and HSV-2 shedding [53]. Though prevalence reduced, genital ulcer has not been completely eliminated implying that HSV-2 could be highly endemic and its sexual transmission is still ongoing in Uganda. It was more common in central and western Uganda compared with other geographical areas of Uganda.

4.2.3 Herpes zoster (Shingles)

Herpes zoster (Shingles) caused by *Varicella zoster* virus is usually a latent infection in immuno-competent persons [6]. However, the virus is quickly reactivated when the immune system is compromised and like Herpes simplex, it has the potential to cause a rapid onset of pneumonia in AIDS patients. Untreated Herpes zoster viral pneumonia can result into death and Herpes zoster is usually an early indicator that the patient is progressing to AIDS [54].

Most studies in the developed countries have reported on Herpes zoster as one of the most frequent AIDS-defining illnesses among HIV-infected persons [2, 27, 55]. In a cohort study in the USA, Herpes zoster accounted for 36% of the opportunistic diseases that appeared in the first 24 weeks of HAART treatment [56]. In developing countries, Herpes zoster is one of the most common opportunistic infections associated with HIV/AIDS [57, 58]. In a population-based cohort in south-western Uganda, the incidence of Herpes zoster was found to be 5.4 per 100 person years of observation [58].

In our recent study, frequency of herpes zoster reduced substantially attributed to increasing availability of HAART. The mean annual prevalence reduced from 1.3% in 2002 to 0.33% in 2013 [59]. These findings are consistent with findings from studies that reported significant reduction in incidence of Herpes zoster after HAART roll-out [60]. The prevalence was more in central and western regions of Uganda compared with other geographical areas. The variance in prevalence of herpes zoster by geographical area could partly be due to differences in the level of natural immunity or endemicity of the infectious agent or other unknown biological factors.

4.3 Bacterial opportunistic infections

4.3.1 Tuberculosis (TB)

Tuberculosis caused by *Mycobacterium tuberculosis* affects about one-third of the world's population and is the leading cause of morbidity and mortality among HIV/AIDS patients in the world [61]. However, it is most common in low- and middle-income countries in which it is responsible for over 75% of mortality among HIV-infected patients [62–65]. A meta-analysis of the published research in sub-Saharan Africa shows that the incidence of tuberculosis varied widely among cohorts of HIV-infected patients in different countries [3]. Studies in Cote d'Ivoire and Kenya found tuberculosis to be the primary cause of death in 32 and 47% of deaths, respectively [62, 66].

Uganda was listed among the 22 high-burden TB countries in the world [67] and studies conducted in eastern Uganda showed that over 80% of the HIV-related morbidity and 30% of the HIV related death were due to TB [68, 69].

In our recent study, the frequency of *M. tuberculosis* has substantially reduced over time consistent with studies elsewhere that reported significant decreasing trends in tuberculosis prevalence attributed to HAART [70–72]. These findings are in agreement with another study that assessed the effect of HAART on TB incidence in Uganda and showed TB reduced from 7.2% at baseline to 5.5% after 1.4 yrs. of follow-up [68]. Though TB had a significant declining trend in this study, it has not been completely eliminated even after introduction of HAART. This could probably be attributed to the fact that TB is endemic in the country and improvements in TB diagnosis with introduction of Gene-Xpert technology [73] that has improved TB detection rates in Uganda. In our recent study, it was also observed that TB was more frequent among HIV-positive patients in Northern and Eastern Uganda compared with other geographical areas probably because of the socioeconomic disparities in the regions.

4.3.2 Mycobacterium avium *complex (MAC)*

M. avium complex are benign in immuno-competent individuals but can cause severe, life-threatening diarrhea, and septicemia in HIV-infected individuals who are severely immune-compromised [56]. Unlike TB, MAC is only environmentally acquired (food, animals, water supplies, and soil) and not transmissible from person to person. MAC accounts for 18–43% of illness in HIV-positive patients and has been implicated as the main cause of a non-specific wasting syndrome in USA [2, 74]. In sub-Saharan Africa, *M. avium* complex is very rare and was only reported in South Africa and Kenya [75, 76]. No information was available on its prevalence among HIV-positive individuals in Uganda.

4.3.3 Bacterial pneumonia

Bacterial pneumonia caused by *Streptococcus pneumonia* is one of the commonest respiratory diseases in HIV-infected patients [6]. Though preventable, the disease is quite common among HIV-positive patients in sub-Saharan Africa [77–79]. Previous studies showed that the risk of bacterial pneumonia were higher among HIV-infected individuals compared with the general population [80, 81].

Though a conjugate pneumococcal vaccine is available [82], it has not been widely accessed by HIV-positive patients. HAART and cotrimoxazole prophylaxis have also been shown to be associated with a significant reduction in the risk of bacterial pneumonia [80, 83].

In our recent study, the frequency of bacterial pneumonia substantially reduced over time. This could probably be attributed to a combination of universal cotrimoxazole prophylaxis introduced in 2003 and HAART in 2004. Prevalence of bacterial pneumonia also varied by geographical area with the highest prevalence observed in Northern and Eastern Uganda. The geographical difference could be due to the socio-economic regional disparities with Northern and Eastern Uganda being more prone to OIs due to poorer living conditions compared with other areas [84].

4.4 Protozoal opportunistic infections

4.4.1 Toxoplasmosis

Toxoplasmosis caused by *Toxoplasma gondii* is a common opportunistic infection in advanced AIDS [6]. A study in Italy reported 15.2% prevalence of cerebral toxoplasmosis among AIDS patients [26], while another study in France reported a 37% prevalence among AIDS patients [27].

However, in sub-Saharan Africa, few studies have been published on this opportunistic infection and perhaps could be under-reported due to lack of surveillance capabilities. A study in Cote d'Ivoire showed only 4% prevalence of cerebral toxoplasmosis of which 60% died [85]. In our recent study, the prevalence of toxoplasmosis was very low (< 1%) (**Figure 6**).

4.4.2 Cryptosporidiosis

Cryptosporidiosis caused by *Cryptosporidium parvum* is usually associated with chronic diarrhea (>1 month) in HIV-positive individuals [24]. Diarrhea has for long been reported to be one of the commonest complication in HIV-positive individuals associated with high mortality rate [86]. Previous studies show up to 60% of people living with HIV experience diarrhea, which negatively affects their quality of life and adherence to HAART [87].

However, diarrhea among HIV-positive individuals may be due to multiple causes including infectious causes (bacterial, viral, protozoal, heliminthic, etc.) or non-infectious causes (ARV drug effects, e.g., ritonavir-boosted protease inhibitors such as lopinavir/ritonavir or nelfinavir) [87–91]. The commonest infectious causes of diarrhea were reported to be helminthic infections (29.5%), bacterial infections (19.2%), and protozoal infections (9.2%) [92]. Enteric viruses have also been reported associated with diarrhea [86]. Prevalence was significantly higher among HIV-positive people when compared with matched controls [87]. Acute diarrhea (<1 month) in adults has been associated with bacterial infections (non-typhoid salmonella), while chronic diarrhea (>1 month) was reported to be associated with cryptosporidial or helminthic infections [93–96]. In Uganda, data on diarrhea disease burden among HIV-positive individuals in different geographical areas and trends were scarce.

Cryptosporidiosis occurs in HIV-positive individuals whose immunity is severely suppressed [6]. It is rare in developed countries probably because of the high hygienic standards [2]. It is associated with communities living in unhygienic conditions with high risk of exposure to the infectious agent [29, 97].

Previous studies in sub-Saharan Africa have reported prevalence of *Cryptosporidium* chronic diarrhea among HIV-infected patients as high as 17% in Kenya [97], 25–32% in Zambia [98], and 28% among HIV patients at Mulago in Kampala, Uganda [99]. Our recent findings show diarrhea mean annual prevalence reduced by 83% (12–2%) between 2002 and 2013 most likely because of HAART [100]. Prevalence was higher in Northern and Eastern Uganda compared with Central and Western Uganda probably because of the socioeconomic disparities between these regions with the latter being relatively more developed compared with the former [84]. However, more studies are required to give more insight on diarrhea causes among HIV-positive patients on HAART in different geographical areas.

4.4.3 Malaria

Although malaria is not diagnostic of AIDS [93], several studies show that malaria tends to occur with increased frequency and severity in HIV-infected adults compared with the general population [3, 101–106]. Previous studies show that HIV increases vulnerability to malaria infection and malaria could enhance the progression of HIV infection to clinical AIDS in the absence of effective treatment [107].

A review of studies on HIV-related opportunistic infections in sub-Saharan Africa showed a relatively higher prevalence of malaria parasitemia among HIV-infected women in Malawi on their first prenatal visit (32–54%) compared with HIV-negative women (19–42%) [3]. A study conducted in Uganda [104] found that most HIV patients seeking treatment for malaria had unexpectedly high levels of HIV infection and more than 30% of adults presenting at district health centers with uncomplicated falciparum malaria were co-infected with HIV. Another study conducted by researchers from Rome's Istituto Superiore di Sanità, University of Milan in Northern Uganda [105] examined the association between HIV and malaria and found high HIV prevalence among patients admitted for malaria at Lacor Hospital (48.8%) compared with that estimated for the general population living in the hospital's catchment's area (17.8%), suggesting an association between HIV and malaria. Other previous studies in Uganda also showed that the risk of clinically diagnosed malaria was significantly higher in HIV-infected individuals compared with HIV-negative controls [101, 106].

In our recent study findings, malaria prevalence among HIV-positive individuals reduced in the period between 2001 and 2003 (80%) and leveled off in the subsequent years. The reduction in malaria prevalence started in the period before HAART and could partly be attributed to universal cotrimoxazole prophylaxis [108, 109]. The study findings reinforce the existing evidence that malaria prevalence has significantly reduced among HIV-positive individuals due to the combined effect of cotrimoxazole prophylaxis and HAART [110–114].

However, the decline in malaria prevalence over time may not be attributed to HAART and cotrimoxazole prophylaxis alone but could also have been caused by the other malaria interventions in Uganda including massive distribution of insecticide-treated mosquito bed nets and introduction of indoor residual spraying especially in Northern Uganda [114, 115]. Though malaria prevalence among HIV-positive patients reduced in the era of HAART, it has not been completely eliminated. In view of the fact that malaria is highly endemic in Uganda and HIV-positive patients are highly vulnerable, malaria prevention/control should therefore remain an integral part of comprehensive HIV/AIDS care in Uganda. Prevalence was highest in Central Uganda, followed by Northern and Eastern regions. Geographical variation in prevalence of malaria could be influenced by malaria endemicity in the different geographical areas.

4.5 Helminthic opportunistic infections

The most common helminthic infections of public health importance are *Ascaris lumbricodes*, *Trichuris trichura*, *Necator americanus*, and *Ancylostoma duodenale*. Globally, it is estimated that about two billion people are infected with intestinal helminthic infections mainly in developing countries [116]. In HIV-positive patients, co-infection with intestinal helminthic infections was associated with dysregulation of the immune response causing inability of the HIV-positive patient to mount an effective immune response [116]. High prevalence of geohelminths can lead to increased prevalence of anemia thereby worsening the health conditions of persons living with HIV/AIDS [117].

In HIV-positive individuals, these parasites compete for food nutrients and cause mal-absorption of certain food nutrients and some of them suck blood (Hook worms) further weakening the body and causing faster progression of HIV disease [118]. The negative effects associated with these helminthic infections have been in terms of diminished physical fitness of the affected individuals who easily succumb to other opportunistic infections in addition to responding poorly to treatment [119].

In our recent study, geohelminths were the most frequent non-AIDS defining opportunistic infections before and after HAART. The study also found out that Northern and Eastern Uganda had the highest burden of the intestinal helminthic infections compared with other regions. The geographical difference could be due to the socioeconomic regional disparities with Northern and Eastern Uganda being relatively poorer compared with other areas [84]. Previous studies showed that poor socioeconomic status was associated with higher risk of geohelminths [120–122].

The high burden of geohelminths even after HAART shows that in high endemic settings, the effect of HAART on these worms is relatively insignificant and alternative or supplementary control efforts are therefore required. A Cochrane review of published literature on testing and treating HIV-positive patients for intestinal helminthic infections showed that regular deworming with a single dose of albendazole is feasible in developing countries and would potentially improve survival and the quality of life of persons living with HIV/AIDs [116]. It is therefore recommended that regular deworming becomes an integral part of comprehensive HIV/AIDS care in Uganda.

4.6 Upper respiratory tract infections (URTI)

Upper respiratory tract infections (URTIs) are contagious infections that affect mainly the nasal sinuses and the throat caused by a variety of bacteria and viruses such as influenza virus, streptococcus bacteria. The most frequent respiratory infections in HIV-infected patients are upper respiratory tract infections presenting as common cold (cough, fever, runny nose), epiglottitis, laryngitis, pharyngitis (sore throat), and sinusitis [123]. In this study, URTIs were the most frequent infections pre-HAART and have remained the most frequent infections even after HAART (**Figure 6**). Previous studies also show that upper respiratory tract infections are more common in HIV-infected persons compared with the general population attributed to the reduced immunity [124].

4.7 HIV-associated opportunistic cancers

Kaposi's sarcoma (KS) is the most reported opportunistic cancer associated with HIV/AIDS and with an infectious cause [24, 125, 126]. In fact, previous studies show that KS is caused by the human herpes virus type 8 (HHV8) [127, 128], and in Uganda, HHV8 has been identified in over 85% of KS tissue specimens [129, 130]. Sero-prevalence studies in Uganda also suggest that HHV8 is endemic in the general population [131, 132]. In our recent study, Kaposi's sarcoma was found rare among study participants. These findings are consistent with other studies elsewhere, which reported lower prevalence of KS in comparison with other OIs among HIV-positive individuals [133–135]. Prevalence was higher in central compared with other regions in Uganda. However, more studies giving insight on the role of HAART on HHV8 disease burden and determinants of its geographical distribution are required.

5. Conclusion

Today, most OIs are less common in people with HIV because of increasing availability of effective antiretroviral treatment. However, there are certain OIs such as intestinal helminthic infections and upper respiratory tract infections whose prevalence has persistently remained high despite increasing access to HAART. Most OIs have not been completely eliminated mainly because some people are not aware that they have HIV and so wait until they experience an OI. Some may delay to access treatment due to late diagnosis or may be on treatment but develop resistance to available drugs.

By end of 2020, around 28million people were accessing effective antiretroviral therapy. Though the global strategy to eliminate HIV by 2020 failed, there is still hope that with sustained global HIV/AIDS eradication efforts, HIV could be eliminated by 2050.

Author details

John Rubaihayo[1]*, Nazarius Mbona Tumwesigye[2] and Josephine Birungi[3]

1 Department of Public Health, Mountains of the Moon University, School of Health Sciences, Fort Portal, Uganda

2 Department of Epidemiology and Biostatistics, Makerere University, School of Public Health, College of Health Sciences, Kampala, Uganda

3 Research and Health System Strengthening, The AIDS Support Organization (TASO), Kampala, Uganda

*Address all correspondence to: jrubaihayo@mmu.ac.ug; rubaihayoj@yahoo.co.uk

References

[1] Colebunders R, Latif AS. Natural history and clinical presentation of HIV-1 infection in adults. AIDS. 1991;**5**:S103-S112

[2] Selik MR, Starcher ET, Curran JW. Opportunistic diseases reported in AIDS patients: Freqiencies, associations and trends. AIDS. 1987;**1**:175-182

[3] Holmes BC, Losina E, Walensky RP, Yazdanpanah Y, Freedberg KA. Review of human immunodeficiency virus type 1–related opportunistic infections in sub-Saharan Africa. Clinical Infectious Diseases. 2003;**36**:652-662

[4] Paton NI, Sangeetha S, Earnest A, Bellamy R. The impact of malnutrition on survival and the CD4 count response in HIV-infected patients starting antiretroviral therapy. HIV Medicine. 2006;**7**:323-330

[5] UNAIDS. UNAIDS DATA 2021. Geneva: WHO; 2021

[6] Staine JG. AIDS Up Date 2007: An Overview of Acquired Immune Deficiency Syndrome. New York: McGraw-Hill co.,Inc; 2008

[7] Pantaleo G, Graziosi C, Fauci SA. The Immunopathogenesis of human immunodeficiency virus infection. The New England Journal of Medicine. 1993;**328**:327-335

[8] WHO. WHO Case Definitions of HIV for Surveillance and Revised Clinical Staging and Immunological Classification of HIV-Related Disease in Adults and Children. Switzerland: World Health Organization; 2007

[9] Calvarese M, Bame S, Bakanume B. Historical analysis of AIDS patients in Uganda using innovative community clinical service: The AIDS support organisation (TASO). Journal of Humanities and Social Sciences. 2007;**1**:1-13

[10] TASO. TASO Services and Programmes Kampala: TASO. 2011. [cited 2011 27/10/2011] Available from: http://www.tasouganda.org/

[11] WHO. Antiretroviral Therapy for HIV Infection in Adults and Adolescents; Recommendations for a Public Health Approach. Geneva: WHO; 2006

[12] Ministry of Health Uganda. Antiretroviral Treatment Policy for Uganda. Kampala: Ministry of Health Uganda; 2003

[13] WHO. Antiretroviral Therapy for HIV Infection in Adults and Adolescents: Recommendations for a Public Health Approach 2010 Revision. Geneva: WHO; 2010

[14] Ministry of Health Uganda. Antiretroviral Treatment Policy. Kampala: Uganda Ministry of Health; 2009

[15] Ministry of Health Uganda. Consolidated Guidelines for Prevention and Treatment of HIV in Uganda. Uganda: Kampala; 2016

[16] Health UMo. National Policy Guidelines for Cotrimoxazole Prophylaxis for People with HIV/AIDS Entebbe. 2003. [07/11/2008] Available from: http://www.aidsuganda.org

[17] Ministry of Health Uganda national policy guidelines for cotrimoxazole prophylaxis for people with HIV/AIDS. Kampala: Ministry of Health, 2005

[18] Ndour M, Sow PS, Coll-Seck AM, Badiane S, Ndour CT, Diakhate N, et al. AIDS caused by HIV1 and HIV2 infection: Are there clinical differences? Results of AIDS surveillance 1986-97 at Fann Hospital in Dakar, Senegal. Tropical Medicine & International Health. 2000;**5**(10):687-691

[19] Malamba SS, Morgan D, Clayton T, Mayanja B, Okongo M, Whitworth J. The prognostic value of the WHO staging system for HIV infection and disease in rural Uganda. AIDS. 1999;**13**:2555-2562

[20] Spacek LA, Shihab HM, Kamya MR, Mwesigire D, Ronald A, Mayanja H, et al. Response to antiretroviral therapy in HIV-infected patients attending a public, urban clinic in Kampala, Uganda. Clinical Infectious Diseases. 2006;**42**:252-259

[21] Morgan D, Mahe C, Mayanja B, Whitworth JA. Progression to symptomatic disease in people infected with HIV-1 in rural Uganda: Prospective cohort study. BMJ. 2002;**324**:193-196

[22] Rubaihayo J, Tumwesigye M, Konde-Lule J, Wamani H, Nakku-Joloba E, Makumbi F. Frequency and distribution patterns of opportunistic infections associated with HIV/AIDS in Uganda. BMC Research Notes. 2016;**9**:501

[23] Schoffelen A, van Lelyveld S, Barth R, Gras L, de Wolf F, Netea M, et al. Lower incidence of pneumocystis jirovecii pneumonia among Africans in the Netherlands host or environmental factors? AIDS. 2013;**27**(7):1179-1184

[24] WHO/UNAIDS. WHO Case Definition of HIV for Surveillance and Revised Clinical Staging and Immunological Classification of HIV-Related Disease in Adults and Children. Geneva: WHO; 2007

[25] Phair J, Munoz A, Detels R, Kaslow R, Rinaldo C, Saah A. The risk of pneumocystis carinii pneumonia among men infected with human immunodeficiency virus type 1. Multicenter AIDS cohort study group. NEJM. 1990;**322**:161-165

[26] Monforte A, Vago L, Lazzarin A, Boldorini R, Bini T, Guzetti S, et al. AIDS defining illnesses in 250 HIV-infected patients; a comparative study of clinical and autopsy diagnoses. AIDS. 1992;**6**(10):1159-1164

[27] Jougla E, Pequignot F, Carbon C, Pavillon G, Eb M, Bourdais JP, et al. AIDS-related conditions: Study of a representative sample of 1203 patients deceased in 1992 in France Internat. Journal of Epidemiology. 1996;**25**:190-197

[28] Stringer JR, Beard CB, Miller RF, Wakefield AE. A new name (pneumocystis jiroveci) for pneumocystis from humans. Emerging Infectious Diseases. 2002;**8**:891-896

[29] Kaplan JE, Hu DJ, Holmes KK, Jaffe HW, Masur H, De Cock KM. Preventing opportunistic infections in human immunodeficiency virus-infected persons: Implications for the developing world. American Journal of Tropical Medicine Hygiene. 1996;**55**(1):1-11

[30] Fisk DT, Meshnick S, Kazanjian PH. Pneumocystis carinii pneumonia in patients in the developing world who have acquired immunodeficiency syndrome. Clinical Infectious Diseases. 2003;**36**:70-78

[31] Bakeera KS, Musoke P, Downing R, Tumwine JK. Pneumocystis carinii in childen with severe pneumonia at Mulago hospital, Uganda. Annals of Tropical Paediatrics. 2004;**24**:227-235

[32] Charurat MN, Blattner W, Hershow R, Buck A, Zorrilla CD, Watts DH, et al. Changing trends in clinical AIDS presentations and survival among HIV-1-infected women. Journal of Women's Health. 2004;**13**(6):719-729

[33] Chang LW, Phipps WT, Kennedy GE, Rutherford G. Antifungal interventions for the primary prevention of cryptococcal disease in adults with HIV. Cochrane Database of Systematic Reviews. 2005, Issue 3. No.: CD004773. DOI: 10.1002/14651858.CD004773.pub2

[34] Hajjeh RA, Conn LA, Stephens DS, Baughman W, Hamill R, Graviss E, et al. Cryptococcosis: Population-based multistate active surveillance and risk factors in human immunodeficiency virus-infected persons. Journal of Infectious Diseases. 1999;**179**(2):449-454

[35] Chariyalertsak S, Sirisanthana T, Saengwonloey O, Nelson KE. Clinical presentation and risk behaviors of patients with acquired immunodeficiency syndrome in Thailand, 1994-1998: Regional variation and temporal trends. Clinical Infectious Diseases. 2001;**32**:955-962

[36] Dromer F, Mathoulin-Pelissier S, Fontanet A, Ronin O, Dupont B, Lortholary O. Epidemiology of HIV-associated cryptococcosis in France (1985-2002): Comparison of pre- and post- HAART eras. AIDS. 2004;**18**:555-562

[37] French N, Gray K, Watera C, Nakiying IJ, Lugada E, Moore M, et al. Cryptococcal infection in a cohort of HIV-1 infected Ugandan adults. AIDS. 2002;**16**:1031-1038

[38] Louie JK, Hsu CL, Osmond DH, Katz MH, Schwarcz SK. Trends in causes of death among persons with acquired immunodeficiency syndrome in the era of highly active antiretroviral therapy, San Francisco, 1994-1998. Journal of Infectious Diseases. 2002;**186**:1023-1027

[39] Aseffa A, Rahlenbeck S, Alemu S. Cryptococcosis in AIDS patients in Ethiopia. The Journal of Infection. 1997;**35**:323-324

[40] Schutte CM, Van der Meyden CH, Magazi DS. The impact of HIV on meningitis as seen at a south African academic hospital (1994 to 1998). Infection. 2000;**28**:3

[41] Kambugu A, Meya DB, Rhein J, O'Brien M, Janoff EN, Ronald AR, et al. Outcomes of cryptococcal meningitis in Uganda before and after the availability of HAART. Clinical Infectious Diseases. 2008;**46**(11):1694-1701

[42] Liechty CA, Solberg P, Were W, Ekwaru JP, Ransom RL, Weidle PJ, et al. Asymptomatic serum cryptococcal antigenemia and early mortality during antiretroviral therapy in rural Uganda. Tropical Medicine & International Health. 2007;**12**(8):929-935

[43] Guimaraes MD, Castilho EA, Fonseca MG. Temporal trends in AIDS associated opportunistic infections in Brazil, 1980-1999. International Conference AIDS. Cadernos de Saude Publica. 2000;**16**(suppl 1):21-36

[44] Warnock DW. Trends in the epidemiology of invasive fungal infections. Japanese Journal of Infectious Diseases. 2007;**48**:1-12

[45] Chariyalertsak S, Sirisanthana T, Saenwonloey O, Nelson KE. Clinical presentation and risk behaviors of patients with acquired immunodeficiency syndrome in Thailand, 1994-98: Regional variation and temporal trends. Clinical Infectious Diseases. 2001;**32**:955-962

[46] Huber F, Nacher M, Azner C, Demar MP, Guedj ME, Vaz T, et al.

AIDS- related Histoplasma capsulatum var capsulatum: 25 years experience in French Guiana. AIDS. 2008;**22**:1047-1053

[47] Cochereau I, Mlika-Cabanne N, Godinaud P, Niyongabo T, Poste B, Ngayiragije A, et al. AIDS related eye disease in Burundi, Africa. British Journal of Ophthalmology. 1999;**83**(3):339-342

[48] Lewallen S, Kumwenda J, Maher D, Harries AD. Retinal findings in Malawian patients with AIDS. The British Journal of Ophthalmology. 1994;**78**:757-759

[49] Freeman EE, Weiss HA, Glynn JR, Cross PL, Whitworth JA, Hayes RJ. Herpes simplex virus 2 infection increases HIV acquisition in men and women: Systematic review and meta-analysis of longitudinal studies. AIDS. 2006;**20**(1):73-83

[50] Kamali A, Nunn AJ, Mulder DW, Dyck EV, Dobbins JG, Whitworth AG. Seroprevalence and incidence of genital ulcer infections in a rural Ugandan population. Sexually Transmitted Infections. 1999;**75**:98-102

[51] Glynn RJ, Biraro S, Weiss HA. Herpes simplex virus type 2: A key role in HIV incidence. AIDS. 2009;**23**:1595-1598

[52] Kamya M, Nsubuga P, Grant R, Hellman N. The high prevalence of genital herpes among patients with genital ulcer disease in Uganda. Sexually Transmitted Diseases. 1995;**22**(6):351-354

[53] Tobian A, Nalugoda F, Grabowski M, Wawer M, Serwadda D, Gray R, et al. Reactivation of herpes simplex virus type 2 after initiation of antiretroviral therapy. The Journal of Infectious Diseases. 2013;**208**:839-846

[54] Vanhems P, Voisin L, Gayet-Ageron A, Trepo C, Cotte L, Peyramond D, et al. The incidence of herpes zoster is less likely than other opportunistic infectionss to be reduced by highly active antiretroviral therapy. Journal of Acquired Immune Deficiency Syndromes. 2005;**38**:111-113

[55] Bonnet F, Lewden C, May T, Heripret C, Jougla E, Bevilacqua S, et al. Opportunistic infections as cause of death in HIV infected patients in the HAART era in France. Scandinavian Journal of Infectious Diseases. 2005;**37**:482-487

[56] Jones JL, Hanson DL, Dworkin MS, Alderton DL, Fleming PL, Kaplan JE, et al. Surveillance for AIDS-defining opportunistic illnesses (1992-97). MMWR. CDC Surveillance Summaries. 1999;**48**(2):1-22

[57] Edhonu-Elyetu Y. Significance of herpes zoster in HIV/AIDS in Kweneng district, Botswana. East African Medicine Journal. 1998;**75**:379-381

[58] Morgan D, Mahe C, Malamba S, Okongo M, Mayanja B, Whitworth J. Herpes zoster and HIV-1 infection in a rural Ugandan cohort. AIDS. 2001;**15**: 223-229

[59] Rubaihayo J, Tumwesigye MN, Konde-Lule J. Trends in prevalence of selected opportunistic infections associated with HIV/AIDS in Uganda. BMC Infectious Diseases. 2015;**15**:187

[60] Moanna A, Rimland D. Decreasing incidence of herpes zoster in the HAART era. Clinical Infectious Diseases. 2013;**57**(1):122-125

[61] WHO. Global Tuberculosis Control Report 2013, Geneva. Switzerland: WHO; 2013

[62] Corbett EL, Marston B, Churchyard GJ, De Cock KM.

Tuberculosis in sub-Saharan Africa: Opportunities, challenges, and change in the era of anti-retroviral treatment. Lancet. 2006;**367**:926-937

[63] Nissapatorn V, Lee C, Tatt QK, Abdullah KA. AIDS-related opportunistic infections in hospital Kuala Lumpur. Japanese Journal of Infectious Diseases. 2003;**56**:187-192

[64] Saldanha D, Gupta N, Shenoy S, Saralaya V. Prevalence of opportunistic infections in AIDS patients in Mangalore, Karnataka. Tropical Doctor. 2008;**38**:172-173

[65] Bellamy R, Sangeetha S, Paton NI. AIDS-defining illnesses among patients with HIV in Singapore, 1985-2001: Results from the Singapore HIV observational cohort study (SHOCS). BMC Infectious Diseases. 2004;**4**:47

[66] Anglaret X, Minga A, Gabillard D, Ouassa T, Messou E, Morris B, et al. AIDS and non-AIDS morbidity and mortality across the spectrum of CD4 cell counts in HIV-infected adults before starting antiretroviral therapy in cote d'Ivoire. Clinical Infectious Diseases. 2012;**54**(5):714-723

[67] WHO. Global Tuberculosis Control: Surveillance, Planning, Financing: WHO Report 2005. WHO/HTM/TB/2005.349. Geneva: WHO; 2005

[68] Moore D, Liechty C, Ekwaru P, Were W, Mwima G, Solberg P, et al. Prevalence, incidence and mortality associated with tuberculosis in HIV-infected patients initiating antiretroviral therapy in rural Uganda. AIDS. 2007;**21**(6):713-719

[69] Mermin J, Were W, Ekwaru JP, Moore D, Dawning R, Behumbiize P, et al. Mortality in HIV-infected Ugandan adults receiving antiretroviral treatment and survival of their HIV-uninfected children: A prospective cohort study. Lancet. 2008;**371**:752-759

[70] Jones JL, Hanson DL, Dworkin MS, Kaplan JE, Ward JW. Trends in AIDS-related opportunistic infections among men who have sex with men and among injecting drug users, 1991-1996. Journal of Infectious Diseases. 1998;**178**:114-120

[71] San-Andres FJ, Rubio R, Castilla J, Pulido F, Palao G, de Pedro I, et al. Incidence of acquired immunodeficiency syndrome–associated opportunistic diseases and the effect of treatment on a cohort of 1115 patients infected with human immunodeficiency virus, 1989-1997. Clinical Infectious Diseases. 2003;**36**:1177-1185

[72] Miranda A, Morgan M, Jamal L, Laserson K, Barreira D, Silva G, et al. Impact of antiretroviral therapy on the incidence of tuberculosis: The Brazilian experience, 1995-2001. PLoS One. 2007;**2**(9):e826

[73] WHO. WHO Tuberculosis Report 2015. 20th ed. Geneva, Switzerland: WHO; 2015

[74] Gona P, Van Dyke RB, Williums PL, Dankner WM, Chernoff MC, Nachman SA, et al. Incidence of opportunistic and other infections in HIV-infected children in the HAART era. Journal of American Medical Association. 2006;**296**(3):292-300

[75] Von Gottberg A, Sacks L, Machala S, Blumberg L. Utility of blood cultures and incidence of mycobacteremia in patients with suspected tuberculosis in a south African infectious disease referral hospital. The International Journal of Tuberculosis and Lung Disease. 2001;**5**(1):80-86

[76] Arthur G, Nduba VN, Kariuki SM, Kimari J, Bhatt M, Gilks CF. Trends in

bloodstream infections among human immunodeficiency virus-infected adults admitted to a Hospital in Nairobi, Kenya, during the last decade. Clinical Infectious Diseases. 2001;**33**:248-256

[77] Gilks CF, Ojoo SA, Ojoo JC, Brindle RJ, Paul J, Batchelor BI, et al. Invasive pneumococcal disease in a cohort of predominantly HIV-1 infected female sex-workers in Nairobi, Kenya. Lancet. 1996;**347**(9003):718-723

[78] French N, Nakiyingi J, Carpenter LM, Lugada E, Moi K, Watera C, et al. 23—Valent pneumococcal polysaccharide vaccine in HIV-1-infected Ugandan adults: Double-blind, randomised and placebo controlled trial. Lancet. 2000;**355**(9221):2106-2111

[79] Miiro G, Kayhty H, Watera C, Tolmie H, Whitworth JA, Gilks CF, et al. Conjugate pneumococcal vaccine in HIV-infected Ugandans and the effect of past receipt of polysaccharide vaccine. The Journal of Infectious Diseases. 2005;**192**(10):1801-1805

[80] Tumbarello M, Tacconelli E, Donati K, Citton R, Leon F, Spanu T, et al. HIV-assocaited bacteremia: How it has changed in the highly active antiretroviral therapy (HAART) era. JAIDS. 2000;**23**(2):145-151

[81] Kohli R, Lo Y, Homel P, Flanigan TP, Gardner LI, Howard AA, et al. Bacterial pneumonia, HIV therapy, and disease progression among HIV-infected women in the HIV epidemiologic research (HER) study. Clinical Infectious Diseases. 2006;**43**:90-98

[82] Dworkin M, Ward J, Hanson D, Jones J, Kaplan J. Pneumococcal disease among human immunodeficiency virus-infected persons:Incidence, risk factors, and impact of vaccination. Clinical Infectious Diseases. 2001;**32**:794-800

[83] Currier J, Williams P, Feinberg J, Becker S, Owens S, Fichtenbaum C. Impact of prophylaxis for Mycobacterium avium complex on bacterial infections in patients with advanced human immunodeficiency virus disease. Clinical Infectious Diseases. 2001;**32**:1615-1622

[84] Uganda Bureau of Statistics (UBOS). Statistical abstract Entebbe: UBOS, 2009;**2019**:24

[85] Grant AD, Djomand G, Smets P, Kadio A, Coulibaly M, Kakou A, et al. Profound immunosuppression across the spectrum of opportunistic disease among hospitalized HIV-infected adults in Abidjan, cote d'Ivoire. AIDS. 1997;**11**(11):1357-1364

[86] Grohmannp G, Glass R, Pereira H, Monroem s, Ainerweber AH, Bryan A. Enteric viruses and diarrhea In Hiv-infected patients. The New England Journal of Medicine. 1993;**329**(1):14-20

[87] MacArthur R, DuPont H. Etiology and pharmacologic Management of Noninfectious Diarrhea in HIV-infected individuals in the highly active antiretroviral therapy era. Clinical Infectious Diseases. 2012;**55**(6):860-867

[88] Guest J, Ruffin C, Tschampa J, DeSilva K, Rimland D. Differences in rates of diarrhea in patients with human immunodeficiency virus receiving Lopinavir-ritonavir or nelfinavir. Pharmacotherapy. 2004;**24**(6):727-735

[89] Johnson M, Grinsztejn B, Rodriguez C, Coco J, DeJesus E, Lazzarin A, et al. 96-week comparison of once-daily atazanavir/ritonavir and twice-daily lopinavir/ritonavir in patients with multiple virologic failures. AIDS. 2006;**20**(5):711-718

[90] Heiser C, Ernst J, Barrett J, French N, Schutz M, Dube M. Probiotics, soluble

fiber and L-glutamine (GLN) reduce nelfinavir (NFV)- or lopinavir/ritonavir (LPV/r)- related diarrhea. Journal of the International Association of Physicians in AIDS Care. 2004;**3**:121-129

[91] Molina J, Andrade-Villanueva J, Echevarria J, Chetchotisakd P, Corral J, David N, et al. Once-daily atazanavir/ritonavir versus twice-daily lopinavir/ritonavir, each in combination with tenofovir and emtricitabine, for management of antiretroviral-naive HIV-1-infected patients: 48 week efficacy and safety results of the CASTLE study. Lancet. 2008;**372**(9639):646-655

[92] Binka A, Mahe C, Watera C, Lugada E, Gilks CF, Whitworth JAG, et al. Diarrhoea, CD4 counts and enteric infections in a community-based cohort of HIV-infected adults in Uganda. Journal of Infection. 2002;**45**(2):99-105

[93] WHO. WHO Case Definitions of HIV for Surveillance and Revised Clinical Staging and Immunological Classification of HIV-Related Diseases in Adults and Children. Geneva, Switzerland: WHO; 2006

[94] Lew E, Poles M, Dieterich D. Diarrheal diseases associated with HIV infection. Gastroenterology Clinics of North America. 1997;**26**:259-290

[95] Lee L, Puhr N, Maloney E, Bean N, Tauxe R. Increase in antimicrobial-resistant salmonella infections in the United States, 1989-1990. The Journal of Infectious Diseases. 1994;**170**:128-134

[96] Sanchez TH, Brooks JT, Sullivan PS, Juhasz M, Mintz E, Dworkin MS, et al. Bacterial diarrhea in persons with HIV infection, United States, 1992-2002. Clinical Infectious Diseases. 2005;**41**(11):1621-1627

[97] Mwachari C, Batchelor BI, Paul J, Waiyaki PG, Gilks CF. Chronic diarrhoea among HIV-infected adult patients in Nairobi, Kenya. Journal of Infection. 1998;**37**:48-53

[98] Kelly P, Baboo KS, Wolff M, Ngwenya B, Luo N, Farthing MJ. The prevalence and aetiology of persistent diarrhoea in adults in urban Zambia. Acta Tropica. 1996;**61**(3):183-190

[99] Tumwine JK, Kekitinwa A, Bakeer-Kitaka S, Ndeezi G, Downing R, Feng X, et al. Cryptosporidiosis and Microsporidiosis in Ugandan children with persistent diarrhea with and without concurrent infection with the human immunodefiency virus. The American Journal of Tropical Medicine and Hygiene. 2005;**73**(5):921-925

[100] Rubaihayo J, Tumwesigye MN, J K-L. trends in prevalence of diarrhoea, Kaposi's sarcoma, bacterial pneumonia, malaria and geohelminths among HIV positive individuals in Uganda. AIDS Research and Therapy 2015;12:20

[101] Whitworth J, Morgan D, Quigley M, Smith A, Mayanja B, Eotu H, et al. Effect of HIV-1 and increasing immunosuppression on malaria parasitaemia and clinical episodes in adults in rural Uganda: A cohort study. The Lancet. 2000;**356**(9235):1051-1056

[102] Verhoeff F, Brabin J, Hart C, Chimsuku L, Kazembe P, Broadhead R. Increased prevalence of malaria in HIV-infected pregnant women and its implications for malaria control. Tropical Medicine & International Health. 1999;**4**(1):5-12

[103] Herrero M, Rivas P, Rallón N, Ramírez-Olivencia G, Puente S. HIV & Malaria. AIDS reviews. 2007;**9**:88-98

[104] Kamya MR et al. Effect of HIV-1 infection on antimalarial treatment

outcomes in Uganda: A population-based study. Journal of Infectious Diseases. 2006;**193**:9-15

[105] Francesconi P, Fabiani M, Dente MG, Okwey R, Ouma J, et al. HIV, malaria parasites, and acute febrile episodes in Ugandan adults: A case–control study. AIDS. 2001;**15**(18):2445-2450

[106] French N, Nakiyingi J, Lugada E, Watera C, Whitworth JA, CF G. Increasing rates of malarial fever with deteriorating immune status in HIV-1–infected Ugandan adults. AIDS. 2001;**15**:899-906

[107] Chandramohan D, Greenwood B. Is there an interaction between human immunodeficiency virus and plasmodium falciparum? Internat J Epidemiol. 1998;**27**:296-301

[108] Manyando C, Njunju E, D'Alessandro U, Van geertruyden J. Safety and efficacy of Co-Trimoxazole for treatment and prevention of plasmodium falciparum malaria: A systematic review. PLoS One. 2013;**8**(2):e56916

[109] Saracino A, Nacarapa EA, Massinga EC, Martinelli D, Scacchetti M, de Oliveira C, et al. Prevalence and clinical features of HIV and malaria co-infection in hospitalized adults in Beira, Mozambique. Malaria Journal. 2012;**11**:241

[110] Skinner-Adams T, McCarthy J, Gardiner D, Hilton P, Andrews K. Antiretrovirals as antimalarial agents. The Journal of Infectious Diseases. 2004;**190**(11):1998-2000

[111] Greenhalgh S, Ndeffo M, Galvani A, Parikh S. The epidemiological impact of HIV antiretroviral therapy on malaria in children. AIDS. 2015;**29**(4):473-482

[112] Nakanjako D, Kiragga A, Castelnuovo B, Kyabayinze D, Kamya M. Low prevalence of plasmodium falciparum antigenaemia among asymptomatic HAART-treated adults in an urban cohort in Uganda. BMC Malaria Journal. 2011;**10**:66

[113] Mermin J, Lule J, Ekwaru JP, Malamba S, Downing R, Ransoma R, et al. Effect of cotrimoxazole prophylaxis on morbidity, mortality, CD4 cell count, and viral load in HIV infection in rural Uganda. Lancet. 2004;**364**:1428-1434

[114] Mermin J, Ekwaru JP, Liechty CA, Were W, Downing R, Ransom R, et al. Effect of co-trimoxazole prophylaxis, antiretroviral therapy, and insecticide-treated bednets on the frequency of malaria in HIV-1-infected adults in Uganda: A prospective cohort study. Lancet. 2006;**367**:1256-1261

[115] Uganda Ministry of Health. Uganda Malaria Control Report 2011 Aide Memoire. Kampala: Ministry of Health, Uganda; 2011

[116] Alexander P, De P. HIV-1 and intestinal helminth review update: Updating a Cochrane review and building the case for treatment and has the time come to test and treat? Parasite Immunology. 2009;**31**:283-286

[117] Woodburn PW, Muhangi L, Hillier S, Ndibazza J, Namujju PB, et al. Risk factors for helminth, malaria, and HIV infection in pregnancy in Entebbe, Uganda. PLoS Neglected Tropical Diseases. 2009;**3**:e473

[118] WHO. Soil-Transmitted Helminth Infections: Facts Sheet. Geneva, Switzerland: WHO media centre; 2015

[119] Muniz PT. The major human helminthiasis and their prevalence

in Africa. African Journal of Clinical Investing. 2008;**118**(4):1311-1321

[120] Walson JL, Stewart BT, Sangare L, Mbogo LW, Otieno PA, Piper BKS, et al. Prevalence and correlates of helminth Co-infection in Kenyan HIV-1 infected adults. PLoS Neglected Tropical Diseases. 2010;**4**(3):e644

[121] Knopp S, Mgeni AF, Khamis IS, Steinmann P, Stothard JR, et al. Diagnosis of soil-transmitted helminths in the era of preventive chemotherapy: Effect of multiple stool sampling and use of different diagnostic techniques. PLoS Neglected Tropical Diseases. 2008;**2**:e331

[122] Taye B, Desta K, Ejigu S, Dori G. The magnitude and risk factors of intestinal parasitic infection in relation to human immunodeficiency virus infection and immune status, at ALERT hospital, Addis Ababa, Ethiopia. Parasitology International. 2014;**2014**(63):550-556

[123] Wallace J, Hansen NI, Lavange L, Glassroth J, Browdy BL, Rosen MJ, et al. Respiratory disease trends in the pulmonary complications of HIV infection study cohort. American Journal of Respiratory and Critical Care Medicine. 1997;**155**(1):72-80

[124] Benito N, Moreno A, Miro JM, A T. Pulmonary infections in HIV-infected patients: An update in the 21st century. The European Respiratory Journal. 2012;**39**:730-745

[125] CDC. Revision of the CDC surveillance case definition for acquired immunodeficiency syndrome. MMWR. CDC Surveillance Summaries. 1987;**36**(1S):3-15S

[126] CDC. Revised classification system for HIV infection and expanded surveillance case definition for AIDS among adolescents and adults. MMWR - Recommendations and Reports. 1992;**41**(RR-17):1-19

[127] Paradžik M, Bučević-Popović V, Šitum M, Jaing C, Degoricija M, McLoughlin K, et al. Association of Kaposi's sarcoma-associated herpesvirus (KSHV) with bladder cancer in Croatian patients. Tumour Biology. 2014;**35**(1):567-572

[128] International agency for research on cancer (IARC). IARC Monograph on the Evaluation of Carcinogenic Risks to Humans: Epstein-Barr Virus and Kaposi's Sarcoma Herpesvirus/Human Herpesvirus 8. Lyon, France: WHO; 1998

[129] Parkin D, Nambooze S, Wabwire-Mangen F, Wabinga H. Changing cancer incidence in Kampala, Uganda, 1991-2006. International Journal of Cancer. 2009;**126**:1187-1195

[130] Chang Y, Ziegler J, Wabinga H, Katangole- Mbidde E, Boshoff C, Schultz T, et al. Kaposi's sarcoma-associated herpesvirus and Kaposi's sarcoma in Africa. Uganda Kaposi's sarcoma study group. Archives of Internal Medicine. 1996;**156**:202-204

[131] Parkin DM, Wabinga H, Nambooze S, Wabwire-Mangen F. AIDS-related cancers in Africa: Maturation of the epidemic in Uganda. AIDS. 1999;**13**:2563-2570

[132] Simpson G, Schulz T, Whitby D, Cook P, Boshoff C, Rainbow L, et al. Prevalence of Kaposi's sarcoma associated herpesvirus infection measured by antibodies to recombinant capsid protein and latent immunofluorescence antigen. Lacent. 1996;**348**:1133-1138

[133] Onyango JF, Njiru A. Kaposis sarcoma in a Nairobi hospital. East African Medical Journal. 2004;**81**(3):120-123

[134] Mbah N, Abdulkareem IH, Panti A. AIDS-associated Kaposi's sarcoma in Sokoto, Nigeria. Nigerian Journal of Clinical Practice. 2008;**11**(3):181-184

[135] Iroezindu M, Ofondu E, Hausler H, VanWyk B. Factors for opportunistic infections in HIV patients receiving antiretroviral therapy in a resource-limited setting in Nigeria. Journal of AIDS Clinic Research. 2013;**S3**:002

Chapter 4

A Deep Learning Approaches for Modeling and Predicting of HIV Test Results Using EDHS Dataset

Daniel Mesafint Belete and Manjaiah D. Huchaiah

Abstract

At present, HIV/AIDS has steadily been listed in the top position as a major cause of death. However, HIV is largely preventable and can be avoided by making strategies to increase HIV early prediction. So, there is a need for a predictive tool that can help the domain experts with early prediction of the disease and hence can recommend strategies to stop the prognosis of the diseases. Using deep learning models, we investigated whether demographic and health survey dataset might be utilized to predict HIV test status. The contribution of this work is to improve the accuracy of a model for predicting an individual's HIV test status. We employed deep learning models to predict HIV status using Ethiopian demography and health survey (EDHS) datasets. Furthermore, we discovered that predictive models based on these dataset may be used to forecast individuals' HIV test status, which might assist domain experts prioritize strategies and policies to safeguard the pandemic. The outcome of the study confirms that a DL model provides the best results with the most promising extracted features. The accuracy of the all DL models can further be enhanced by including the big dataset for predicting the prognosis of the disease.

Keywords: deep learning, prediction, CNNLSTM, CNNRNN, EDHS, HIV/AIDS test result

1. Introduction

HIV is the world's most critical community health and development problem. Although millions of people have died as a result of AIDS since the pandemic began in 1981, around 36 million individuals now have HIV. An estimated 19 million people living with HIV are enrolled in and getting treatment through regular care programs [1].

Local HIV/AIDS epidemics require immediate investigation and development of relevant intervention plans, as well as methodologies. Behavioral and socio-demographic characteristics are key contributors to the spread of HIV and require a study on the nature and the influence of the HIV pandemic in a specific community [2]. Although the fact that HIV testing is an efficient technique for determining the test status of people, even has challenges and limitations. As a result, strong prediction models are critical for managing and monitoring the local HIV pandemic.

Ethiopian demographic and health survey (EDHS-CSA) [3] generates a massive amount of dataset that may be analyzed to extract important evidence. The development of the deep learning (DL) model supports the processing of huge datasets and the extraction of underlying dataset patterns that support decision making.

Deep learning methods have recently achieved noteworthy success in a variety of research disciplines, including speech recognition [4], natural language processing [5], recommendation systems [6], and computer vision [7]. This approach is very useful in the health sector for disease prediction and classification. Deep learning algorithms are one of the most recent breakthroughs in HIV statistical dataset prediction tools and identification approaches, allowing for faster processing of large datasets. These algorithms can also be used to predict disease. These techniques work well and can be used to predict HIV test results.

In this paper, we use numerous deep learning application models to construct an HIV status prediction system. On the Ethiopian demographic and health survey dataset (EDHS), six DL models have been developed and are being deployed. These deep learning models were tested using well-known metrics such as accuracy, precision, recall, AUC, and F1 scores.

Our contributions are presented below concerning the core goal of predicting HIV test status:

- Identification of the best performing deep learning algorithm for the task at hand among well-known and widely utilized ones.

- To conduct an HIV test prediction research using deep learning application models with the EDHS dataset.

- We created the HIV/AIDS dataset by applying various techniques such as dataset acquisition, dataset labeling and compared the findings using cutting-edge methodologies, and we got good findings.

To the best of our understanding, no research has been conducted using deep learning models to predict HIV test status using the EDHS dataset. This is the first time that a deep learning model has been used in the health sector to predict HIV test results using only 20 attributes. This work may motivate researchers to validate models using other HIV/AIDS datasets.

The major goal of this study is to propose the development of a more accurate prognostic tool for HIV/AIDS test result prediction. This research comprises six DL models that were used to conduct detailed analyses on the EDHS dataset. The algorithm comparison is presented in a logical and well-organized manner, allowing DL to produce more effective and prominent findings.

The remaining section is structured as follows. Section 2 discusses relevant research studies. The proposed techniques are presented in Section 3. Section 4 describes an experimental design and results from the analysis. Section 5 is devoted to comparative analysis, while Section 6 is focused on concluding remarks.

2. Related work

Various scholars have previously done a great amount of study on health topics. This section provides an overview of previous research in the prediction of HIV epidemics using advanced ML algorithms and big dataset technologies. We highlighted some of the most important and significant work done by various researchers in this field.

McSharry et al. [8] used ML approaches to successfully discover HIV predictors through screening on the PHIA dataset. The study aims to analyze the HIV disease trial at various levels of society, detect HIV predictors, and forecast the risk of the disease. For the prediction tasks, six ML models were utilized in the study. The primary finding of this study is that the XGBoost algorithm greatly outperformed the other algorithms in terms of identifying HIV-positive. Another ML methodology presented by Orel et al. [9] examined more than 3,200 parameters of the current Demographic Health Surveys from ten African nations. This study trained four ML models and chose the best one through the f1 score. The primary goal of the study is to identify PLHIV at a rate of more than 95\% and to identify the number of positive persons at a rate greater than 95%. The authors emphasized the significance of attribute extraction strategies in mining information for prediction. Using four separate datasets from UCI, Lu et al. [10] employed one-hot coding to translate the protease cleavage site dataset for prediction using two DL models, RNN and LSTM. Finally, the DL model results are compared to SVM and RF. The author Wang et al. [11] created a convenient model to explain the prevalence of HIV and forecast its occurrence in Guangxi. From 2005 to 2016, the HIV incidence statistics datasets were utilized in the study. They trained the HIV incidence using four models, including LSTM, ARIMA, ES, and GRNN. Following training, all models are assessed using the most popular prediction task evaluation criteria. According to the findings of the studies, LSTM and ARIMA outperform ES and GRNN. The LSTM model, on the other hand, proved more successful than other models. Ahlström et al. [12] provided an algorithmic prediction of HIV status. The author investigated whether a dataset from a national electronic registry might be utilized to predict HIV status using machine learning techniques. The study employed multiple techniques to train prediction models, which were then verified using a dataset from Danish households. They trained the models to simulate various clinical. Steiner et al. [13] evaluate the DL models for drug resistance prediction using the HIV-1 sequencing dataset. DL algorithms are combined with HIV genotypic and phenotypic datasets and studies by the author to study the classification performance of the fundamental evolutionary methods of HIV treatment resistance. They assessed the effectiveness of three DL models using a publicly accessible HIV sequencing dataset.

As a result, we have observed several research projects being conducted in the field of HIV/AIDS prediction. All of the available approaches have been shown to perform on various datasets and produce promising results. These concerns inspire us to investigate deep learning methods for predicting HIV test status to improve prediction performance.

3. Proposed methodology

We discuss the proposed work in this part, which encompasses several phases such as pre-processing, normalizing features, and a deep learning-based prediction technique with parameter settings. **Figure 1** depicts the architecture for the proposed deep learning models for predicting HIV test status in people using the EDHS dataset.

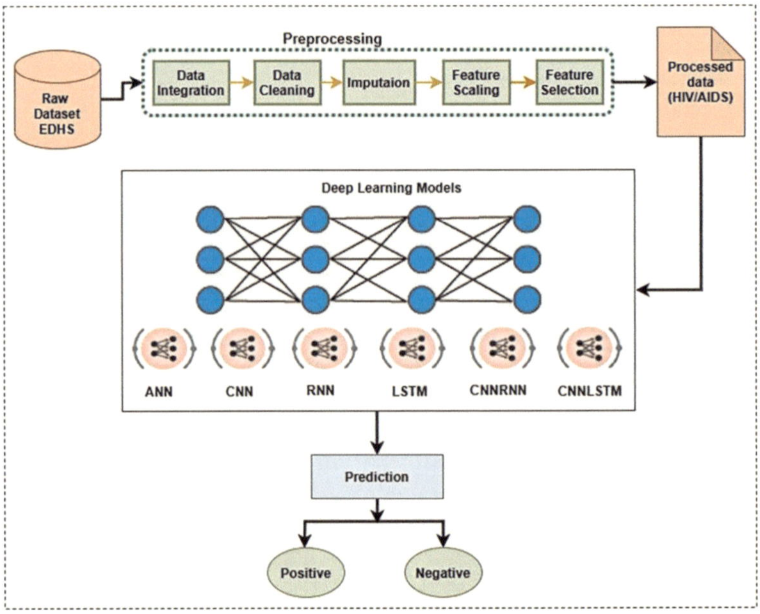

Figure 1.
The proposed deep learning approach's architecture.

3.1 Dataset

The HIV/AIDS dataset [3] has been collected from the EDHS repository from Central Statistics Agency (CSA) and DHS program https://dhsprogram.com that has been used for both training and testing purposes it is available on https://github.com/danielmesafint/Datasets. We collect this dataset as it is from the above sources and we create the HIV/AIDS dataset by considering the criteria to create a dataset from the secondary dataset, the techniques we were used to create our dataset are dataset acquisition, dataset cleaning, dataset labeling and more. The EDHS dataset has more features or attributes, it includes various demographic and health-related datasets. After the creation of our dataset, HIV/AIDS contains 83,100 instances and 33 attributes. The output level has two classes, where "0" represents Negative results (HIV-) and "1" represents Positive results (HIV+). The preprocessing section has explained how we process the EDHS dataset.

3.2 Preprocessing

As an initial step in the pre-processing stage, the original input dataset is analyzed, making the raw dataset ready for use in the prediction process [14]. In the years 2000, 2005, 2011, and 2016, four separate datasets were used to compile the dataset. The size of the dataset is reduced as a result of preprocessing. As a result, there is a scarcity of datasets, which has a negative impact on the prediction of HIV test results. As a result, the dataset integration technique is used to combine all separate dataset sets. The tight coupling method is used for integration. There are 83,100 dataset instances collected; 4,223 of these instances are incorrect, owing to user entry errors, storage or transmission corruption, or different dataset dictionary definitions of similar items in different stores; these datasets are unreliable, inaccurate, or irrelevant. To address this issue, we use dataset cleaning techniques to identify and remove crude and incorrect instances. The dataset cleaning technique used in this process is: to remove duplicate techniques and delete all formatting techniques. After cleaning, the dataset set is uniform. There is also an issue of incompleteness with some features or variables, such as R_SeA, Had_Sex, and Con_Use, and we use the imputation technique to fill in the missing values. Some of the dataset entries in the dataset have not been completed (that is not having values present for every single variable in the dataset set). At this phase, we do two simple approaches to imputation: dropping rows with null values and dropping features with high nullity. Otherwise, the most frequent value for numerical variables and the mean for quantitative variables were used to handle missing results.

Because the nominal dataset cannot be used in a DL model, all nominal attributes, including the label class (Negative/Positive), were converted to numerical binary values with "0" and "1." The Attribute AGE is classified as 1–7. (the original value of the Age should be grouped into 1 to 7). Furthermore, depending on the form of the attribute, the unsupervised discretization filter discretized all continuous numeric attributes using different bins range accuracy. The dataset discretization technique is used to perform this transformation.

The EDHS dataset has several features, each with a unique set of numerical values, which complicates the computing procedure. As a result, a normalizing methodology is utilized to normalize dataset D^{hiv} in the range of "0" to "1", as well as to reduce numerical complexity during the HIV test status prediction computational process. Normalization may be accomplished using a variety of approaches. The well-known min-max normalizing approach is employed in the proposed system [15]. Using the following equation, this approach maps to a numeric value, D, of the initial dataset D^{hiv} into D_{norm} with an interval of [0, 1]

$$D_{norm} = \frac{D^{hiv} - D_{min}}{D_{max} - D_{min}} X \left[n\_max - n\_min\right] + n\_min \tag{1}$$

In this case, D_{norm}, D^{hiv}, D_{max}, and D_{min} represent the normalized dataset value, the original dataset value, the minimal and maximum value in the complete dataset, respectively, while *n_max* and *n_min* represent the range of the transformed dataset. We use the values $n\_max = 1$ and $n\_min = 0$. Using this strategy, all of the feature values fall inside the range [0, 1].

3.3 Feature selection

The EDHS-HIV/AIDS dataset were having 33 (thirty-three) variables but from these variables, we are using 20 variables as a final feature. The feature selection technique is applied to select the features. For this study, we apply the backward feature selection (BFS) technique of wrapper-based methods [16].

BFS algorithm aims to reduce the dimensionality of the initial feature subspace from *N* to *K-features* with a minimum reduction in the model performance to improve upon computational efficiency and reduce generalization error. The primary idea is to sequentially remove features from the given features list consisting of *N* features to reach the list of *K-features*. At each stage of removal, the feature that causes the least performance loss gets removed.

We use the hit and trial method for different values of *K-features* and evaluate all subsets of features using their obtaining accuracy and making the final decision. Based on this, we select the 20 best features and the selected features are presented in **Table 1**. Moreover, the selected feature helps to reduce the over-fitting of the DL models, making the training time fast, reducing the complexity, and easier to interpret our models, and then it helps to make a better prediction power.

After preprocessing we use a total of 78,877 (83,100–4223) instances and 20 (from 33) features. **Table 1** shows the statistical descriptions of the selected features.

3.4 Deep learning models

The study's goal is to create an HIV test status prediction model by employing six deep learning models that have not been used before in HIV test result prediction. Recently, different deep learning techniques and their combinations are widely used for demographic and health dataset prediction or classification based on some obtained parameters.

In this work, we create and test prediction models for HIV status based on demographic and health survey datasets. To assess the study, we trained four DL models, including Artificial Neural Network (ANN), Convolutional Neural Network (CNN), Recurrent Neural Network (RNN), Long Short Term Memory (LSTM), and two hybrid DL Models such as CNNRNN and CNNLSTM.

Features	MIN	MEAN	MAX	Descriptions
Sex	1.000000	1.502419	2.000000	Gender of the person
Age	1.000000	3.259434	7.000000	Age of the person
Reg	1.000000	5.177661	15.000000	Region where is lived
M_Sta	0.000000	0.885908	5.000000	Marital status of a person
W_Ind	1.000000	3.196857	5.000000	Standard of Living
H_Sex	1.000000	1.222080	2.000000	Did you have Sex?
R_SeA	0.000000	0.607065	1.000000	Recent sexual activity
N_S_Part	1.000000	1.121004	3.000000	How many sex partners do you have?
C_Use	0.000000	0.346349	1.000000	Can you use a condom?
R_Use_Con	0.000000	0.762203	1.000000	Refuse to use a condom?
R_Nhave_Sex	0.000000	0.735561	1.000000	Refuse not to have sex?
HIV_Mosq	0.000000	0.401831	1.000000	Did get HIV by Mosquito?
H_STI	0.000000	0.285557	1.000000	Did you hear HIV transmission?
H_O_STI	0.000000	0.317876	1.000000	Did you hear other means of transmission?
H_AIDS	0.000000	0.966567	1.000000	Did you hear about AIDS?
E_T_HIV	0.000000	0.399634	1.000000	Did you test HIV before?
P_T_HIV	0.000000	0.384085	1.000000	Where do you test?
S_Test	0.000000	0.244282	1.000000	Sample test?
T_in_LAB	0.000000	0.914153	1.000000	Laboratory test
F_T_Resu	0.000000	0.203449	1.000000	Final results

Table 1.
The statistical descriptions of the selected features using backward feature selection methods.

ANN [17] is commonly used for prediction and modeling tasks. Because of its self-learning and self-adapting abilities, ANN is an interesting choice for estimating underlying dataset relationships. It is made up of different neurons, input, output, hidden layers, and activation functions. CNN [18] is a neural network type that is often utilized in image categorization research. It has layers like pooling, convolutional, classification, and fully-connected layer. CNN, contrasting ML, acquires characteristics on its own. The dimension of the inputs is lowered in the pooling layer. RNN [19] is a type of feed-forward NN that includes internal memory. RNN employs the same procedure for each input; however, the result of the input dataset is reliant on the previous result. RNN processes inputs using its internal memory. LSTM [19] is a variant of the RNN. It is simpler to recall the previous dataset in the LSTM. The LSTM networks address the RNN vanishing gradient problem. CNNRNN [20] is a hybrid model that uses a different convolutional layer and a single recurrent layer to process the input sequence of characters. CNNLSTM [21] is a hybrid of CNN and LSTM layers that provides the benefits of both models.

3.5 Performance evaluation metrics

Before building a prediction model, all models must be assessed using several evaluation parameters [22]. We've so far used accuracy scores to evaluate our prediction models. But sometimes accuracy score isn't all enough to evaluate a model properly as the accuracy score doesn't tell exactly which class (positive or negative) is being wrongly predicted by our models in case of a low accuracy score. To clarify this, we perform precision score; recall score, f1 score, AUC, and log-loss for both models. And then we compare our models using these calculated metrics to see exactly where one model excels over the other. We utilized 10-fold CV and an 80:20 train-test split technique to validate the utilized dataset.

$$\text{Acc} = \frac{TP + TN}{TP + TN + FP + FN} \tag{2}$$

$$\text{Precision} = \frac{TP}{TP + FP} \tag{3}$$

$$\text{Recall} = \frac{TP}{TP + FN} \tag{4}$$

As shown in Eqs. (2)-(4), where true positive (TP) is the number of HIV-positive persons who are actually positive. The number of predicted negative persons that are actually negative is represented by the true negative (TP). The amount of people who are labeled as positive but are actually negative is known as false positive (FP). The number of labeled negative persons who are actually positive is defined as false negative (FN). These metrics are frequently computed to measure the predictive quality of models.

$$\text{F1} - \text{score} = 2 * \frac{Precision * Recall}{Precision + Recall} \tag{5}$$

The F1 score may be calculated by dividing the product of recall and precision by the total of recall and precision, as shown in Eq. (5).

$$\text{AUC} = \int_{-\infty}^{\infty} y(t)dx(t) \quad (6)$$

$$\text{Log loss} = (x+a)^n = \sum_{i=0}^{n} y_i \bullet (\log(P_i) + (1-y) \bullet \log(1-P_i)) \quad (7)$$

As Eq. (7), where n is the samples count, yi is the label of the actual class, and pi is the probability of ith sample fits one class. The model performance is measured using log-loss, which computes the prediction as a probability value between "0" and "1". A better predictor must have a lower error value of log-loss, for the goal of lowering it to "0" in the case of a perfect predictor.

4. Experiment setups and result discussion

This part presents the experimental setting and experimental findings and analysis.

4.1 Experimental setting

We carried out our model experiments on Microsoft Windows 10 with an Intel® Core™ i7- 9700 CPU running at 3.00 GHz, 8 processors, 16 GB RAM, and a 1 TB hard disc. The Python language version 3.6 tool with Keras [23] and Tenser-flow was utilized.

To evaluate a model's performance, we need some dataset (input) for which we know the ground truth (label). For this problem, we don't know the ground truth for the test set but we do know for the train set. So the idea is to train and evaluate the model performance on HIV/AIDS dataset. One thing we do is to split the train set into two groups, in the case we use the 80:20 ratio, the ratio is done randomly. That means we would train the model on 80% of the training dataset and we reserve the rest 20% for evaluating the model since we know the ground truth for this 20% dataset. Then we compare our model prediction with this ground truth (for 20% dataset). That's we observe how our model would perform on the unseen dataset. This is the first model evaluation technique. This process is used by the sklearn library in a train-test split method [24].

The parameters setting: For ANN we have 3 hidden dense layers with 32, 16, and 8 perceptrons and the last layer is activation functions with sigmoid. For CNN we have 2 hidden CNN layers with 512 and 256 perceptrons with MaxPooling1D function followed by 2 fully connected layers with 2048 and 1024 perceptrons. And the last layer is activation functions with the sigmoid. For RNN the input layer is Simple RNN with 512 perceptrons followed by 2 fully connected layers with 2048 and 1024 perceptrons. And the last layer is activation functions with the sigmoid. For LSTM the input layer is LSTM with 512 perceptrons followed by 2 fully connected layers with 2048 and 1024 perceptrons. And the last layer is activation functions with the sigmoid. For CNNLSTM the input layer is Conv1D with 512 perceptrons followed by MaxPooling1D layer, and the output of them is connected to the LSTM layers with 512 perceptrons. And the last hidden layers are dense layers with 2048 and 1024 perceptrons. For CNNRNN the input layer is Conv1D with 512 perceptrons followed by the MaxPooling1D layer, and the output of them is connected to the RNN layers with 512 perceptrons. And the last hidden layers are dense layers with 2048 and 1024 perceptrons. Batch Normalization and Dropout layers have been added to all the models to improve the accuracy and help to avoid overfitting. For all models the Learning rate is 0.001, the Loss function is Binary Cross entropy, the Decay is 0.0001, and the optimizer is ADAM [25].

4.2 Experimental result analysis

This subsection presents a detailed analysis of the experimental findings achieved using the proposed approach on HIV/AIDS datasets with standard performance metrics.

As a predictor, six DL models were constructed and used. Predictions were then made, and the performance was assessed. The first experiment is conducted with a train-test split.

For performance evaluation, in terms of goodness-of-fit, the HIV test result prediction model performances are compared. The model compared in this proposed method is; the RNN model, achieving an accuracy of 0.870, the precision of 0.871, recall of 0.876, f1-score of 0.876, and AUC of 0.94. As shown in **Table 2**, all DL models' accuracy results were at least 0.834 or above. With 0.870, the RNN model had the best evaluation performance. RNN was implemented considering several parameters such as dropout, batch-size, epochs, optimizers, etc. The performance of the RNN was based on those parameters. Thus, the performance of RNN is slightly better than the other DL models. The CNNLSTM hybrid model was shown to be the second-best model with 86.2%.

Performance measure metrics values were found to be more than 83.0%. Precision is the proportion of accurately predicted positive findings to the total number of expected positive findings. A perfect precision in information retrieval experiments should be 1. The greatest precision score in this study was obtained using RNN, which was 0.871. A ratio of accurately predicted positive findings to all results is defined as recall. A recall score, like accuracy, must be one for the categorization process to be perfect. With 0.876, the best recall value was attained using the RNN model. F1-score calculated as the weighted average of accuracy and recall scores. This criterion considers both FP and FN. A high F1-score indicates that the predictor has few FP and few FN. In this scenario, the predictor identifies serious threats while avoiding false alarms. When the value of an F1-score is 1, it is deemed perfect. The best F1-score got with RNN was 0.876, as with any other assessment criterion. In classification analysis, The AUC is used to determine the best algorithms used to predict target classes. In general, a score value of AUC 0.5 indicates that no variance, a score between 0.6 and 0.8 is held as allowable, a score of 0.8–0.9 is regarded as excellent, and a value of

Model	Accuracy in training	Accuracy of testing	Precision	Recall	F1-score	AUC	Log-loss
ANN	0.881	0.8629	0.858	0.858	0.858	0.94	0.3137
CNN	0.879	0.856	0.856	0.856	0.856	0.94	0.3201
RNN	0.910	0.870	0.871	0.876	0.876	0.94	0.2909
LSTM	0.870	0.844	0.844	0.844	0.844	0.92	0.3587
CNNRNN	0.881	0.862	0.862	0.862	0.862	0.93	0.3130
CNNLSTM	0.863	0.834	0.835	0.835	0.835	0.93	0.3707

Table 2.
The evaluation outcomes of all DL models using the train-test split method.

greater than 0.9 is regarded as exceptional [26]. The AUC values of all DL models were outstanding since all of the outcomes were more than 0.9. All DL models may be used to predict HIV test results based on their AUC values.

True positive rates are critical in health investigations since recall indicates the percentage of actual positives identified [27]. A recall is a significant assessment criterion in this study since it is computed by dividing the number of properly-recognized HIV-positive samples by the total number of HIV test results. Besides, the AUC score plays an important role in health research since it has a relevant interpretation for health prediction [28]. Accuracy is a study criterion that indicates how near the sample parameters are to population characteristics. We can demonstrate that the study is generalizable, dependable, and valid by testing the correctness of the models [29]. As a result, just these three assessment indicators were examined in this study. The remaining ones were computed to compare the findings to earlier studies. The AUC values using the train test split strategy are shown in **Figures 2–7**.

In addition to the metrics listed above, we calculated prediction accuracy to assess the efficacy of the proposed approach. **Figures 8–13** depict the prediction accuracy of the proposed technique on the HIV/AIDS dataset in terms of each DL model. Because of

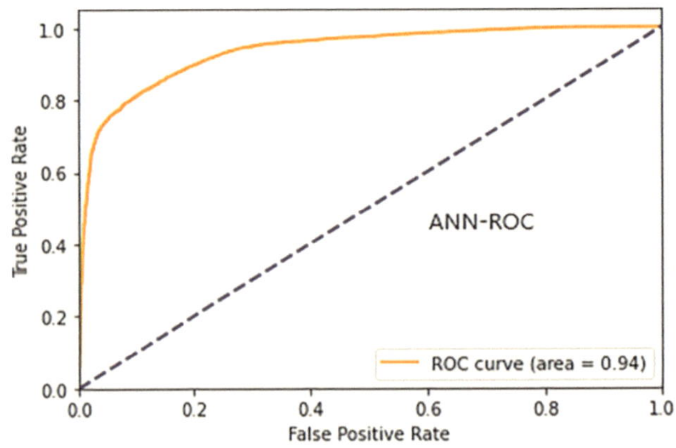

Figure 2.
ANN models AUC using the train-test split strategy.

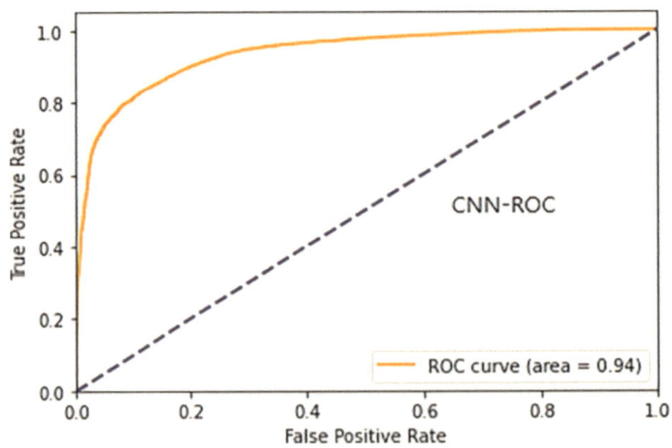

Figure 3.
CNN models AUC using the train-test split strategy.

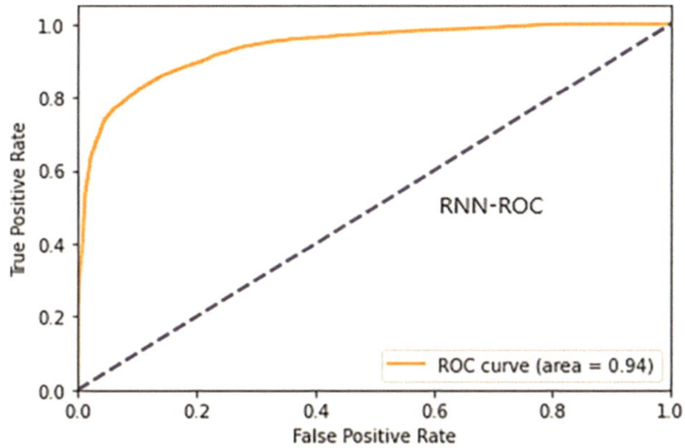

Figure 4.
RNN models AUC using the train-test split strategy.

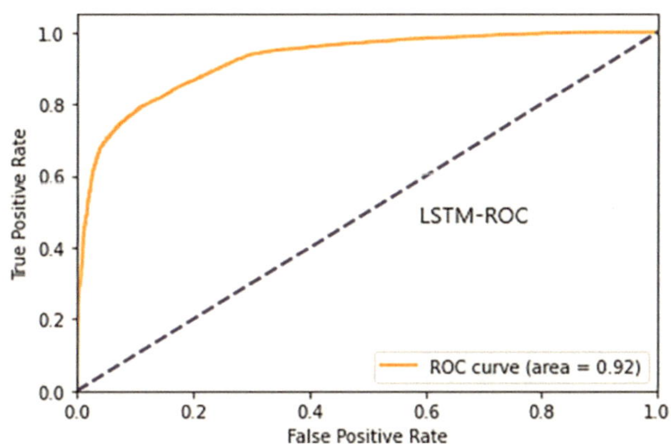

Figure 5.
LSTM models AUC using the train-test split Strategy.

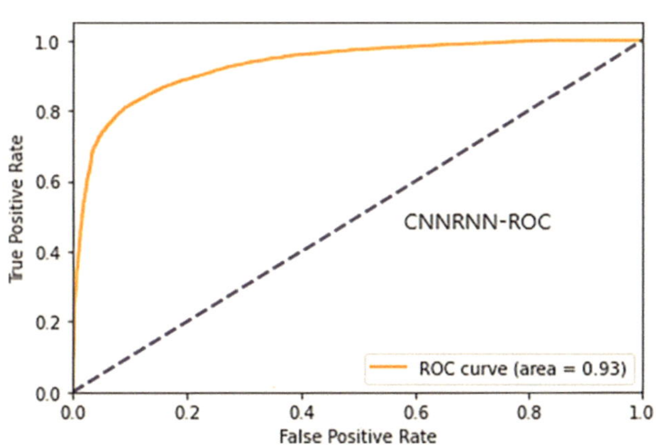

Figure 6.
CNNRNN models AUC using the train-test split strategy.

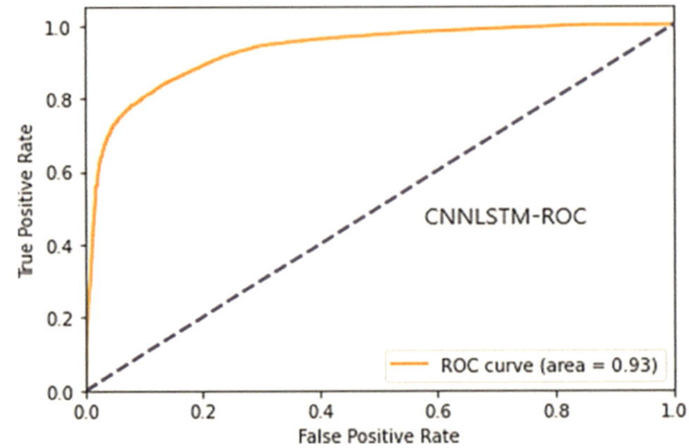

Figure 7.
CNNLSTM models AUC using the train-test split strategy.

the flawless prediction accuracy of the HIV/AIDS dataset, a substantial difference is not there among lines related to the training and test dataset, as shown in **Figures 8–13**.

We also used the log-loss error function to evaluate our work. As shown in **Figures 14–19** the training sample loss is near to 0, while the stated loss with the test sample is 0.3707 (refer to **Table 2**) implying that more research on this specific dataset is required to reduce the error. As demonstrated in Loss Figures, the proposed technique outperforms all DL models by scoring the least number of errors in the test instances, with the ANN, CNN, RNN, LSTM, CNNLSTM, and CNNRNN scoring 0.3137, 0.3201, 0.2929, 0.3587, 0.3130, and 0.3707, correspondingly (refer **Table 2**). It is noticed that a distance between the training and the test lines indicates whether or not the model is over-fitting.

The second experimental result for this work is a 10-fold CV. **Table 3** demonstrates the assessment results of all DL models using a 10-fold CV technique.

Concerning the predictive performances, we discovered that the best comprehensive recognized models on AUC score for predicting HIV test status were 89.72 by ANN. The main reason behind ANN outperforming better results is its activation function unlike CNN, RNN, and LSTM. Moreover, ANN works better for numerical datasets unlike CNN, RNN, and LSTM which work on image data and time-series data

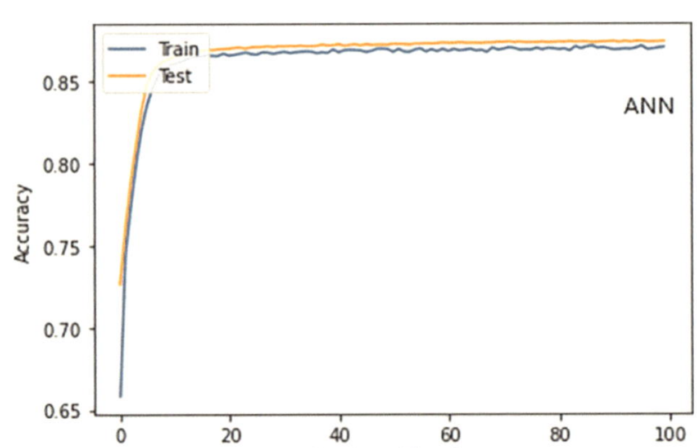

Figure 8.
The prediction accuracy on the model ANN.

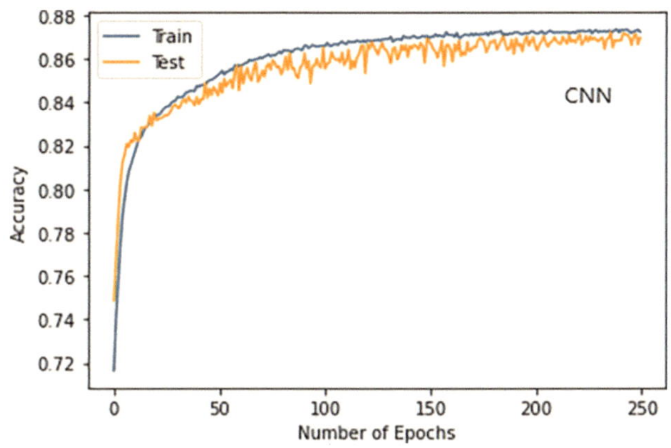

Figure 9.
The prediction accuracy on the model CNN.

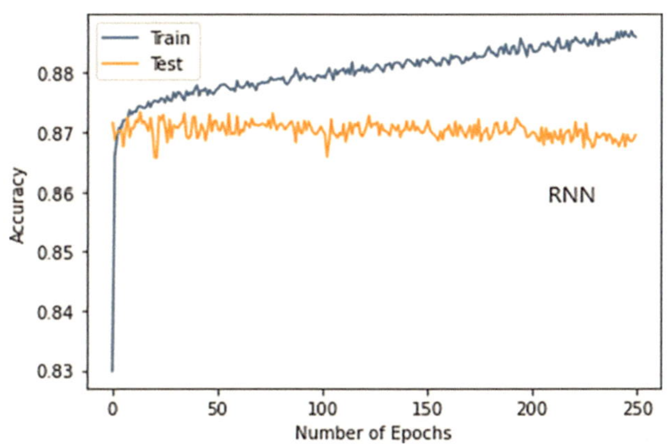

Figure 10.
The prediction accuracy on the model RNN.

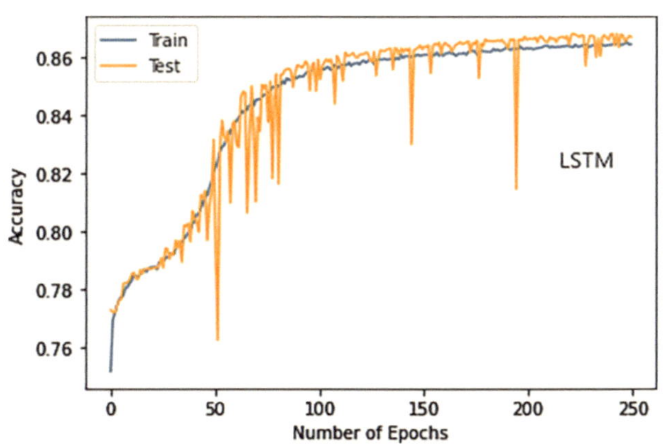

Figure 11.
The prediction accuracy on the model LSTM.

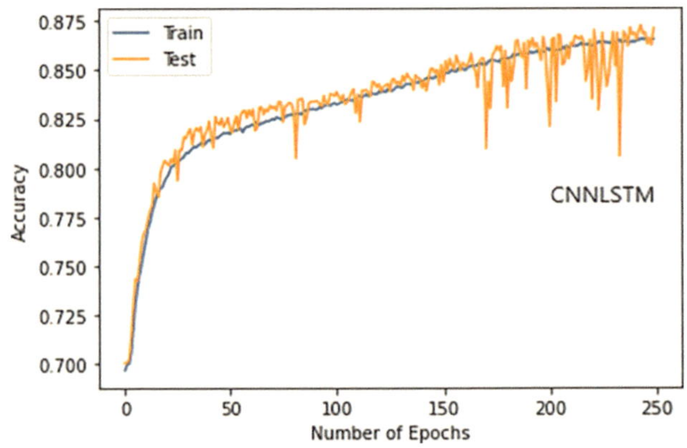

Figure 12.
The prediction accuracy on the model CNNLSTM.

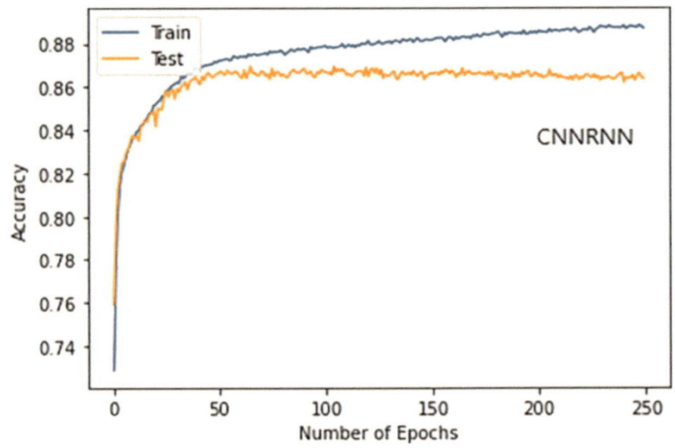

Figure 13.
The prediction accuracy on the model CNNRNN.

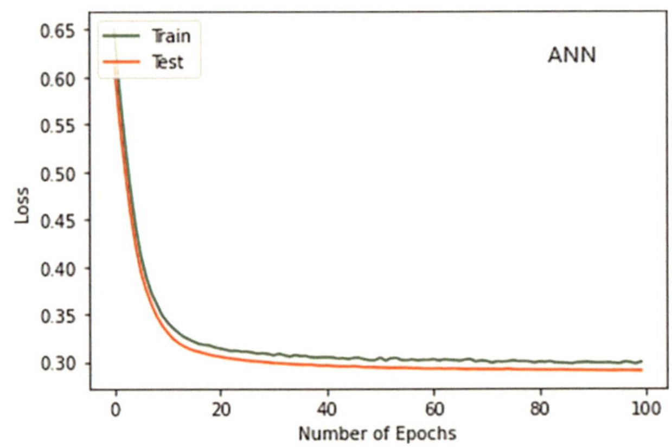

Figure 14.
Prediction Loss on the model ANN.

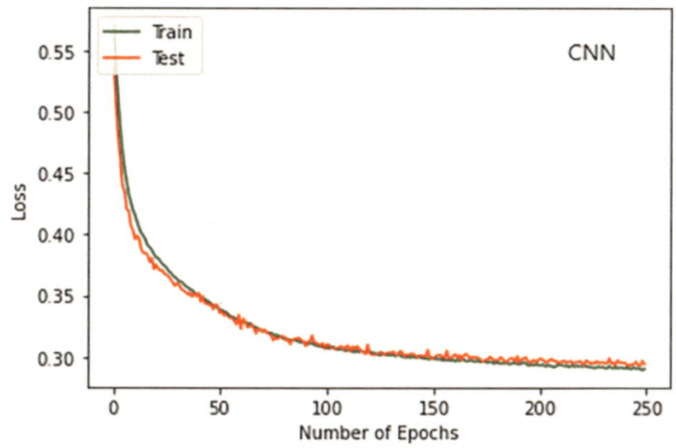

Figure 15.
Prediction loss on the model CNN.

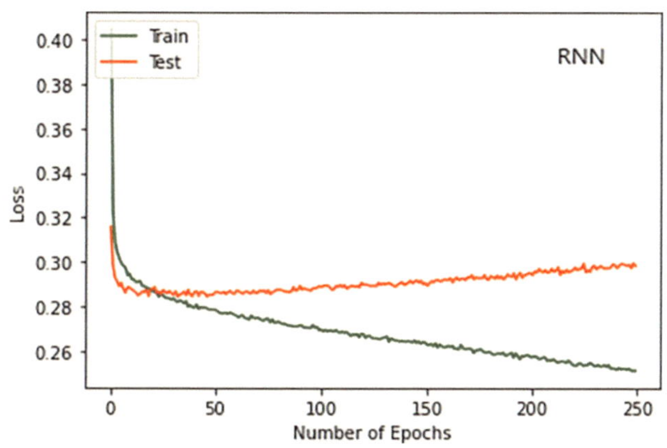

Figure 16.
Prediction loss on the model RNN.

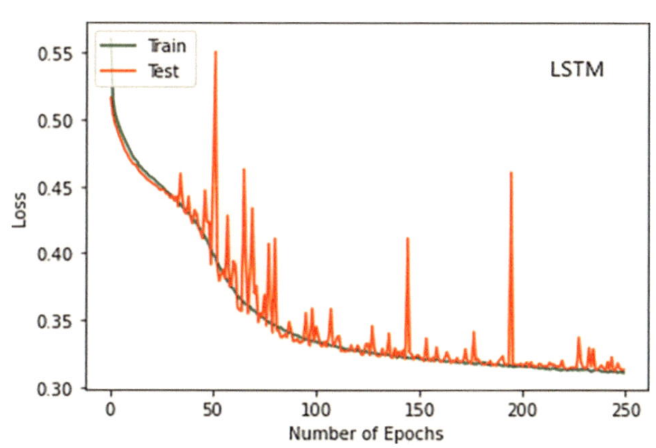

Figure 17.
Prediction loss on the model LSTM.

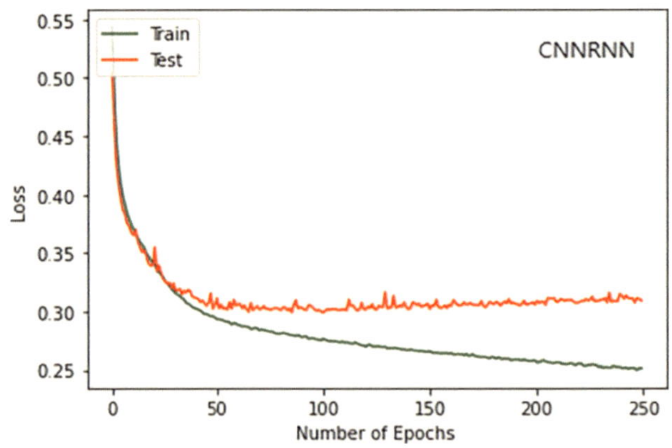

Figure 18.
Prediction loss on the model CNNRNN.

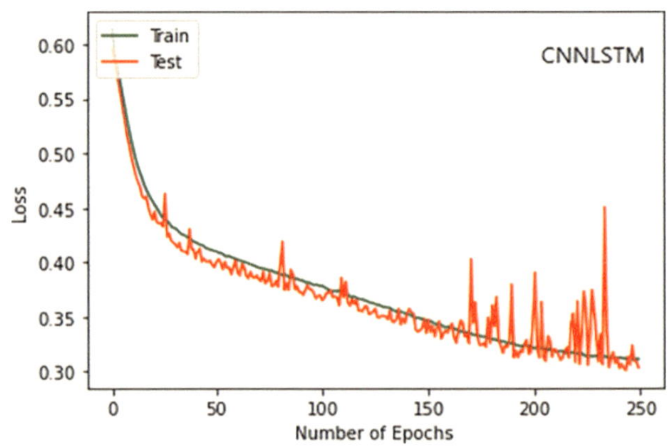

Figure 19.
Prediction loss on the model CNNLSTM.

Model	Accuracy	Precision	Recall	F1-score	AUC
ANN	0.855	0.844	0.857	0.851	89.72
CNN	0.834	0.833	0.845	0.841	87.52
RNN	0.847	0.821	0.822	0.834	87.62
LSTM	0.821	0.830	0.836	0.831	86.46
CNNRNN	0.801	0.800	0.822	0.826	83.78
CNNLSTM	0.792	0.800	0.821	0.801	83.77

Table 3.
The outcomes of all DL models were evaluated using a 10-fold cross-validation methodology.

respectively. It was discovered that predicting HIV test status from the EDHS dataset was considered a difficult activity. Nonetheless, the best HIV test status prediction outcomes using ANN obtained reasonable accuracy of 85.5%, precision of 84.4%, recall of 85.7%, and f1-score of 85.1%.

References	Dataset	Methods	Best Results	Accuracy	F1-score	AUC
McSharry et al. [8]	Population-based HIV Impact Assessment	Machine Learning	XGBoost	—	0.789	—
Orel et al. [9]	DHS dataset	Machine Learning	SVM	0.80	—	—
Ahlström et al. [12]	Danish National Hospital Registry	Machine Learning	LR	—	—	88.4
Lu et al. [13]	UCI ML repository	Deep Learning		—	0.927	—
Steiner et al. [22]	HIV Drug Resistance Dataset	Deep Learning	MLP	0.826	0.732	0.90
Betechuoh et al. [30]	Antenatal Survey	Deep Learning	ANN	0.840	—	0.86
Proposed method	EDHS –HIV/AIDS	Deep learning	RNN	0.87	0.87	0.94

Table 4.
The proposed model comparison with some of the most recent related research works.

5. Comparison

This section of the study compares the proposed method to certain selected recent research in terms of performance measures. **Table 4** compares the proposed method's assessment metrics to those of six other recent research works. The hyphen (-) in the table's specific cells indicates that the researchers did not consider metrics in their study. As shown in **Table 4**, the best results were obtained with various models. Nonetheless, we have not employed ML in our research. We created six DL models and achieved higher accuracy, f1-scores, and AUC when compared to earlier similar efforts. In the considered HIV/AIDS dataset, the suggested technique obtains improved prediction performance, with 0.87 in total accuracy and f1-score and 0.94 in AUC score.

6. Conclusion

In this work, deep learning models based on the EDHS dataset were used to predict HIV test results. Six deep learning models were used to analyze HIV/AIDS dataset. The dataset was normalized in the first stage of the study then utilized as an input for the DL models. Following that, prediction is performed, and the models' results were evaluated using precision, recall, accuracy, AUC, and F1-scores. We used 10 fold CV and train test split techniques to assess the models. In a 10-fold CV technique, the ANN deep learning model produced the most meaningful results, with an accuracy of 85.5%, a recall of 85.7%, and an AUC score of 87.72%. Despite its popularity, this validation did not produce the best validation results. In the train-test split technique, the greatest accuracy, precision, recall, and AUC values were obtained with the RNN model, which was 87%, 87%, 87%, and 94%, respectively. The accuracy of all DL models produced in the study was greater than 83%. Precision and recall values can be inferred in the same way.

Finally, we discovered evidence that DL models may be used to predict HIV test status using demographic and health survey datasets. Our findings on the role of DHS in predicting HIV test status for people improve our knowledge of the consequences of HIV epidemics. Based on the findings of our study, we believe that the health domain should investigate the use of DL models that analyze individual HIV test status to enhance and re-evaluate health policies and intervention mechanisms.

Acknowledgements

The authors would like to thank anonymous reviewers for their valuable recommendations for improving the article.

Funding

Not applicable.

Author contributions

This is a collaborative work with both authors that contribute throughout.

Conflict of interest

The authors declare that they have no conflict of interest.

Ethical standard

This article does not contain any studies with human participants or animals performed by any of the authors.

Data availability

The authors declare that all data supporting the findings of this study are available on https://github.com/danielmesafint/Datasets

Author details

Daniel Mesafint Belete* and Manjaiah D. Huchaiah
Department of Computer Science, Mangalore University, India

*Address all correspondence to: danielmesafint1985@mail.com;
drmdhmu@gmail.com

References

[1] WHO. HIV/AIDS fact sheet. 2017. Available from: http://www.who.int/features/factfiles/hiv/en/

[2] Huerga H et al. Who needs to be targeted for HIV testing and treatment in KwaZulu-Natal? Results from a population-based survey. Journal of Acquired Immune Deficiency Syndrome. 2016;**73**(4):411-418. DOI: 10.1097/QAI.0000000000001081

[3] CSA, Demographic and Health Survey. 2018. [Online]. Available from: http://www.csa.gov.et/survey-report/category/2-demographic-and-health-survey [Accessed: October 28, 2018]

[4] Nassif AB, Shahin I, Attili I, Azzeh M, Shaalan K. Speech recognition using deep neural networks: A systematic review. IEEE Access. 2019;**7**:19143-19165

[5] Ramabhadran B, Khudanpur S, Arisoy E. Will We Ever Really Replace the N-gram Model? On the Future of Language Modeling for HLT. In: Proceedings of the NAACL-HLT, Montreal. Canada: Omni Press Inc.; 2012. pp. 1-10

[6] Aljunid MF, Huchaiah MD. Multi-model deep learning approach for collaborative filtering recommendation system. CAAI Transactions on Intelligence Technology. 2020;**5**(4):268-275

[7] Ciregan D, Meier U, Schmidhuber J. Multi-column deep neural networks for image classification. In: IEEE Conference on Computer Vision and Pattern Recognition. Providence, RI, USA: IEEE; 2012. pp. 3642-3649

[8] McSharry PE, Mutai C, Ngaruye I, Musabanganji E. Use of machine learning techniques to identify HIV predictors for screening in sub-Saharan Africa. BMC Medical Research Methodology. 2021;**1**:1-11

[9] Orel E, Esra R, Estill J, Marchand-Maillet S, Merzouki A, Keiser O. Machine learning to identify socio-behavioural predictors of HIV positivity in east and Southern Africa. medRxiv. BMJ. 2020:1-29

[10] Lu X, Wang L, Jiang Z. The application of deep learning in the prediction of HIV-1 protease cleavage site. In: 5th International Conference on Systems and Informatics (ICSAI). Nanjing, China: IEEE; 2018. pp. 1299-1304

[11] Wang G, Wei W, Jiang J, Ning C, Chen H, Huang J, et al. Application of a long short-term memory neural network: A burgeoning method of deep learning in forecasting HIV incidence in Guangxi, China. Epidemiology & Infection. 2019;**147**(194):1-7

[12] Ahlstrom MG, Ronit A, Omland LH, Vedel S, Obel N. Algorithmic prediction of HIV status using nation-wide electronic registry dataset. E Clinical Medicine. 2019;**17**:100203

[13] Steiner MC, Gibson KM, Crandall KA. Drug resistance prediction using deep learning techniques on HIV-1 sequence dataset. Viruses. 2020;**12**(5):560

[14] Garcia S, Luengo J, Herrera F. Dataset Preprocessing in Dataset Mining. Intelligent Systems Reference Library book series. Vol. 72. Singapore: Springer; 2015

[15] Jain YK, Bhandare SK. Min max normalization based dataset perturbation method for privacy protection. International Journal of Computer & Communication Technology. 2011;**2**(8):45-50

[16] Manjaiah D, Belete DM. Wrapper based feature selection techniques on EDHS-HIV/AIDS dataset. European Journal of Molecular& Clinical Medicine. 2020;7(8):2642-2657

[17] Han J, Kamber M, Pei J. Dataset mining concepts and techniques third edition. The Morgan Kaufmann Series in Dataset Management Systems. 2011; **5**(4):83-124

[18] Wu J. Introduction to Convolutional Neural Networks. Vol. 5, No. 23. China: National Key Lab for Novel Software Technology, Nanjing University; 2017. pp. 1-30

[19] Sherstinsky A. Fundamentals of recurrent neural network (rnn) andlong short-term memory (lstm) network. Physica D: Nonlinear Phenomena. 2020; **404**:132306

[20] Xiao Y, Cho K. Efficient character-level document classification by combining convolution and recurrent layers. Computer Science - Computation and Language. 2016;**65**:1-10

[21] Rahman M, Islam D, Mukti RJ, Saha I. A deep learning approach based on convolutional LSTM for detecting diabetes. Computational Biology and Chemistry. 2020;**88**:107329

[22] Xie Y, Zhu C, Zhou W, Li Z, Liu X, Tu M. Evaluation of machine learning methods for formation lithology identification: A comparison of tuning processes and model performances. Journal of Petroleum Science and Engineering. 2018;**160**:182-193

[23] Chollet F. Keras. 2018. Available from: https://keras.io/ [Accessed: June 10, 2021]

[24] Pedregosa F, Varoquaux G, Gramfort A, Michel V, Thirion B, Grisel O, et al. Scikit-learn: Machine learning in python. Journal of machine Learning Research. 2011;**12**: 2825-2830

[25] Kingma DP, Ba J. Adam: A method for stochastic optimization. In: 3rd Int. Conf. for Learning Representations. Vol. 1. 2014. pp. 1-15

[26] Mandrekar JN. Receiver operating characteristic curve in diagnostic test assessment. Journal of Thoracic Oncology. 2010;**5**(9):1315-1316

[27] Avati A, Jung K, Harman S, Downing L, Ng A, Shah NH. Im-proving palliative care with deep learning. BMC Medical Informatics and Decision Making. 2018;**18**(4):55-64

[28] Kamarudin AN, Cox T, Kolamunnage-Dona R. Time-dependentroc curve analysis in medical research: Current methods and applications. BMC Medical Research Methodology. 2017;**17**(1):1-19

[29] Pierce R. Evaluating information: Validity, reliability, accuracy, triangulation. In: Research Methods in Politics: A Practical Guide. Edmonton, AB, Canada: Sage Publications; 2008

[30] Betechuoh BL, Marwala T, Tettey T. Autoencoder networks for HIV classification. Current Science. 2006; **91**(11):1467-1473

Section 3

Testing for HIV

Chapter 5

Streamlining Laboratory Tests for HIV Detection

Ramakrishna Prakash and Mysore Krishnamurthy Yashaswini

Abstract

HIV is a retrovirus that primarily infects CD4 presenting cells of the human immune system, such as macrophages and dendritic cells. People die of AIDS because the disease remains undetected for long periods of time. HIV diagnostic testing has come a long way since it was introduced in the early 1980s. Early diagnosis is key to successful treatment of HIV. Assay selection is based on initial screening results and clinical information provided by the physician, both of which are essential for the laboratory's ability to make accurate diagnoses. Detecting HIV with high specificity and sensitivity in the early stages of infection requires simple, accurate and economical methods. In this chapter we have described the indications & criteria's for HIV testing, HIV diagnosis by utilizing variety of immunological and molecular methods, like ELISA, rapid diagnostics, Western blotting, indirect immunoassays, and nucleic acid-based tests. Diagnostic laboratories must use testing algorithms to ensure the accuracy of results and the optimal use of lab resources. Participation in laboratory quality assurance programs are also essential to ensure that diagnostic laboratories provide accurate, timely and clinically relevant test results. HIV testing is the first step in maintaining a healthy life and preventing HIV transmission.

Keywords: generations, HIV antibody test, HIV diagnosis, HIV testing algorithm, quality assurance, Western Blot

1. Introduction

Early detection and diagnosis is key to ending the HIV/AIDs pandemic by 2030. The need for timely and quality programs to enhance rapid, timely, accurate and relevant tests as the initial step in reducing HIV and maintaining the quality of life is a fundamental process. This chapter describes the known tests for HIV Infection. The author bases his discussion on significant systematic review of literature of HIV diagnostic tests. The aim is to explain and provide rationale for the use of tests available. The chapter also describes, and discusses the various indications, criteria for HIV testing, detection and identifies phases and stages of laboratory detection. A variety of immunological and molecular methods are outlined and discussed. These include the simplest from point of care such as ELISA diagnostic tests, rapid tests and brands. It also extends the discussion to more advanced tests including indirect immunoassays, nucleic based assays and the Western blot confirmatory tests. The laboratory algorithms are discussed to promote quality assurance in practice. The

IntechOpen

paper discusses the difficulties encountered during the early window period of infection and suggests appropriate detection tools. The staging and the dynamics of HIV viremia post infection and its implications for detection is discussed. The classifications of tests from first generation to forth generation is described and recommendations made on their appropriate usage for early and sustained quality in detection of infection. The challenges of detection during the acute and the window period post infection is discussed and suggestions made. Establishing several testing stages is discussed to support quality HIV detection and ideal screening and confirmatory tests for each stage are recommended. The review has a potential benefit to improve HIV [1, 2].

2. Indications for HIV testing

HIV testing should be considered in the following situations. The healthcare team should be aware of the screening recommendations [3].

- All the patients in the age group 13 and above.
- Patients with risky sexual behavior
- Occupational exposure of patients or healthcare workers
- Before providing pre-exposure prophylaxis
- Signs and symptoms suggestive of HIV
- Patients sharing needles for substance abuse
- Pregnant women

3. Criteria's for HIV testing

There are ample of tests which can detect HIV starting from the point of care testing to confirmatory test. The test algorithm to be followed has been released by the Centre for Disease Control (CDC) and Association of Public Health Laboratories (APHL) as well as the national organizations in every country [4, 5].

3.1 Clinical laboratory improvement amendments (CLIA)

Centers for Medicare and Medicaid Services (CMS) has regulated for all the clinical laboratory testing to be done through the CLIA. As per this amendments, a three-level test complexity criteria has been established for HIV testing procedures. The criteria are as follows [4, 5]:

- **Waived:** These are the tests which are simple to perform with low-risk, it can be performed by any person with minimal training and the specimens do not require any centrifugation for testing.

- **Moderate Complexity:** These are the tests which are simple to perform but requires the use of plasma or serum samples as well as participation in an external quality assessment or proficiency testing program.

- **High Complexity:** These are the tests which need multiple steps to be performed as well as well-trained laboratory technician to perform the test, it also needs the participation in an external quality assessment or proficiency testing program and internal quality control regularly.

3.2 Fiebig staging system

The Fiebig staging system (2003) defines six stages on initial HIV infection. Stage I is defined as the emergence of HIV RNA and Stage VI is defined as full Western blot reactivity. The markers which appear as per timeline after HIV infection are HIV RNA after 10 to 11 days, p24 antigen after 4 to 10 days after emergence of HIV RNA, IgM antibodies after 3 to 5 days later, IgG antibodies after 2 to 6 weeks after HIV RNA emergence [6].

4. Tests used for the diagnosis of HIV

HIV tests were classified as first, second, third and fourth generation tests based on the substrate used for testing. First generation HIV antibody tests were developed using separate HTLV III and lymphadenopathy virus (LAV) isolates proteins isolated from virus-infected tissue cultures as antigenic targets. Initially window period was up to 12 weeks or more post-infection. These assays detected only IgG antibody of HIV-1. Second generation HIV test were based on the recombinant antigens for HIV-1 p24. The window period was up to 4 to 6 weeks post-infection. Third generation HIV test can detect IgM antibody in addition to second generation tests. Fourth generation tests is a test which can detect both HIV-specific antigen p24 and HIV antibodies. This test reduced window period to approximately 2 weeks [7]. Fifth generation HIV test detects both HIV-specific antigen p24 and HIV antibodies with increased sensitivity in detection of p24 and it also identifies the individual HIV1 and HIV2 markers. The different generations of HIV tests are shown in **Table 1**.

Assay progression	**Indirect ELISA (HIV-1/2)**	**Sandwich ELISA HIV-1/2, IgG & IgM**		**Sandwich ELISA HIV-1/2, IgG & IgM + P24**	
Generations	1st	2nd	3rd	4th	5th
Source of Antigen	Virus Infected Cell Lysate	Lysate & Recombinant	Recombinant & Synthetic peptides	Recombinant & Synthetic peptides	Recombinant & Synthetic peptides
Window period	8–10 weeks	4–6 weeks	2–3 weeks	2 weeks	2 weeks

Source: Alexander [8].

Table 1.
Different generations of HIV tests.

With the invention of new HIV tests, the distinction between the different generations of ELISA test has been obscure. So the generation nomenclature is being modified as:

- IgG- sensitive tests for first and second generation antibody assays.
- IgM/IgG-sensitive tests for third generation assays
- Antigen-antibody immunoassays for fourth generation assays [5, 9–11].
- Laboratory-based assays and point-of-care assays are being used now instead of rapid HIV tests [10, 12].

4.1 Non-specific tests

The non-specific tests for HIV diagnosis are [13]:

- **Total and differential leucocyte count:** Lymphocyte count can decrease may be up to less than 400 per cubic mm with leucopenia.
- **T-lymphocyte subset assays:** Reversal of CD4:CD8 T-cell ratio up to around 0.5:1 from the normal ratio of 2:1.
- **Platelet count:** Thrombocytopenia will be seen in full blown HIV patients.
- **IgG and IgA levels:** Both levels will be raised in blood.
- **Skin tests for CMI:** Cell mediated immunity (CMI) will be diminished which can be evidenced by any skin allergy test.

4.2 Specific tests for HIV infection

These are the tests which are specifically done for testing of HIV.

4.2.1 Virus isolation

This is a time-consuming procedure which is not routinely done. The viruses are present in the lymphocytes in the peripheral blood and also seen in lymphocytes in bone marrow, plasma and other body fluids. The procedure used to cultivate HIV virus is called as **Cocultivation.** In this both infected and noninfected mononuclear cells will be co-cultivated. The culture may become positive for HIV p24 antigen and HIV reverse transcriptase by 7–14 days or by 28 days. This test will be useful when the viral load is high especially in the initial stage of the disease [14].

4.2.2 Serologic tests

These tests include demonstration of antigens and antibodies in the serum. The tests have been classified as:

1. HIV antigen-antibody laboratory-based tests.

2. HIV antigen-antibody point-of-care tests.

3. HIV antibody laboratory-based tests.

4. HIV antibody point-of-care tests.

5. HIV 1 and 2 differentiation tests.

6. HIV-1 Western Blot test.

7. HIV Nucleic acid diagnostic tests.

8. In-home HIV tests.

4.2.2.1 HIV antigen-antibody laboratory-based tests

These immunoassay tests are the preferred screening tests which detect HIV-1 p24 (capsid) antigen and antibodies (IgM and IgG) to HIV-1 and HIV-2. (**Figure 1A–C**) These antigen-antibody test detect HIV infection much earlier than the antibody-based tests. If found positive in these tests, then it may require a confirmatory test. Limitation of these tests are cross-reactivity to HIV-1 p24 antigen seen in HIV-2 infected persons. Examples are ADVIA Centaur HIV Ag/Ab Combo (CHIV) Assay, ARCHITECT HIV Ag/Ab Combo, BioPlex 2200 HIV Ag-Ab Assay, Elecsys HIV Combi PT, GS HIV Combo Ag/Ab EIA, & VITROS HIV Combo Test [10, 16].

4.2.2.2 HIV antigen-antibody point-of-care tests

This assay is a single use, rapid test which is a point-of-care test for the detection of HIV-1 p24 antigen, antibodies to HIV-1 (group 0), and antibodies to HIV-2. This test does not differentiate HIV-1 and HIV-2 antibodies. This test is less sensitive for acute or recent HIV infection when compared to laboratory-based HIV-1/2 antigen-antibody tests. Example: Abbott Determine HIV-1/2 Ag/Ab Combo [17–19].

4.2.2.3 HIV antibody laboratory based tests

Laboratory-based HIV antibody tests were the first to be used for screening HIV since 20 years which has been replace by HIV antigen-antibody tests. These tests can detect the IgM/IgG-sensitive assays for HIV IgM antibodies in 23–25 days after HIV infection. Window period is around 90 days. The positive result in this tests would require an confirmatory test. Examples are: ADVIA Centaur HIV 1/O/2 Enhanced, Avioq HIV-1 Microelisa System, Genetic Systems (GS) HIV-1/HIV-2 Plus O EIA, VITROS Anti-HIV 1 + 2 Assay [5, 6, 10, 12].

4.2.2.4 HIV antibody point-of-care tests

Single-use, point-of-care tests can yield result in 40 min. These tests can detect antibodies to HIV-1 or HIV-2 or both but they will not be able to differentiate between HIV-1 and HIV-2. These tests are primarily used for testing (1) emergency situations (2) pregnant women whose HIV status in not known (3) occupational, and (4) in patients for whom follow-up for HIV result will not be possible. Examples are: Chembio DPP HIV 1/2 Assay, Chembio HIV 1/2 STAT-PAK Assay, Chembio SURE

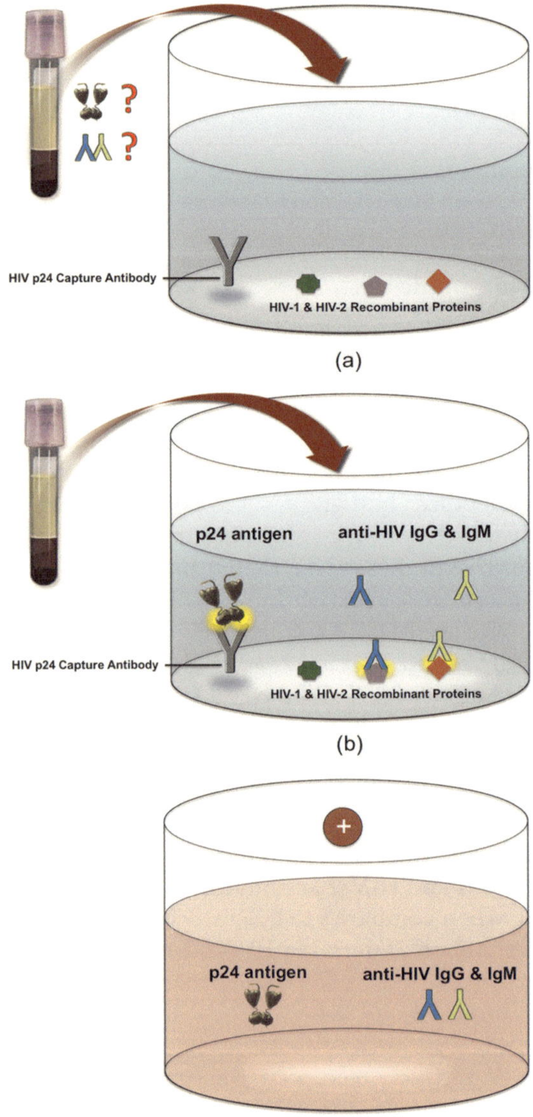

Figure 1.
(a) Components of HIV-1/2 antigen-antibody immunoassay. (b) Patient sample reacting with components in HIV-1/2 antigen-antibody immunoassay. (c) Reactive HIV-1/2 antigen-antibody immunoassay. Source: Illustration: David H. Spach, MD [15].

CHECK HIV 1/2 Assay, INSTI HIV-1/HIV-2 Antibody Test, OraQuick ADVANCE Rapid HIV-1/2 Antibody Test, Reveal G4 Rapid HIV-1 Antibody Test (Reveal G4), Uni-Gold Recombigen HIV-1/2 [9, 20, 21].

4.2.2.5 HIV 1 and 2 differentiation tests

These tests will be able to differentiate between HIV-1 and HIV-2. These tests utilize multiple recombinant or synthetic peptides to detect HIV-1 antibodies and HIV-2

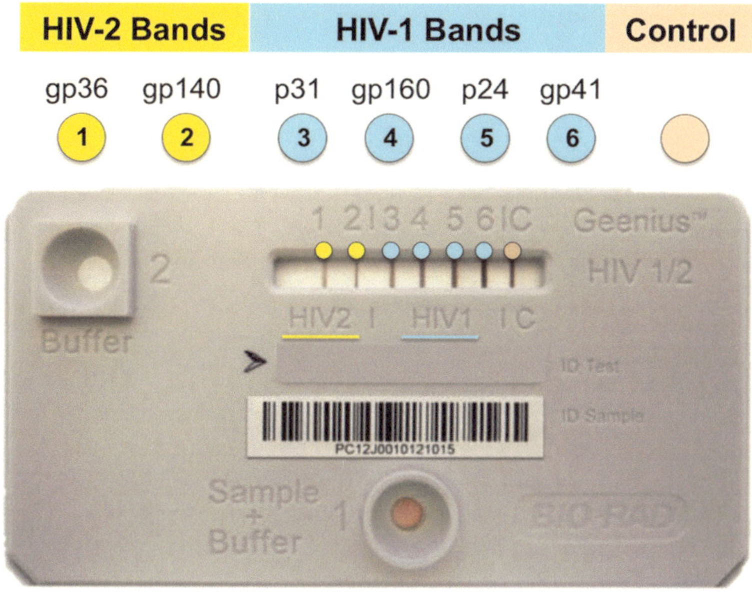

Figure 2.
Geenius HIV 1/2 supplemental assay. Source: modified from [15].

antibodies. These immunochromatographic tests will contain 7 lines which consists of 6 HIV peptides and one control. A minimum of 2 envelope peptides (gp160 and gp41) or 1 envelope peptide plus either the p24 or the polymerase peptide p31 for HIV-1 reactive or HIV-2 envelope peptides gp36 and gp140 should be present for HIV-2 reactive test. (**Figure 2**) Example: Geenius HIV 1/2 Supplemental Assay [15, 22].

The Geenius HIV 1/2 Supplemental Assay is a single-use immunochromatographic test that utilizes multiple recombinant or synthetic peptides to detect HIV-1 antibodies (p31, gp160, p24, and gp41) and HIV-2 antibodies (gp36 and gp140). The test cassette as shown here contains seven test lines, including the six HIV peptides and one control.

4.2.2.6 HIV-1 Western blot test

Western blot test is used as supplemental tests for those tests which are reactive by rapid tests. It can detect the human antibodies for three HIV-1 gene regions: env (gp41, gp120/160), pol (p31, p51, p66), and gag (p15, p17, p24, p55) (**Figure 3A-D**).

This graphic shows the relationship of the HIV-1 genes and products with the corresponding band on the HIV-1 Western blot.

CDC and the Association of State and Territorial Public Health Laboratory Directors (ASTPHLD) have published the criteria for interpretation of Western blot tests [23].

Positive: A positive Western blot indicates the presence of at least two of the following bands: p24, gp41, and gp120/160.

Negative: A negative Western blot is defined by the absence of any bands.

Indeterminate: An indeterminate Western blot results from the presence of any bands, but not meeting positive criteria. Possible causes of an indeterminate Western blot include early HIV infection, HIV-2, pregnancy, or cross-reactivity with other antibodies, such as in persons who have recently received an influenza immunization or who have autoimmune disorder.

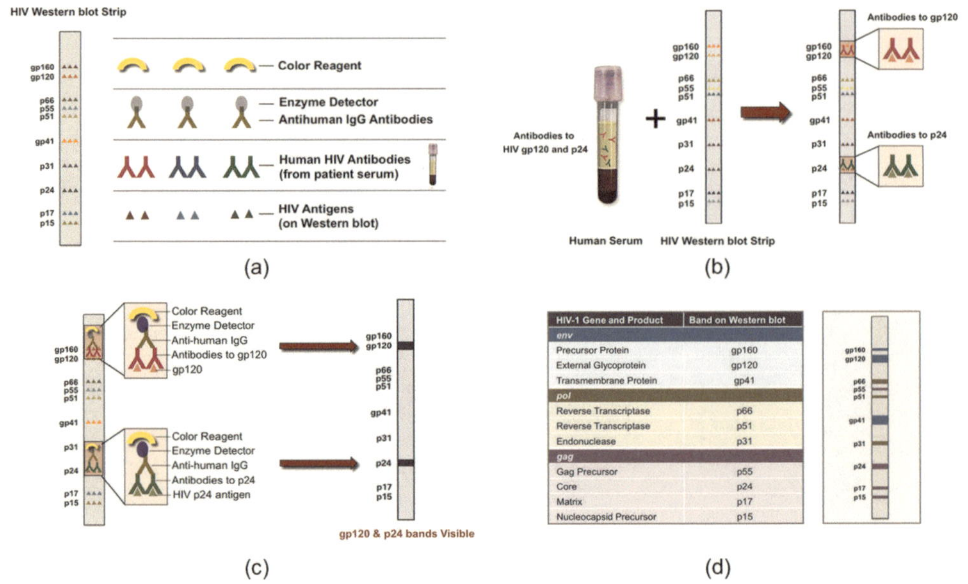

Figure 3.
(a) Components used in the HIV-1 Western blot; (b) HIV-1 antibodies bound to HIV-1 antigens on Western blot test strip. (c) Addition of secondary anti-human antibody linked to enzyme signal. (d) HIV-1 Western blot genes. Source: Illustration: David H. Spach, MD [15].

4.2.2.7 HIV nucleic acid diagnostic tests

HIV RNA nucleic acid test (NAT) is used in case of 1. Reactive HIV-1/2 antigen-antibody immunoassay but a nonreactive or indeterminate HIV-1/HIV-2 differentiation test, 2. HIV-1/2 antigen-antibody immunoassay is negative but there is high suspicion of acute HIV, and 3. Confirmative test for chronic HIV-1 infection. The limitation of these tests are cost, time taken to perform the test is 3 hours and the expert is required to perform the test. Example: APTIMA HIV-1 RNA Qualitative Assay [9, 24–26].

4.2.2.8 In-home HIV tests

This test can be performed at home by the client itself within 40 minutes by simply collecting an oral sample and performing the test as per kit literature. A confirmatory test will be required if this test is reactive. Example OraQuick In-Home HIV test [27].

5. HIV laboratory testing algorithms

There are several algorithms published for HIV laboratory testing among which CDC, NACO (National AIDS Control Organization) and APHL are some of them (**Figure 4**) [28].

This graphic shows the HIV testing algorithm as recommended in 2014 and 2018 by the Centers for Disease Control and Prevention (CDC) and Association of Public Health Laboratories (APHL). Source: Centers for Disease Control and Prevention and Association of Public Health Laboratories [4, 5].

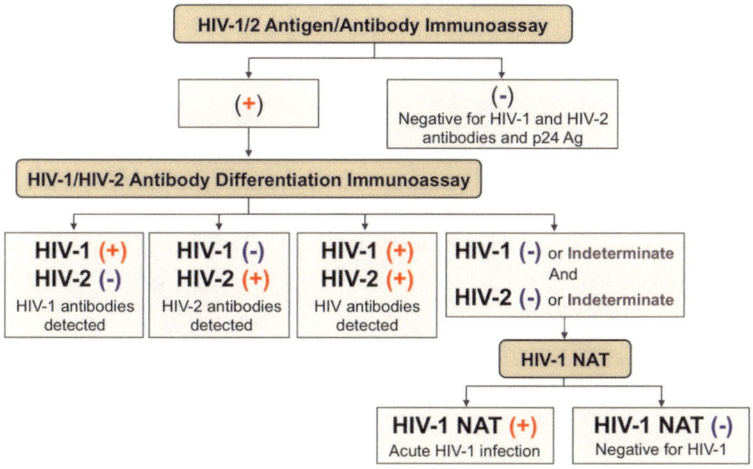

Figure 4.
CDC and APHL Recommended Laboratory Testing for the Diagnosis of HIV Infection.

6. Interpretation of HIV test results

- If any HIV-1/2 antigen-antibody immunoassay test is NONREACTIVE, then the test result should be interpreted as not infected with HIV-1 or HIV-2. If acute HIV is suspected, then there will be a need to perform HIV-1 RNA test.

- If any HIV-1/2 antigen-antibody immunoassay test is REACTIVE, then the test should be checked with HIV-1/HIV-2 differentiation assay result to check for whether the person is reactive to HIV-1 or HIV-2.

- If any HIV-1/2 antigen-antibody immunoassay is reactive and HIV-1/ HIV-2 differentiation test is indeterminate for HIV-1 and nonreactive for HIV-2, then it is indeterminate result. HIV-1 NAT should be done in this case.

7. Staging of HIV and tests recommended

Days following HIV acquisition which of the HIV diagnostic tests can show positivity for infection are shown in **Figure 5** [14, 29].

This graphic shows the HIV testing algorithm as recommended in 2014 and 2018 by the Centers for Disease Control and Prevention (CDC) and Association of Public Health Laboratories (APHL).

The stages of HIV infection and the tests that are recommended are [5, 30].

- Eclipse Phase: This is the first phase of HIV infection during which no diagnostic test will be able to detect HIV infection. HIV nucleic acid test (NAT) is the test which can detect HIV infection at the earliest.

- Window Period: The time between HIV infection and the accurate detection of HIV infection by any laboratory test. This period can vary depending the type of test done to detect HIV infection. CDC has recommended around 45 days

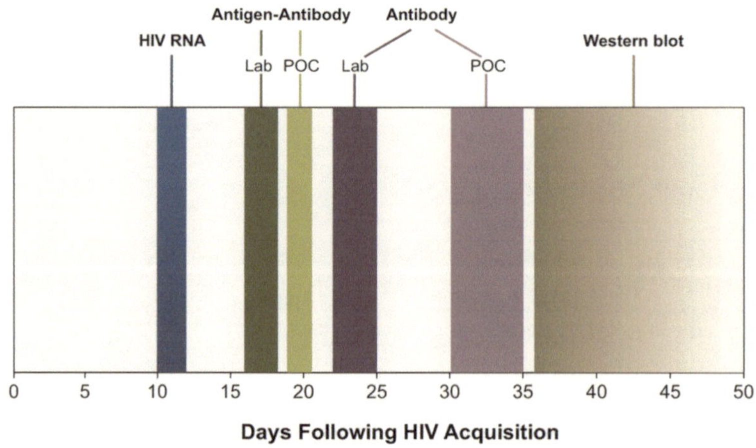

Figure 5.
Timing of positivity for HIV diagnostic tests.This figure shows estimates for the mean number of days for HIV diagnostic tests to become positive after acquisition of HIV. Abbreviation: POC = point-of-careSource: modified from Centers for Disease Control and Prevention and Association of Public Health Laboratories [5].

window period for the HIV 1/2 antigen–antibody tests and 90 days for all HIV antibody tests and all HIV point-of-care tests.

- Seroconversion Window Period: The time interval between HIV infection and the detection of anti-HIV antibodies by any laboratory test. This period also can vary depending on the type of HIV test used.

- Acute HIV infection: The time interval between the detection of HIV RNA and anti-HIV antibodies.

- Recent Infection: The time interval from the HIV infection to 6 months of infection when anti-HIV antibodies are rising.

- Early Infection: The time interval which includes both acute HIV infection and recent HIV infection.

- Established HIV Infection: The full-blown HIV infection when the anti-HIV IgG antibody response is fully detectable.

8. Performance of diagnostic tests

8.1 An ideal screening tests

An ideal screening test should be able to accurately identify individuals with the HIV infection and rule out infection in individuals without HIV infection.

The characteristics that define a screening test are [31]

- The disease should be a health problem.

- The disease should be treatable.
- The disease should be diagnosable.
- The disease should have a test for diagnosis.
- The test should be acceptable.
- The test should cost-effective.

8.2 Sensitivity and specificity

Sensitivity and specificity refers to the diagnostic ability of a given test. Sensitivity refers to the percentage of individual who are correctly identified as having disease if they are infected with HIV. A very high sensitivity is desirable for the initial screening test so that if we get a non-reactive result we can be 100% sure that the person is not having HIV infection [32]. Specificity refers to the percentage of individuals who are correctly identified as not having disease if the person does not have HIV infection. A very high specificity is desirable for the confirmation test as a reactive result means the person is suffering from HIV infection [33].

8.3 Positive predictive value and negative predictive value

The predictive value of a test refers to the accuracy of the test. Positive predictive value refers to the proportion of patients who are correctly diagnosed as reactive. Negative predictive value refers to the proportion of patients who are correctly diagnosed as non-reactive [32].

8.4 False negative and false positive HIV test

False negative HIV test result refers to the non-reactive report in a person who is possessing HIV infection.

A false negative HIV antigen–antibody test result can be seen in [34–46]:

- Common causes
    - o acute HIV infection,
    - o from error in laboratory reporting,
    - o person on antiretroviral therapy,
- Rare causes
    - o Immunosuppression.
    - o Hypogammaglobulinemia.
    - o Immunosuppressant medications.
    - o Chronic HIV.

A false negative p24 antigen test can be seen in the window period and in chronic HIV. A false negative HIV RNA tests can be seen in first one to two weeks after HIV infection and chronic HIV.

False positive HIV test result refers to the reactive report in a person who is not possessing HIV infection.

A false positive HIV test result can be seen in [47, 48]

- Polyclonal cross-reactivity
- Recent Influenza vaccination
- Autoimmune disorders
- Trial HIV-1 vaccination
- Gammaglobulin therapy
- Prior blood transfusions
- HTLV-1/2 infection
- Recent viral infection
- Collagen vascular diseases
- Laboratory error in reporting

A false positive HIV NATs can be seen in persons receiving chimeric antigen receptor (CAR) T-cell therapy.

9. Special diagnostic situation

9.1 Diagnosis of Acute HIV-1

HIV RNA is the most reliable test for diagnosis of acute HIV-1 infection as this test can detect HIV in about 17 days after HIV infection which is much earlier when compared to all other methods of testing [49, 50].

9.2 Diagnosing HIV in persons receiving preexposure prophylaxis

Diagnosis of HIV infection in persons receiving preexposure prophylaxis is difficult due to delayed seroconversion, indeterminate results in HIV differentiation tests, and low viraemia [51].

9.3 Diagnosing HIV in HIV exposed infants and children

Antibody tests or antigen-antibody immunoassays will not be useful in diagnosis of HIV in infants or children as they may have maternal HIV antibodies. Nucleic acid tests like HIV RNA, HIV DNA polymerase chain reaction or RNA qualitative or quantitative tests will be better option for HIV diagnosis in infants. Qualitative HIV proviral DNA PCR assays detects cell-associated virus as they are less affected by the antiretroviral drugs [52].

9.4 Diagnosis of HIV-2

Diagnosis of HIV-2 should be done using a HIV-1/2 antigen-antibody immunoassay followed by HIV-1/HIV-2 differentiation test. Confirmation of HIV-2 can be done by HIV-2 DNA/RNA Qualitative and Quantitative assays. Western blot can give a negative, indeterminate or positive HIV-1 result in HIV-2 infected individuals. Western blot will be indeterminate with the presence of gag and pol bands but the env bands will be absent in HIV-2 infection [53–57].

10. Laboratory quality assurance

The laboratory should participate in quality assurance program to ensure the quality of reports. The quality control should be monitored in preanalytical, analytical and post-analytical stages with Internal QC (quality control), external QC as well as test kit controls [58].

11. Conclusions

Testing an individual having HIV infection is important using the appropriate test at the appropriate time. Differentiation of HIV-1 and HIV-2 can be done using the differentiation assays. Diagnosis of HIV-2 and infection in infants and children requires Nucleic acid tests. Quality assurance needs to be maintained in all the labs which do HIV testing as the entire process has to be done in an appropriate manner to get the perfect results.

Acknowledgements

I would like to acknowledge the head of the department of Microbiology, Dr. Lakshminarayana S A for his encouragement and support in writing this chapter.

Conflict of interest

"The authors declare no conflict of interest."

Author details

Ramakrishna Prakash* and Mysore Krishnamurthy Yashaswini
Rajarajeswari Medical College and Hospital, Bengaluru, India

*Address all correspondence to: prakashssmc@gmail.com

References

[1] Global AIDS Strategy 2021–2026. Available from: https://www.unaids.org/en/Global-AIDS-Strategy-2021-2026. [Accessed: April 04, 2022]

[2] Li Z, Purcell DW, Sansom SL, Hayes D, Hall HI. Vital signs: HIV transmission along the continuum of care – United States, 2016. MMWR. Morbidity and Mortality Weekly Report. 2019;**68**(11):267-272

[3] Huynh K, Kahwaji CI. HIV Testing. Treasure Island (FL): StatPearls Publishing; 2021

[4] National Center for HIV/AIDS, Viral Hepatitis, and TB Prevention (U.S.). Division of HIV/AIDS Prevention; Association of Public Health Laboratories. 2018 Quick reference guide: Recommended laboratory HIV testing algorithm for serum or plasma specimens. Available from: https://stacks.cdc.gov/view/cdc/50872

[5] Branson BM, Owen SM, Wesolowski LG, Bennett B, Werner BG, Wroblewski KE, Pentella MA. Laboratory testing for the diagnosis of HIV infection: Updated recommendations. Corporate Authors (s): Centers for Disease Control and Prevention (U.S.); Association of Public Health Laboratories; National Center for HIV/AIDS, Viral Hepatitis, and TB Prevention (U.S.). Division of HIV/AIDS Prevention, 2014. Available from: https://stacks.cdc.gov/view/cdc/23447

[6] Fiebig EW, Wright DJ, Rawal BD, Garrett PE, Schumacher RT, Peddada L, et al. Dynamics of HIV viremia and antibody seroconversion in plasma donors: Implications for diagnosis and staging of primary HIV infection. AIDS. 2003;**17**(13):1871-1879. DOI: 10.1097/00002030-200309050-00005

[7] Chappel RJ, Wilson KM, Dax EM. Immunoassays for the diagnosis of HIV: Meeting future needs by enhancing the quality of testing. Future Microbiology. 2009;**4**:963-982. DOI: 10.2217/fmb.09.77

[8] Alexander TS. Human immunodeficiency virus diagnostic testing: 30 years of evolution. Clinical and Vaccine Immunology. 2016;**23**(4):249-253

[9] Branson BM. State of the art for diagnosis of HIV infection. Clinical Infectious Diseases. 2007;**45**(Suppl. 4): S221-S225

[10] Hurt CB, Nelson JAE, Hightow-Weidman LB, Miller WC. Selecting an HIV test: A narrative review for clinicians and researchers. Sexually Transmitted Diseases. 2017;**44**:739-746

[11] Branson BM, Mermin J. Establishing the diagnosis of HIV infection: New tests and a new algorithm for the United States. Journal of Clinical Virology. 2011; **52**(Suppl. 1):S3-S4

[12] Delaney KP, Wesolowski LG, Owen SM. The evolution of HIV testing continues. Sexually Transmitted Diseases. 2017;**44**:747-749

[13] Baveja CP. Retroviruses: HIV in Textbook of Microbiology. 5th ed. New Delhi: Arya Publishers; 2017. pp. 509-522

[14] Masciotra S, McDougal JS, Feldman J, Sprinkle P, Wesolowski L, Owen SM. Evaluation of an alternative HIV diagnostic algorithm using specimens from seroconversion panels and persons with established HIV infections. Journal of Clinical Virology. 2011;**52**(Suppl. 1):S17-S22

[15] David H, Spach DH. HIV Diagnostic testing. In: Spach DH, Wood BR, Kalapila

AG, Budak JZ, editors. National HIV Curriculum 2nd ed. University of Washington Infectious Diseases Education & Assessment Program. 31 Aug 2020. [Accessed: March 15, 2022]. Available from: https://www.hiv.uw.edu/go/screening-diagnosis/diagnostic-testing/core-concept/all

[16] Delaney KP, Hanson DL, Masciotra S, Ethridge SF, Wesolowski L, Owen SM. Time Until Emergence of HIV Test Reactivity Following Infection With HIV-1: Implications for Interpreting Test Results and Retesting After Exposure. Clinical Infectious Diseases. 2017;**64**: 53-59

[17] U.S. Food and Drug Administration. Alere Determine HIV-1/2 Ag/Ab Combo

[18] Masciotra S, Luo W, Youngpairoj AS, et al. Performance of the Alere Determine™ HIV-1/2 Ag/Ab Combo Rapid Test with specimens from HIV-1 seroconverters from the US and HIV-2 infected individuals from Ivory Coast. Journal of Clinical Virology. 2013; **58**(Suppl. 1):e54-e58

[19] Masciotra S, Luo W, Westheimer E, et al. Performance evaluation of the FDA-approved Determine™ HIV-1/2 Ag/Ab Combo assay using plasma and whole blood specimens. Journal of Clinical Virology. 2017;**91**:95-100

[20] Kuhar DT, Henderson DK, Struble KA, et al. Updated US Public Health Service guidelines for the management of occupational exposures to human immunodeficiency virus and recommendations for postexposure prophylaxis. Infection Control and Hospital Epidemiology. 2013;**34**:875-892

[21] Centers for Disease Control and Prevention. Advancing HIV prevention: New strategies for a changing epidemic–United States, 2003. MMWR. Morbidity and Mortality Weekly Report. 2003;**52**: 329-332

[22] U.S. Food and Drug Administration. Geenius HIV 1/2 Supplemental Assay

[23] Centers for Disease Control (CDC). Interpretation and use of the Western blot assay for serodiagnosis of human immunodeficiency virus type 1 infections. MMWR. Morbidity and Mortality Weekly Report. 1989;**38**(Suppl. 7):1-7

[24] U.S. Food and Drug Administration. APTIMA HIV-1 RNA Qualitative Assay [U.S. FDA]

[25] Giachetti C, Linnen JM, Kolk DP, et al. Highly sensitive multiplex assay for detection of human immunodeficiency virus type 1 and hepatitis C virus RNA. Journal of Clinical Microbiology. 2002; **40**:2408-2419

[26] Pierce VM, Neide B, Hodinka RL. Evaluation of the Gen-Probe Aptima HIV-1 RNA qualitative assay as an alternative to Western blot analysis for confirmation of HIV infection. Journal of Clinical Microbiology. 2011;**49**: 1642-1645

[27] U.S. Food and Drug Administration. OraQuick In-Home HIV Test

[28] Branson BM, Stekler JD. Detection of acute HIV infection: We can't close the window. Journal of Infectious Diseases. 2012;**205**(4):521-524

[29] Owen SM, Yang C, Spira T, et al. Alternative algorithms for human immunodeficiency virus infection diagnosis using tests that are licensed in the United States. Journal of Clinical Microbiology. 2008;**46**:1588-1595

[30] Panel on Antiretroviral Guidelines for Adults and Adolescents. Guidelines for the use of antiretroviral agents in

adults and adolescents with HIV. Department of Health and Human Services. Considerations for antiretroviral use in special patient populations: Acute and recent (early) HIV infection. 2019

[31] WHO Recommendations on the Diagnosis of HIV Infection in Infants and Children. Geneva: World Health Organization; 2010. Annex 4, Characteristics of a screening test. Available from: https://www.ncbi.nlm.nih.gov/books/NBK138555/

[32] Altman DG, Bland JM. Diagnostic tests 2: Predictive values. BMJ. 1994;**309**:102

[33] Altman DG, Bland JM. Diagnostic tests. 1: Sensitivity and specificity. BMJ. 1994;**308**:1552

[34] Manak MM, Jagodzinski LL, Shutt A, et al. Decreased seroreactivity in individuals initiating antiretroviral therapy during acute HIV infection. Journal of Clinical Microbiology. 2019; **57**:e00757

[35] Kassutto S, Johnston MN, Rosenberg ES. Incomplete HIV type 1 antibody evolution and seroreversion in acutely infected individuals treated with early antiretroviral therapy. Clinical Infectious Diseases. 2005;**40**: 868-873

[36] Hare CB, Pappalardo BL, Busch MP, et al. Seroreversion in subjects receiving antiretroviral therapy during acute/early HIV infection. Clinical Infectious Diseases. 2006;**42**:700-708

[37] de Souza MS, Pinyakorn S, Akapirat S, et al. Initiation of antiretroviral therapy during acute HIV-1 infection leads to a high rate of nonreactive HIV serology. Clinical Infectious Diseases. 2016;**63**:555-561

[38] Sullivan PS, Schable C, Koch W, et al. Persistently negative HIV-1 antibody enzyme immunoassay screening results for patients with HIV-1 infection and AIDS: Serologic, clinical, and virologic results. Seronegative AIDS Clinical Study Group. AIDS. 1999; **13**:89-96

[39] Spivak AM, Brennan TP, O'Connell KA, et al. A case of seronegative HIV-1 infection. The Journal of Infectious Diseases. 2010;**201**: 341-345

[40] Spivak AM, Sydnor ER, Blankson JN, Gallant JE. Seronegative HIV-1 infection: A review of the literature. AIDS. 2010;**24**:1407-1414

[41] Ellenberger DL, Sullivan PS, Dorn J, et al. Viral and immunologic examination of human immunodeficiency virus type 1-infected, persistently seronegative persons. The Journal of Infectious Diseases. 1999;**180**: 1033-1042

[42] Donnell D, Ramos E, Celum C, et al. The effect of oral preexposure prophylaxis on the progression of HIV-1 seroconversion. AIDS. 2017;**31**: 2007-2016

[43] Smith DK, Switzer WM, Peters P, et al. A strategy for PrEP clinicians to manage ambiguous HIV test results during follow-up visits. Open Forum Infectious Diseases. 2018;**5**:180

[44] Padeh YC, Rubinstein A, Shliozberg J. Common variable immunodeficiency and testing for HIV-1. The New England Journal of Medicine. 2005;**353**:1074-1075

[45] Jurriaans S, Sankatsing SU, Prins JM, et al. HIV-1 seroreversion in an HIV-1-seropositive patient treated during acute infection with highly active

antiretroviral therapy and mycophenolate mofetil. AIDS. 2004;**18**: 1607-1608

[46] Roy MJ, Damato JJ, Burke DS. Absence of true seroreversion of HIV-1 antibody in seroreactive individuals. Journal of the American Medical Association. 1993;**269**:2876-2879

[47] Klarkowski D, O'Brien DP, Shanks L, Singh KP. Causes of false-positive HIV rapid diagnostic test results. Expert Review of Anti-Infective Therapy. 2014; **12**:49-62

[48] Theppote AS, Carmack AE, Riedel DJ. False positive HIV testing after T-cell receptor therapy. AIDS. 2020;**34**:1103-1105

[49] Cornett JK, Kirn TJ. Laboratory diagnosis of HIV in adults: A review of current methods. Clinical Infectious Diseases. 2013;**57**:712-718

[50] Cohen MS, Gay CL, Busch MP, Hecht FM. The detection of acute HIV infection. The Journal of Infectious Diseases. 2010;**202**(Suppl. 2):S270-S277

[51] Sivay MV, Li M, Piwowar-Manning E, et al. Characterization of HIV Seroconverters in a TDF/FTC PrEP Study: HPTN 067/ADAPT. Journal of Acquired Immune Deficiency Syndromes. 2017;**75**:271-279

[52] Management of Infants Born to People with HIV Infection. In: Recommendations for the Use of Antiretroviral Drugs During Pregnancy and Interventions to Reduce Perinatal HIV Transmission in the United States [Internet]. 2021. Available from: https://clinicalinfo.hiv.gov/en/guidelines/perinatal/diagnosis-hiv-infection-infants-and-children#:~:text=Diagnosis%20of%20HIV%20in%20Infants,age%204%20to%206%20months [Accessed: April 15, 2022]

[53] Peruski AH, Wesolowski LG, Delaney KP, et al. Trends in HIV-2 diagnoses and use of the HIV-1/HIV-2 differentiation test – United States, 2010-2017. MMWR. Morbidity and Mortality Weekly Report. 2020;**69**:63-66

[54] Panel on Antiretroviral Guidelines for Adults and Adolescents. Guidelines for the use of antiretroviral agents in adults and adolescents with HIV. Department of Health and Human Services. Considerations for antiretroviral use in special patient populations: HIV-2 infection. 2019

[55] Centers for Disease Control and Prevention. HIV-2 Infection Surveillance–United States, 1987–2009. MMWR. Morbidity and Mortality Weekly Report. 2011;**60**:985-988

[56] O'Brien TR, George JR, Epstein JS, Holmberg SD, Schochetman G. Testing for antibodies to human immunodeficiency virus type 2 in the United States. MMWR - Recommendations and Reports. 1992; **41**:1-9

[57] Campbell-Yesufu OT, Gandhi RT. Update on human immunodeficiency virus (HIV)-2 Infection. Clinical Infectious Diseases. 2011;**52**:780-787

[58] Consolidated Guidelines on HIV Testing Services. 5Cs: Consent, Confidentiality, Counselling, Correct Results and Connection 2015. Geneva: World Health Organization; 2015, Quality assurance of HIV testing. Available from: https://www.ncbi.nlm.nih.gov/books/NBK316025/ [Accessed: April 15, 2022]

Chapter 6

Challenges in Platelet Functions in HIV/AIDS Management

Gordon Ogweno

Abstract

The interest in platelet functions in HIV/AIDS is due to the high incidence of microvascular thrombosis in these individuals. A lot of laboratory data have been generated regarding platelet functions in this population. The tests demonstrate platelet hyperactivity but decreased aggregation, though results are inconsistent depending on the study design. Antiretroviral treatments currently in use display complex interactions. Many studies on platelet functions in these patients have been for research purposes, but none have found utility in guiding drug treatment of thrombosis.

Keywords: HIV, AIDS, platelet functions, light transmission aggregometry, flow cytometry, microparticles, combined antiretroviral, antiplatelets

1. Introduction

There is increasing focus on platelet functions in people living with HIV/AIDS. This is because of the high incidence of cardiovascular events in these individuals that is 10 times higher than general population [1] independent of traditional risk factors such as age, hyperlipidemia, and ethnic/racial differences. Acquired platelet dysfunctions are often observed in association with HIV/AIDS. Of the available tests for platelet functions [2, 3], none fully captures the complexity involved in this population group.

The results of the functional assays are modified by the viral count, CD4/CD8 ratio, and immunological response and whether or not on antiretroviral treatment. The effects of combined antiretroviral therapy (cART) on platelet functions are complex. Despite achieving viral suppression, these drugs have been demonstrated to have independent effects on platelet functions.

2. Platelet count and indices in HIV/AIDS

Complete blood count and microscopic examination of formed elements are often the first investigations in suspected hemostatic disorders in clinical situations. Platelet count and morphological changes have impact on bleeding or thrombosis.

 IntechOpen

2.1 HIV-associated thrombocytopenia

Globally, the prevalence of HIV-associated thrombocytopenia is 4–40% [4] though there are geographical, racial as well as ethnic differences from the same locality [5] and stage of disease. Indeed, thrombocytopenia has been considered as a marker of disease progression and improvement [6]. Whereas platelet counts improve with initiation of combined antiretroviral therapy (cART) viral suppression [7], beneficial effect does not apply to zidovudin (AZT) [8].

Despite thrombocytopenia, very low rates of clinical hemorrhage have been reported, estimated at only 3.2% among HIV thrombocytopenic patients [9] even with platelet count as low as 50×10^9/L [10] casting doubt on the clinical relevance of the laboratory results. As a result of lack of clear correlation between HIV-associated thrombocytopenia and clinical significance, some authors have questioned benefit of treatments purely directed toward improvement of platelet count [11].

2.2 HIV-associated thrombocytosis

The prevalence of HIV-associated thrombocytosis, defined as platelet count of more than 400×10^9/L [12], is low but depends on the population studied and concurrent medications. Reported prevalence of thrombocytosis in pediatric group who were also HIV-positive cART naive was found at 6% [13], though could be higher at 14% (more than thrombocytopenia at 7% in same cohort) for children on co-trimoxazole prophylaxis [14]. Whether these findings were independent or dependent on co-administered drugs remains undetermined.

Thrombocytosis is an emerging toxic complication accounting for 9% on stable cART depending on the regimen [7] up from 5.8% in treatment-naïve individuals [7]. It remains undetermined the relationship between HIV-associated thrombocytosis and accelerated thrombosis.

2.3 Platelet ultrastructure in HIV/AIDS

Despite the thrombocytopenia being associated with HIV, peripheral blood film smears of platelets are either unremarkable or hypogranular, which are of different sizes appearing as fragments [15].

Ultrastructure of platelets from HIV individuals, apart from showing normal features of hyperactivated aggregates having membrane pseudopodia/filopodia formation, in addition have shriveled aggregates with irregular and torn membrane surfaces, membrane blebbing and shedding of vesicles [16, 17]. The most distinctive features are alteration of granular structure though data are limited.

3. Tests based on platelet aggregation

3.1 Light transmission aggregometry (LTA)

Most studies on platelet aggregation in HIV have used single or fewer than the recommended panel of agonists with conflicting results [18]. Application of escalating agonist concentrations has uncovered dose-response patterns [19]. In this study, while epinephrine demonstrated greater potency indicating hyperresponsiveness, responses with collagen, TRAP, and ADP showed lesser maximum aggregation indicating lesser efficacy and hyporesponsiveness. The agonist dose-response curve is, however, modified by cART viral suppression, especially abacavir-containing regimens [20] depending on agonist [21]. It must be remembered that although cART is a commonly mentioned modifier, the effects of fever associated with HIV are neither reported nor analyzed in these studies. Hyperthermic conditions such as fever are associated with reduced platelet aggregation [22].

3.2 Whole blood platelet aggregometry-multiple electrode aggregometry (MEA) and impedance aggregometry

A study comparing whole blood platelet aggregation using MEA found hyporeactivity in both HIV-treated and untreated individuals [23], similar to findings by impedance aggregometry [24]. It is worth noting that co-infection with HBV (6 vs. 4%) and HCV (0 vs. 2%) and low CRP levels [23] could have obscured the overall response. Co-infection with other viruses modulates platelet responses in HIV [25].

3.3 Thromboelastography (TEG)/ Thromboelastometry (ROTEM)

Few studies have been performed using thromboelastography (TEG) in HIV individuals. Of the few studies done, MA amplitude was low despite higher normal fibrinogen levels in both cART-treated [21] and untreated HIV subjects [23]. These study results of hypocoagulability are not in keeping with other tests, probably reflecting lack of sensitivity of TEG as a platelet function assay.

4. Platelet activation

Activated platelets are characterized by surface expression of activation-specific molecules such as P-selectin or CD62P, active GPIIbIIIa (PAC-1), phosphatidyleserine (PS) externalization; platelet-leukocyte aggregates (PLA); platelet microparticle formation (PMP), in addition to granule secretion such as platelet factor 4(PF4), β-thromboglobulin, and intracellular calcium flux [26].

4.1 Flow cytometry for membrane surface glycoprotein expression

A number of studies have documented platelet hyperactivity in HIV characterized by increased plasma membrane surface expression of CD62P, PAC-1, PS, CD63, [27], but paradoxically decreased GPIbα [28]. The levels positively correlate with viral loads but not CD4 count [29].

Although activation markers are higher in HIV sero-positive individuals who are cART naïve compared to healthy controls [30], with cART treatment levels decrease but do not normalize to pre-treatment levels [20, 31]. The persistent levels are related to inflammatory markers in virally suppressed individuals [32].

4.2 Intracellular signal transduction test—VASP

There is evidence of altered signal transduction affecting protein synthesis, degranulation, and activation functioning in HIV platelets. Experimental data show that HIV platelets had upregulation of ABCC4 (ATP-binding cassette subfamily 4), increase in cAMP, decrease in vasodilator-stimulated phosphoprotein (VASP), which correlated with increased membrane expression of CD62P and integrin αIIbβ3 (GPIIbIIIa) [33]. It must be noted that VASP is only sensitive to PY12 inhibitors, and not much data are available from HIV patients.

5. Platelet secretion

5.1 Alpha granules

People living with HIV have increased secretion of alpha granule contents such as RANTES, sP-selectin, and sCD40L [34], despite viral suppression [33]. The persistence of these chemokines, especially anomalous secretion of RANTES, despite cART treatment [28] remains unexplained to date.

5.2 Dense granules

HIV platelets have low basal dense granule content and diminished secretion response as evidenced by low mepacrine uptake and release [33]. Although platelet mepacrine uptake and release have been considered among dense granule assays, it is not as specific as serotonin and lummiaggregometry for ATP [35, 36]. Despite this knowledge, the measurements of platelet serotonin and ATP remain largely undescribed in people living with HIV.

5.3 Concept of "platelet exhaustion" in HIV

Although HIV-associated platelets display increased baseline expression of surface activation markers compared to healthy controls [32], there is evidence of refractoriness to further agonist stimulation. This behavior has been referred to as "platelet exhaustion" in many publications [25, 28, 32, 37, 38].

Platelet "exhaustion" as a concept was postulated in references to previous observations, before HIV era, where activated platelets continued to circulate [39, 40] and were shown to be activated [41] but with decreased aggregation [42, 43]. They were considered refractory to further agonist stimulation [44] owing to acquired storage pool granule depletion [45, 46].

In HIV, stimulation with increased agonist concentration leads to lesser response at each corresponding dose [21]. Specifically, decreased thrombin dose-response curve for granule content and secretions for P-selectin, PFA/CXCL4,TXA and RANTES in HIV platelets less than healthy controls [32]. The decreased P-selectin and PAC-1 secretory responses correspond to impaired c-AMP, ABCC4 and VASP signal transduction mechanisms [33]. Furthermore, HIV platelets display decreased mepacrine uptake and release [33], and wheat germ agglutinin staining (WGA) [32] indicating reduction of dense and alpha granule contents respectively.

Despite many studies mentioning "platelet exhaustion" in HIV, however the results in support are neither consistent for all agonists nor confirmed by other tests. In patients who are cART naïve, stimulation with AA, ADP or collagen, the dose-response curves for CD62P are higher than the uninfected controls [30]. None of the LTA aggregation tests have been accompanied by corresponding Lummiaggregometry test which could have better characterized platelet ATP dense granule secretion [47, 48]. Platelet lumiaggregometry testing remains largely un-described in HIV.

Furthermore, the studies are on people who are already infected by HIV, but platelet responses prior to HIV infection remains unknown.

From the foregoing, evidence in support for "platelet exhaustion" in HIV is suggestive but inconclusive. Although decreased dose-response to thrombin has been described, however response to epinephrine was enhanced in some studies. The maintained response to epinephrine casts doubt on granule exhaustion, since true storage pool disorder do not respond to epinephrine [49] or variable [50]. Indeed HIV platelets maintain both alpha and dense granule secretions to collagen and ADP agonists stimulation [51]. Perhaps a better term to use could be "anergy," refractory or "tired" platelets.

6. Platelet adhesion

HIV platelets have enhanced adherence to fibrinogen-coated surfaces [32, 33]. However, testing by this method is technically difficult and not available in clinical situations.

Although platelet PFA-100/200 testing is always recorded as aggregation in most studies, in actual fact it is marker of adhesion [2, 52]. The few tests of PFA-100 in HIV compared those on cART treatment with untreated [31], or in addition to [53] all of which showed shorter closure time in treatment-naïve individuals. The short closure times were neither normalized with aspirin nor with cART. The results are strongly indicative of influence of vWF as a third dimension in platelet function testing [54, 55].

7. vWF-ADAMTS-13 axis in HIV/AIDS

People living with HIV (PLWHIV) despite having very low platelet counts do not have issues of bleeding [56–58]. Instead, HIV-associated thrombotic complications [59] are an emerging issue of concern [60]. Although congenital thrombotic thrombocytopenic purpura (TTP) is very rare, acquired TTP is on the increase and associated with HIV estimated to be 15–40 times than the HIV negative in the general population [61]. It has been reported that HIV is responsible for 80% of TTP cases [62].

TTP is characterized by reduced or absent ADAMTS-13 and elevated vWF antigen as well as activity [63] especially the Unusually Ultralarge vWF multimers [64]. Elevated vWF Ag and high-molecular-weight vWF multimers [65] with reduced ADAMTS-13 have been detected in acute and chronic HIV [66, 67] and those with confirmed thrombosis [68]. Unusually, ultralarge vWF multimers that have increased adhesion to platelet GPIbα-V-IX receptors [69] compensates for hemostasis in the presence of the low platelet count in HIV.

8. Platelet microparticles

It has been demonstrated that blood from HIV individuals have abundant circulating platelet microparticles [70], and this is despite viral suppression [71, 72]. The levels were associated with increased cellular ROS, caspases, eNOS [72], and mitochondrial membrane depolarization [73] indicative of apoptosis [74] . Further, co-existence of platelet microparticles with increased LPS and platelet P-selectin and TF [29] are strong indicators that they are products of platelet activation.

9. Mechanisms of platelet activation in HIV

9.1 Direct effect of HIV

Recently, in mice, HIV particles were shown to be endocytosed by platelets by binding to TLR-7&9 leading to increased secretion of alpha (PFA-4) and dense granules (serotonin), and membrane expression of P-selectin [75]. Additionally, HIV interacts directly with platelets CLEC-2 and DC-SIGN receptors [76] *via* its trans-activating factor (Tat) [77]. The consequence is increased intracellular calcium flux, translocation of P-selectin (CD62P) from the alpha granules to the membrane surface, secretion of chemokine CD154, and release of platelet microparticles [77]. The process is by enhancing platelet NOX-2 oxidative stress [78].

9.2 Gut microbiol translocation

HIV preferentially infects CD4-T lymphocytes present in the gut leading to reduction in number and function [79]. The consequence is loss of gut epithelial immune protection and disruption of gut epithelial barrier allowing luminal indigenous intestinal bacteria to translocate out of the mucosa and into circulation [80]. Once in circulation, bacterial products such as lipopolysaccharides (LPS) interact with platelet toll-like receptors 4 (TLR4) [81]. The microbial products induce signal transduction mechanisms that eventually lead to facilitating platelet membrane receptor expression [82, 83]. The phenomenon of gut microbial translocation has been used to explain enhanced platelet reactivity despite therapy with antiplatelets such as ticagrelor in myocardial infarction [84]. However, some studies have disputed the role of LPS in platelet activation instead of reporting attenuation of receptor expression and aggregation in the presence of agonists [85] contradicting earlier findings. The paradoxical result may be due to the absence or presence of other factors such as soluble CD14 that prime TLR4 sensing of LPS [86], extent of TLR expression [87] or the different LPS isoforms [88], and experimental conditions [89] as well as clinical condition [89].

9.3 Immune complexes, cytokines, and inflammatory markers

9.3.1 Cytokines

HIV infection is associated with elaboration of cytokines from inflammatory cells, and these have been shown to induce platelet activation [90, 91] The platelet activation is not limited to interleukins only, since tumor necrosis factor in blood leads to dose- and time-dependent increase in platelet expression of GPIIbIIIa, PS, and mitochondrial dysfunction [92]. The role of TNF-α in platelet activation and apoptosis are well supported by empirical evidence [93].

9.3.2 Immune complexes

Platelets express FcRIIA (CD32a) or simply FcR receptor that recognizes the constant region of IgG in immune complexes [94]. The consequence of platelet-immune complex binding leads to platelet activation [95], aggregation and release of contents from alpha and dense granules [94], and microparticle formation [96]. The platelet activation from immune complexes is dependent on membrane GP IIbIIIa [97]. However, the immune complex-induced platelet aggregation is dependent on dose and charge [98].

Cross-reactive antibodies between HIV epitopes and platelet receptors have been described [99, 100].

9.3.3 Neutrophil extracellular traps (NETS)

When neutrophils encounter viruses such as HIV, they respond by releasing reactive oxygen species and net-like structures called neutrophil extracellular traps [101, 102]. The NETs, composed of DNA, histones, myeloperoxidase, citrinulated histones, and elastases, are the potent inducers of platelet aggregation and activation [103–105].

9.3.4 Platelet-leukocyte complexes

There is often cross-talk between platelets and leukocytes associated with bidirectional priming and activation of each other [106, 107]. These two cells interact through platelets such as P-selecti-PSGL-1, GPIb-vWF-CD18, integrin IIaIIIb-fibrinogen-MAC-1 neutrophil linkages that lead to the formation of platelet-leukocyte aggregates (PLA) [108] linked by P-selectin-PSGL. These PLA conjugates have been found in HIV patients involving T-cells associated with CD42b and CD62P [109]. Elevated PLA together with other immune markers is positively correlated with increased platelet CD36, CD62P, and platelet aggregation but inversely with CD4 count [110].

9.3.5 vWF-GPIbα in platelet activation in HIV

There is evidence of endothelial damage [111] and increased vWF levels in HIV patients [66–68, 112, 113]. Apart from the high vWF Ag levels, of significant is the persistently high functionally active Ultralarge vWF multimers (ULvWFM) in HIV individuals [65] that causes adhesion even at low platelet counts [114]. Correspondingly, as HIV disease progresses, platelet expression of the integrin GPIbα decreases paradoxically unlike the other surface receptors indicating consumption [28].

9.4 Platelet apoptosis

There are similarities in markers of platelet activation and apoptosis [115]. In both processes, there is phosphatidyleserine (PS) exposure on the membrane [116] and microparticles [117]. However, specific features of platelet apoptosis include mitochondrial membrane leakage characterized by changes in membrane depolarization ($\Delta\psi m$) and increase in cytosolic caspases 3&8, [118, 119]. Indeed, features of platelet apoptosis and activation have been demonstrated in HIV patients [25, 32, 38]. It should be noted that the few studies demonstrating occurrence of full spectra of apoptosis in HIV individuals were confounded by cART viral suppression [32] and dengue co-infection [25] and therefore, whether results were specific to HIV in itself largely remains undetermined.

Some of the consequences of platelet apoptosis include thrombocytopenia [120, 121]. This is because, apart from the fact that apoptotic platelet eventually disintegrates [74], the surface exposure of PS acts as "eat me" signal for engulfment by the macrophages thus removing the altered cells from circulation shortening survival [122–124].

10. Antiretrovirals and platelet functions in HIV

Despite the success attained by cART in viral suppression and recovery of platelet counts [125, 126], their effects on platelet function remain variable. In general, platelet surface markers such as CD62P, PAC-1 and CD40L, soluble sCD62P, sCD40L as well as platelet-secreted chemokines such as RANTES persist despite cART viral suppression [27] with some variations between the individual drugs and study designs.

Platelet signal transduction and secretory effects are enhanced by HIV, but these effects are accentuated by cART. This was demonstrated by Pastori et al.'s [78] study in which levels of sCD40L, platelet sNOX-dp, and 8-iso-PGF2-α were elevated, the effects of PIs greater than NNRTI. The mechanism appears to be induction of oxidative stress, ROS, and arachidonic pathways that synergistically augment AA platelet activation. cART causes mitochondrial toxicities [127] *via* ROS release and inner membrane depolarization that eventually lead to apoptosis that persists even with viral suppression [32].

Abacavir is unique among cART [51] since it is a guanosine analogue and induces platelet activation *via* its effects on NO-cGMP signal transduction pathway [20]. *In vitro*, incubation of platelets with abacavir inhibits cAMP pathway and dose-dependently increases surface expression of P-selectin, an observation that is augmented by ADP agonist [128]. Compared with TDF and TAF, abacavir enhances platelet aggregation and increases agonist-induced platelet activation *in vivo* (CD62P, PAC-1) [31]. It has been shown that it induces both alpha and dense platelet granule secretions thereby increasing membrane CD62P [128] levels as well as increasing PAC-1 [129]. It also alters metabolic enzymes that lead to increase in PAF from leukocytes [130]. This likely explains its association with cardiovascular events where enhanced platelet hyperactivity plays a central role [131, 132].

Despite other studies reporting levels of platelets MP remaining unchanged [29] or increased [71] after initiating antiretrovirals, one study found MP TF levels decreased with cART treatment [133]. The difference could be attributed to monocyte phenotypes [134] and level of activation and attendant TF expression with cART [135]. This is because platelets undergo decryption [136] and transfer TF to monocytes using microparticles as vehicles [137, 138].

The effects of cART on platelets are complicated by other factors such as TNF-α, a known platelet activator and apoptosis inducer. Although TNF levels are often elevated in HIV infection, levels persist despite cART [139] even if used over 24-month period [34]. Whereas cART treatment decreases circulating bacterial LPS levels in HIV patients, platelet reactivity is increased instead [23] suggesting intrinsic effects of the drugs independent of bacterial translocation.

11. Antiplatelets in HIV/AIDS

People living with HIV/AIDS are at increased risk of cardiovascular events [140, 141], especially coronary heart disease [142, 143] and ischemic stroke [144, 145], than the general population. The increased risk is due to HIV infection alone and accentuated by cART [146, 147].

Although there is evidence of enhanced platelet activation in association with HIV [27], studies of antiplatelet therapy in these patients have yielded inconsistent results, perhaps owing to drug interactions [148]. It should be noted that the studies so far done were on patients concurrently taking cART.

In a study of HIV-1 infected patients who had been on 6-month cART, it was found that 325 mg of oral aspirin-attenuated platelet aggregation to agonists, activation markers [37]. In the same study, although levels of urinary thromboxane were decreased in both HIV-positive cART untreated and treated, it was least responsive to aspirin. Furthermore, despite aspirin administration, suppression of platelet hyperactivity did not decline to baseline levels indicating the contributory effects of cART. Apart from the small sample size and short duration of therapy, other limitations of this pilot study are that it evaluated only one antiplatelet drug, and it did not perform subgroup analysis among the different cART drugs (NNRTI, PI, Raltegravir, and abacavir) as well as the racial and ethnic differences.

Although aspirin and R406 (thromboxane analogue) but not ticagrelor inhibits platelet engulfment, they do not inhibit CD62P expression or PMA complex formation [149]. Other studies have confirmed the suboptimal effects of aspirin on platelets agonist (collagen and epinephrine)-induced aggregation, surface expression of CD62P, CD40L, and PAC-1 from individuals with HIV taking ABC [53]. This study identified subjects taking abacavir-containing cART as poor responders. While cART is currently standard of care in the treatment of HIV, there are no data on effects of antiplatelets in PLWH before adoption of practice.

Clopidogrel reduces thrombogenicity and platelet hyperreactivity better than aspirin in PLWH on cART [21]. The question whether dual antiplatelet therapy compared to single agent may have a better reduction in platelet hyperreactivity in HIV concurrently taking cART was evaluated in the EVERE$_2$ST-HIV [18]. This study evaluated the extent of platelet inhibition patients with acute coronary patients on dual antiplatelet therapy undergoing PCI utilizing various platelet function assays [18]. The findings were that P2Y12 inhibitors (clopidogrel, prasugrel, and ticagralor) and aspirin were all associated with residual platelet reactivity on light transmission aggregometry (LTA), VerifyNow, and VASP assays. Furthermore, HIV infection was an independent risk factor for the high on antiplatelet reactivity that was increased by combined antiretroviral therapy (cART). Of the cART, protease inhibitors had greater effects than the NNRTIs. The residual platelet reactivity in PLWHIV despite viral suppression and dual antiplatelet therapy can probably be accounted by the active immune mechanisms and drug interactions [148].

Overall, few studies have evaluated the effects of antiplatelets in persons living with HIV. The available studies suffer from small sample sizes and have not been performed in populations not taking cART. Furthermore, the different classes of antiplatelets have not been evaluated. Of the studies done so far, the results do demonstrate neither efficacy nor improved outcomes with either aspirin or clopidogrel.

12. Conclusion

Infection with HIV is associated with reduced platelet count; extent of thrombocytopenia inversely correlates with viral load and disease progression. Despite thrombocytopenia, cardiovascular events are on the increase. There is associated platelet hyperactivity, as evidenced by increased surface expression of CD62P, CD40L, platelet microparticles, and platelet leukocyte aggregates. There is enhanced secretion of chemokines such as RANTES. Combined antiretroviral drugs independently and synergistically with HIV enhance platelet hyperactivity that persists despite viral suppression. Data on the effects of antiplatelets in this population can at best be described as clinical equipoise.

Other declarations

Autor's ORCID identifier: 0000-0001-6466-172X.

Author details

Gordon Ogweno
Department of Medical Physiology, School of Medicine, Kenyatta University, Nairobi, Kenya

*Address all correspondence to: ogweno.gordon@ku.ac.ke

References

[1] Ahonkhai AA, Gebo KA, Steiff MB, Moore RD, Segal JB. Venous thromboembolism in patients with HIV/AIDS. A case-control study. Journal of Acquired Immune Deficiency Syndromes. 2008;**48**(3):310-314. DOI: 10.1097/QAI.0b013e318163bd70

[2] Lordkipanidzé M. Platelet function tests. Seminars in Thrombosis and Hemostasis. 2016;**42**(3):258-267. DOI: 10.1055/s-0035-1564834

[3] Mansouritorghabeh H, De Laat B, Roest M. Current methods of measuring platelet activity : Pros and cons. Blood Coagulation & Fibrinolysis. 2020;**31**:426-433. DOI: 10.1097/MBC.000000000 0000941

[4] Getawa S, Aynalem M, Bayleyegn B, Adane T. The global prevalence of thrombocytopenia among HIV-infected adults: A systematic review and meta-analysis. International Journal of Infectious Diseases. 2021;**105**:495-504. DOI: 10.1016/j.ijid.2021.02.118

[5] Sloand EM, Klein HG, Banks SM, Vareldzis B, Merritt S, Pierce P. Epidemiology of thrombocytopenia in HIV infection. European Journal of Haematology. 1992;**48**(3):168-172. DOI: 10.1111/j.1600-0609.1992.tb00591.x

[6] Passos AM, Treitinger A, Spada C. An overview of the mechanisms of HIV-related thrombocytopenia. Acta Haematologica. 2010;**124**(1):13-18. DOI: 10.1159/000313782

[7] Li B et al. Manifestations and related risk factors of thrombocyte abnormalities in HIV-positive patients before and after the initiation of art. Infection and Drug Resistance. 2021;**14**:4809-4819. DOI: 10.2147/IDR.S334046

[8] Marchionatti A, Parisi MM. Anemia and thrombocytopenia in people living with HIV/AIDS: A narrative literature review. International Health. 2021;**13**(2):98-109. DOI: 10.1093/inthealth/ihaa036

[9] Ongondi M, Amayo EO, Lule GN, Rajab JA. Thrombocytopenia in HAART NAIVE HIV infected patients attending the Comprehensive Care Clinic at Kenyatta National Hospital. East African Medical Journal. 2016;**93**(9):406-408

[10] Dominguez A, Gamallo G, Garcia R, Lopez-Pastor A, Peña JM, Vazquez JJ. Pathophysiology of HIV related thrombocytopenia: An analysis of 41 patients. Journal of Clinical Pathology. 1994;**47**(11):999-1003. DOI: 10.1136/jcp.47.11.999

[11] Miguez-Burbano MJ, Jackson J, Hadrigan S. Thrombocytopenia in HIV disease: Clinical relevance, physiopathology and management. Current Medicinal Chemistry. Cardiovascular and Hematological Agents. 2005;**3**(4):365-376. DOI: 10.2174/1568016057743 22364

[12] Mathur A, Samaranayake S, Storrar NPF, Vickers MA. Investigating thrombocytosis. BMJ. 2019;**366**(July): 1-6. DOI: 10.1136/bmj.l4183

[13] Ellaurie M. Thrombocytosis in pediatric HIV infection. Clinical Pediatrics (Phila). 2004;**43**(7):627-629. DOI: 10.1177/000992280404300707

[14] Mateveke-Kuona P, Bwakura MF, Dzangare J, Pazvakavambwa I. Haematological features in children

less than 12 years on co-trimoxazole prophylaxis seen in opportunistic infection clinics at Harare and Parirenyatwa Teaching Hospitals. The Central African Journal of Medicine. 2010;**56**(9/12):51-56

[15] Bamberg R, Johnson J. Segmented neutrophil size and platelet morphology in HIV/AIDS patients. Clinical Laboratory Science. 2002;**15**(1):18-22

[16] Pretorius E, Smit E, Oberholzer HM, Steyn E, Briedenhann S, Franz RC. Investigating the ultrastructure of platelets of HIV patients treated with the immuno-regulator, Canova. Histology and Histopathology. 2009;**24**:399-405

[17] Jackson BS, Nunes Goncalves J, Pretorius E. Comparison of pathological clotting using haematological, functional and morphological investigations in HIV-positive and HIV-negative patients with deep vein thrombosis. Retrovirology. 2020;**17**(1):1-13. DOI: 10.1186/s12977-020-00523-3

[18] Hauguel-Moreau M et al. Platelet reactivity in human immunodeficiency virus infected patients on dual antiplatelet therapy for an acute coronary syndrome: The EVERE2ST-HIV study. European Heart Journal. 2017;**38**(21):1676-1686. DOI: 10.1093/eurheartj/ehw583

[19] Satchell CS et al. Platelet function and HIV : A case – Control study. AIDS. 2010;**24**:649-657. DOI: 10.1097/QAD.0b013e328336098c

[20] Satchell CS et al. Increased platelet reactivity in HIV-1 – Infected patients receiving abacavir-containing antiretroviral therapy. JID. 2011;**204**:1202-1210. DOI: 10.1093/infdis/jir509

[21] Brien MPO et al. Targeting thrombogenicity and inflammation in chronic HIV infection. Science Advances. 2019;**5**:eaav5463

[22] Etulain J et al. Hyperthermia inhibits platelet hemostatic functions and selectively regulates the release of alpha-granule proteins. Journal of Thrombosis and Haemostasis. 2011;**9**(8):1562-1571. DOI: 10.1111/j.1538-7836.2011.04394.x

[23] Haugaard AK, Lund TT, Birch C, Trøseid M, Ullum H, Gerstoft J. Discrepant coagulation profile in HIV infection : Elevated D-dimer but impaired platelet aggregation and clot initiation. AIDS. 2013;**27**:2749-2758. DOI: 10.1097/01.aids.0000432462.21723.ed

[24] Muñoz RP et al. Whole blood platelet aggregometry in HIV-infected patients on treatment with abacavir *. OJIM. 2012;**2012**:62-66. DOI: 10.4236/ojim.2012.22013

[25] Hottz ED, Quirino-teixeira AC, Valls-de-souza R, Zimmerman GA, Bozza FA, Bozza PT. Platelet function in HIV plus dengue coinfection associates with reduced inflammation and milder dengue illness. Scientific Reports. 2019;**9**(1):1-13. DOI: 10.1038/s41598-019-43275-7

[26] Kannan M, Ahmad F, Saxena R. Platelet activation markers in evaluation of thrombotic risk factors in various clinical settings. Blood Reviews. 2019;**37**:100583. DOI: 10.1016/j.blre.2019.05.007

[27] Nkambule BB et al. Platelet activation in adult HIV-infected patients on antiretroviral therapy: A systematic review and meta-analysis. BMC Medicine. 2020;**18**:357. DOI: 10.1186/s12916-020-01801-9

[28] Holme PA, Muller F, Solum NO, Brosstad F, Land Q, Aukrust PAL. Enhanced activation of platelets with abnormal release of RANTES

in human immunodeficiency virus type 1 infection. The FASEB Journal. 1998;**12**:79-89

[29] Mayne E et al. Increased platelet and microparticle activation in HIV infection : Upregulation of P-selectin and tissue factor expression. Journal of Acquired Immune Deficiency Syndromes. 2012;**59**(4):340-346

[30] Nkambule BB, Davison GM, Ipp H. The evaluation of platelet function in HIV infected, asymptomatic treatment-naïve individuals using flow cytometry. Thrombosis Research. 2015;**135**(6):1131-1139. DOI: 10.1016/j.thromres.2015.01.031

[31] Francisci D, Falcinelli E, Belfiori B, Petito E, Guglielmini G, Malincarne L. In vivo platelet activation and platelet hyperreactivity in abacavir- treated HIV infected patients. Thrombosis and Haemostasis. 2013;**110**(8):349-357. DOI: 10.1160/TH12-07-0504

[32] Mesquita EC et al. Persistent platelet activation and apoptosis in virologically suppressed HIV-infected individuals. Scientific Reports. 2018;**8**(1):1-10. DOI: 10.1038/s41598-018-33403-0

[33] Marcantoni E et al. Platelet transcriptome profiling in as a mediator of platelet activity. JACC: Basic to Translational Science. 2018;**3**:9-22. DOI: 10.1016/j.jacbts.2017.10.005

[34] Landrø L, Ueland T, Otterdal K, Frøland SS, Aukrust P. Persistently raised plasma levels of platelet-derived inflammatory mediators in HIV-infected patients during highly active anti-retroviral therapy. Journal of Thrombosis and Haemostasis. 2011;**9**(5):1075-1077. DOI: 10.1111/j.1538-7836.2011.04242.x

[35] Mumford AD et al. A review of platelet secretion assays for the diagnosis of inherited platelet secretion disorders. Thrombosis and Haemostasis. 2015;**114**(1):14-25. DOI: 10.1160/TH14-11-0999

[36] Pai M et al. Diagnostic usefulness of a lumi-aggregometer adenosine triphosphate release assay for the assessment of platelet function disorders. American Journal of Clinical Pathology. 2011;**136**(3):350-358. DOI: 10.1309/AJCP9IPR1TFLUAGM

[37] O'Brien M et al. Aspirin attenuates platelet activation and immune activation in HIV-1-infected subjects on antiretroviral therapy: A pilot study. Journal of Acquired Immune Deficiency Syndromes. 2013;**63**(3):280-288. DOI: 10.1097/QAI.0b013e31828a292c

[38] Gama WM et al. Increased levels of reactive oxygen species in platelets and platelet-derived microparticles and the risk of respiratory failure in HIV/AIDS patients. Memórias do Instituto Oswaldo Cruz. 2020;**115**:e200082. DOI: 10.1590/0074-02760200082

[39] O'Brien JR. "Exhausted " platelets continue to circulate. The *Lancet*. 1978;**312**(8103):1316-1317. DOI: 10.1016/s0140-6736(78)92087-1

[40] Pareti FI, Capitanio A, Mannucci L, Ponticelli C, Mannucci PM. Acquired dysfunction due to the circulation of 'exhausted' platelets. The American Journal of Medicine. 1980;**69**(2):235-240. DOI: 10.1016/0002-9343(80)90383-6

[41] Boneu B, Bugat R, Boneu A, Eche N, Sie P, Combes P-F. Exhausted platelets in patients with malignant solid tumors without evidence of active consumption coagulation. European Journal of Cancer & Clinical Oncology. 1984;**20**(7):890-903

[42] Evans RJ, Gordon JL. Refractoriness in blood platelets: Effect of prior

exposure to aggregating agents on subsequent aggregation responses. British Journal of Pharmacology. 1974;**51**(1):123

[43] Fong BJSC, Kaplan BS. Ipairment of platelet aggregation in Hemolytic uremic syndrome: Evidence for platelet 'exhaustion'. Blood. 1982;**60**(3):564-571

[44] O'Brien JR, Etherrington M, Jameson S. Refractory state of platelet aggregation with major operations. The *Lancet*. 1971;**2**(7727):741-743. DOI: 10.1016/s0140-6736(71)92107-6

[45] Pareti F, Capitanio A, Mannucci P. Acquired storage pool disease in platelets during disseminated intravascular coagulation. Blood. 1976;**48**(4):511-515. DOI: 10.1182/blood.v48.4.511.511

[46] Zahavi J, Marder VJ. Acquired 'storage pool disease' of platelets associated with circulating antiplatelet antibodies. The American Journal of Medicine. 1974;**56**(6):883-890. DOI: 10.1016/0002-9343(74)90819-5

[47] Hughes CE. How to perform aggregometry and lumi-aggregometry in mouse platelets. Platelets. 2018;**29**(7):638-643. DOI: 10.1080/09537104.2018.1478074

[48] Jurk K, Shiravand Y. Platelet phenotyping and function testing in thrombocytopenia. Journal of Clinical Medicine. 2021;**10**(5):1114. DOI: 10.3390/jcm10051114

[49] Fritsma GA. Platelet function testing: Aggregometry and lumiaggregometry. Clinical Laboratory Science. 2007;**20**(1): 32-37. DOI: 10.29074/ascls.20.1.32

[50] Weiss HJ, Lages B. The response of platelets to epinephrine in storage pool deficiency - evidence pertaining to the role of adenosine diphosphate in mediating primary and secondary aggregation. Blood. 1988;**72**(5):1717-1725. DOI: 10.1182/blood.v72.5.1717.1717

[51] Taylor KA et al. Pharmacological impact of antiretroviral therapy on platelet function to investigate human immunodeficiency virus - associated cardiovascular risk. British Journal of Pharmacology. 2019;**176**:879-889. DOI: 10.1111/bph.14589

[52] Paniccia R, Priora R, Liotta AA, Abbate R. Platelet function tests: A comparative review. Vascular Health and Risk Management. 2015;**11**:133-148. DOI: 10.2147/VHRM.S44469

[53] Falcinelli E et al. Effect of aspirin treatment on abacavir-associated platelet hyperreactivity in HIV-infected patients. International Journal of Cardiology. 2018;**263**:118-124. DOI: 10.1016/j.ijcard.2018.04.052

[54] Castaman G et al. The impact of bleeding history, von Willebrand factor and PFA – 100 â on the diagnosis of type 1 von Willebrand disease : Results from the European study MCMDM-1VWD. British Journal of Haematology. 2010;**151**:245-251. DOI: 10.1111/j.1365-2141.2010.08333.x

[55] Gianetti J, Parri MS, Della Pina F, Marchi F, Koni E, De Caterina A, et al. Von willebrand factor antigen predicts response to double dose of aspirin and clopidogrel by PFA-100 in patients undergoing primary angioplasty for ST elevation myocardial infarction. The Scientific World Journal. 2013:313492. DOI: 10.1155/2013/313492

[56] Franzetti M et al. Changes in the incidence of severe thrombocytopenia and its predisposing conditions in HIV-infected patients since the introduction

of highly active antiretroviral therapy. Journal of Acquired Immune Deficiency Syndromes. 2014;**67**(5):493-498. DOI: 10.1097/QAI.0000000000000347

[57] Nascimento FG, Tanaka PY. Thrombocytopenia in HIV-infected patients. Indian Journal of Hematology and Blood Transfusion. 2012;**28**(2):109-111. DOI: 10.1007/s12288-011-0124-9

[58] Vannappagari V, Nkhoma ET, Atashili J, Laurent SS, Zhao H. Prevalence, severity, and duration of thrombocytopenia among HIV patients in the era of highly active antiretroviral therapy. Platelets. 2011;**22**(8):611-618. DOI: 10.3109/09537104.2011.582526

[59] Ahmed S, Siddiqui RK, Siddiqui AK, Zaidi SA, Cervia J. HIV associated thrombotic microangiopathy. Postgraduate Medical Journal. 2002;**78**:520-525

[60] Dentali F, Nicolini E, Ageno W. Venous and arterial thrombosis associated with HIV infection. Seminars in Thrombosis and Hemostasis. 2012;**38**(5):524-529. DOI: 10.1055/s-0032-1306434

[61] Meiring M, Webb M, Goedhals D, Louw V. HIV-associated thrombotic thrombocytopenic purpura - what we know so far. European Oncology & Haematology. 2012;**8**(2):89-91. DOI: 10.17925/eoh.2012.08.02.89

[62] Gunther K, Garizio D, Dhlamini B. The pathogenesis of HIV-related thrombotic thrombocytopaenic purpura – Is it different? ISBT Science Series. 2006;**1**(1):246-250. DOI: 10.1111/j.1751-2824.2006.00041.x

[63] De La, Rubia J, Contreras E, Del Río-Garma J. Thrombotic thrombocytopenic purpura. Medicina Clínica (Barcelona). 2011;**136**(12):534-540. DOI: 10.1016/j.medcli.2010.02.011

[64] Tsai H-M. Deficiency of ADAMTS13 causes thrombotic thrombocytopenic Purpura. Arteriosclerosis, Thrombosis, and Vascular Biology. 2003;**23**:388-397. DOI: 10.1161/01.ATV.0000058401.34021.D4

[65] Aukrust P et al. Persistently elevated levels of von Willebrand factor antigen in HIV infection. Downregulation during highly active antiretroviral therapy. Thrombosis and Haemostasis. 2000;**84**:183-187

[66] Graham SM et al. Von willebrand factor adhesive activity and ADAMTS13 protease activity in HIV-1-infected men. International Journal of Medical Sciences. 2019;**16**(2):276-284. DOI: 10.7150/ijms.28110

[67] Graham SM et al. Elevated plasma von Willebrand factor levels are associated with subsequent ischemic stroke in persons with treated HIV infection. Open Forum Infectious Diseases. 2021;**1**:1-9. DOI: 10.1093/ofid/ofab521

[68] van den, Dries LWJ et al. von Willebrand factor is elevated in HIV patients with a history of thrombosis. Frontiers in Microbiology. 2015;**6**:1-8. DOI: 10.3389/fmicb.2015.00180

[69] Varga-Szabo D, Pleines I, Nieswandt B. Cell adhesion mechanisms in platelets. Arteriosclerosis, Thrombosis, and Vascular Biology. 2008;**28**(3):403-413. DOI: 10.1161/ATVBAHA.107.150474

[70] Kelly C et al. Circulating microparticles are increased amongst people presenting with HIV and advanced immune suppression in Malawi and correlate closely with arterial stiffness: A nested case control study.

Wellcome Open Research. 2021;**6**:264. DOI: 10.12688/wellcomeopenres.17044.1

[71] Corrales-Medina VF et al. Increased levels of platelet microparticles in HIV-infected patients with good response to highly active antiretroviral therapy. Journal of Acquired Immune Deficiency Syndromes. 2010;**54**(2):217-218

[72] Hijmans JG et al. Circulating microparticles are elevated in treated HIV-1 infection and are deleterious to endothelial cell function. Journal of the American Heart Association. 2019;**8**:e011134. DOI: 10.1161/JAHA.118.011134

[73] van der, Heijden WA et al. Long-term treated HIV infection is associated with platelet mitochondrial dysfunction. Scientific Reports. 2021;**11**(1):1-12. DOI: 10.1038/s41598-021-85775-5

[74] Gyulkhandanyan AV, Mutlu A, Freedman J, Leytin V. Markers of platelet apoptosis: Methodology and applications. Journal of Thrombosis and Thrombolysis. 2012;**33**(4):397-411. DOI: 10.1007/s11239-012-0688-8

[75] Banerjee M et al. Platelets endocytose viral particles and are activated via TLR (toll-like receptor) signalling. Arteriosclerosis, Thrombosis, and Vascular Biology. 2020;**40**:1635-1650. DOI: 10.1161/ATVBAHA.120.314180

[76] Chaipan C et al. DC-SIGN and CLEC-2 mediate human immunodeficiency virus type 1 capture by platelets. Journal of Virology. 2006;**80**(18):8951-8960. DOI: 10.1128/jvi.00136-06

[77] Wang J, Zhang W, Nardi MA, Li Z. HIV-1 Tat-induced platelet activation and release of CD154 contribute to HIV-1-associated autoimmune thrombocytopenia. Journal of Thrombosis and Haemostasis. 2011;**9**(3):562-573. DOI: 10.1111/j.1538-7836.2010.04168.x

[78] Pastori D et al. HIV-1 induces in vivo platelet activation by enhancing platelet NOX2 activity. The Journal of Infection. 2015;**70**(6):651-658. DOI: 10.1016/j.jinf.2015.01.005

[79] Hsue PY. Mechanisms of cardiovascular disease in the setting of HIV infection. The Canadian Journal of Cardiology. 2019;**35**(3):238-248. DOI: 10.1016/j.cjca.2018.12.024

[80] Shan L, Siliciano RF. Unraveling the relationship between microbial translocation and systemic immune activation in HIV infection. The Journal of Clinical Investigation. 2014;**124**(6):2368-2371. DOI: 10.1172/JCI75799

[81] Lopes Pires ME, Clarke SR, Marcondes S, Gibbins JM. Lipopolysaccharide potentiates platelet responses via toll-like receptor 4-stimulated Akt-Erk-PLA2 signalling. PLoS One. 2017;**12**(11):1-22. DOI: 10.1371/journal.pone.0186981

[82] Nocella C et al. Lipopolysaccharide induces platelet activation in HIV patients: The role of different viral load patterns. HIV Medicine. 2021;**22**(6):434-444. DOI: 10.1111/hiv.13059

[83] Zhang G et al. Lipopolysaccharide stimulates platelet secretion and potentiates platelet aggregation via TLR4/MyD88 and the cGMP-dependent protein kinase pathway. Journal of Immunology. 2009;**182**(12):7997-8004. DOI: 10.4049/jimmunol.0802884

[84] Zhang X et al. Gut microbiota induces high platelet response in patients with ST segment elevation myocardial infarction after ticagrelor treatment.

eLife. 2022;**11**:e70240. DOI: 10.7554/eLife.70240

[85] Martyanov AA et al. Effects of bacterial lipopolysaccharides on platelet function: Inhibition of weak platelet activation. Scientific Reports. 2020;**10**(1):1-10. DOI: 10.1038/s41598-020-69173-x

[86] Damien P et al. LPS stimulation of purified human platelets is partly dependent on plasma soluble CD14 to secrete their main secreted product, soluble-CD40-ligand. BMC Immunology. 2015;**16**(1):1-7. DOI: 10.1186/s12865-015-0067-2

[87] Aslam R et al. Platelet toll-like receptor expression modulates lipopolysaccharide-induced thrombocytopenia and tumor necrosis factor-α production *in vivo*. Blood. 2006;**107**(2):637-641. DOI: 10.1182/blood-2005-06-2202

[88] Berthet J et al. Human platelets can discriminate between various bacterial LPS isoforms via TLR4 signaling and differential cytokine secretion. Clinical Immunology. 2012;**145**(3):189-200. DOI: 10.1016/j.clim.2012.09.004

[89] Jonathan S, Rajendran V, Dash P, Ketan P, Darius W. Effect of ultrapure lipopolysaccharides derived from diverse bacterial species on the modulation of platelet activation. Scientific Reports. 2019;**9**:18258. DOI: 10.1038/s41598-019-54617-w

[90] Lumadue JA, Lanzkron SM, Kennedy SD, Kuhl DT, Mt BS, Kickler TS. Cytokine induction of platelet activation. American Journal of Clinical Pathology. 1996;**106**:795-798

[91] Burstein SA et al. Cytokine-induced alteration of platelet and hemostatic function. Stem Cells. 1996;**14**(Suppl 1): 154-162

[92] Davizon-Castillo P et al. TNF-a–driven inflammation and mitochondrial dysfunction define the platelet hyperreactivity of aging. Blood. 2019;**134**(9):727-740. DOI: 10.1182/blood.2019000200

[93] Çevİk Ö, Adigüzel Z, Baykal AT, Şener A. Tumor necrosis factor-alpha induced caspase-3 activation-related iNOS gene expression in ADP-activated platelets. Turkish Journal of Biology. 2017;**41**:31-40. DOI: 10.3906/biy-1509-64

[94] Arman M, Krauel K. Human platelet IgG Fc receptor Fc c RIIA in immunity and thrombosis. Journal of Thrombosis and Haemostasis. 2015;**13**:893-908. DOI: 10.1111/jth.12905

[95] Goette NP, Glembotsky AC, Lev PR, Grodzielski M. Platelet apoptosis in adult immune thrombocytopenia : Insights into the mechanism of damage triggered by auto- antibodies. PLoS One. 2016;**11**(8):e0160563. DOI: 10.1371/journal.pone.0160563

[96] Larson A, Egberg N, Lindahl L. Platelet activation and binding of complement components to platelets induced by immune complexes. Platelets. 1994;**5**:149-155

[97] Zhi H, Dai J, Liu J, Zhu J, Newman DK, Gao C. Platelet activation and thrombus formation over IgG immune complexes requires integrin α IIb β 3 and Lyn kinase. PLoS One. 2015;**10**(8):e0135738. DOI: 10.1371/journal.pone.0135738

[98] Schattner BM et al. Activation of human platelets by immune complexes prepared with cationized human IgG. Blood. 1993;**82**(10):3045-3051

[99] Li Z, Nardi MA, Karpatkin S. Role of molecular mimicry to HIV-1 peptides in HIV-1-related immunologic thrombocytopenia. Blood. 2005;**106**(2): 572-576. DOI: 10.1182/blood-2005-01-0243

[100] Zhang W, Nardi MA, Borkowsky W, Li Z, Karpatkin S. Role of molecular mimicry of hepatitis C virus protein with platelet GPIIIa in hepatitis C-related immunologic thrombocytopenia. Blood. 2009;**113**(17):4086-4093. DOI: 10.1182/blood-2008-09-181073

[101] Saitoh T et al. Neutrophil extracellular traps mediate a host defense response to human immunodeficiency virus-1. Cell Host & Microbe. 2012;**12**(1):109-116. DOI: 10.1016/j.chom.2012.05.015

[102] Barr FD, Ochsenbauer C, Wira CR, Rodriguez-Garcia M. Neutrophil extracellular traps prevent HIV infection in the female genital tract. Mucosal Immunology. 2018;**11**(5):1420-1428. DOI: 10.1038/s41385-018-0045-0

[103] Fuchs TA et al. Extracellular DNA traps promote thrombosis. Proceedings of the National Academy of Sciences of the United States of America. 2010;**107**(36):15880-15885. DOI: 10.1073/pnas.1005743107

[104] Elaskalani O, Abdol Razak NB, Metharom P. Neutrophil extracellular traps induce aggregation of washed human platelets independently of extracellular DNA and histones. Cell Communication and Signalling. 2018;**16**(1):1-15. DOI: 10.1186/s12964-018-0235-0

[105] Zhou P et al. Interactions between neutrophil extracellular traps and activated platelets enhance procoagulant activity in acute stroke patients with ICA occlusion. eBioMedicine. 2020;**53**:102671. DOI: 10.1016/j.ebiom.2020.102671

[106] Zarbock A, Polanowska-Grabowska RK, Ley K. Platelet-neutrophil-interactions: Linking hemostasis and inflammation. Blood Reviews. 2007;**21**(2):99-111. DOI: 10.1016/j.blre.2006.06.001

[107] Stark K. Platelet-neutrophil crosstalk and netosis. HemaSphere. 2019;**3**(S2):89-91. DOI: 10.1097/HS9.0000000000000231

[108] Carestia A, Kaufman T, Schattner M. Platelets: New bricks in the building of neutrophil extracellular traps. Frontiers in Immunology. 2016;**7**:271. DOI: 10.3389/fimmu.2016.00271

[109] Green SA et al. Activated platelet – T-cell conjugates in peripheral blood of patients with HIV infection : Coupling coagulation / inflammation and T cells. AIDS. 2015;**29**:1297-1308. DOI: 10.1097/QAD.0000000000000701

[110] Nkambule BB, Davison G, Ipp H. Platelet leukocyte aggregates and markers of platelet aggregation, immune activation and disease progression in HIV infected treatment naive asymptomatic individuals. Journal of Thrombosis and Thrombolysis. 2015;**40**(4):458-467. DOI: 10.1007/s11239-015-1212-8

[111] Francisci D et al. HIV type 1 infection, and not short-term HAART , induces endothelial dysfunction. AIDS. 2009;**23**:589-596. DOI: 10.1097/QAD.0b013e328325a87c

[112] Jong E, Louw S, Van Gorp ECM, Meijers JCM, Ten Cate H, Jacobson BF. The effect of initiating combined antiretroviral therapy on endothelial cell activation and coagulation markers in South African HIV-infected individuals. Thrombosis

and Haemostasis. 2010;**104**(6):1228-1234. DOI: 10.1160/TH10-04-0233

[113] Van Den Dries LWJ, Gruters RA, Van Der Borden SBCH. von Willebrand factor is elevated in HIV patients with a history of thrombosis. Frontiers in Microbiology. 2015;**6**:180. DOI: 10.3389/fmicb.2015.00180

[114] Reininger AJ. The function of ultra-large von Willebrand factor multimers in high shear flow controlled by ADAMTS13. Hämostaseologie. 2015;**35**:225-233

[115] Mutlu A, Gyulkhandanyan AV, Freedman J, Leytin V. Concurrent and separate inside-out transition of platelet apoptosis and activation markers to the platelet surface. British Journal of Haematology. 2013;**163**(3):377-384. DOI: 10.1111/bjh.12529

[116] Reddy EC, Rand ML. Procoagulant phosphatidylserine-exposing platelets *in vitro* and *in vivo*. Frontiers in Cardiovascular Medicine. 2020;**7**:1-11. DOI: 10.3389/fcvm.2020.00015

[117] Böing AN, Hau CM, Sturk A, Nieuwland R. Platelet microparticles contain active caspase 3. Platelets. 2008;**19**(2):96-103. DOI: 10.1080/09537100701777295

[118] Gyulkhandanyan AV et al. Mitochondrial inner membrane depolarization as a marker of platelet apoptosis : Disclosure of nonapoptotic membrane depolarization. Clinical and Applied Thrombosis/Hemostasis. 2017;**23**(2):139-147. DOI: 10.1177/1076029616665924

[119] Leytin V, Allen DJ, Mutlu A, Gyulkhandanyan AV, Mykhaylov S, Freedman J. Mitochondrial control of platelet apoptosis: Effect of cyclosporin a, an inhibitor of the mitochondrial permeability transition pore. Laboratory Investigation. 2009;**89**(4):374-384. DOI: 10.1038/labinvest.2009.13

[120] Thushara RM, Hemshekhar M, Kemparaju K, Rangappa KS, Girish KS. Biologicals, platelet apoptosis and human diseases : An outlook. Critical Reviews in Oncology/Hematology. 2015;**93**(3):149-158. DOI: 10.1016/j.critrevonc.2014.11.002

[121] Von Gunten S, Wehrli M, Simon H. Cell death in immune thrombocytopenia_ novel insights and perspectives. Seminars in Hematology. 2013;**50**(1):S109-S115. DOI: 10.1053/j.seminhematol.2013.03.016

[122] Rand ML, Wang H, Bang KWA, Poon KSV, Packhams MA, Freedman J. Procoagulant surface exposure and apoptosis in rabbit platelets : Association with shortened survival and steady-state senescence. Journal of Thrombosis and Haemostasis. 2004;**2**:651-659

[123] Lebois M, Josefsson EC, Lebois M, Josefsson EC. Regulation of platelet lifespan by apoptosis. Platelets;**27**(6):497-504. DOI: 10.3109/09537104.2016.1161739

[124] Dasgupta SK et al. Platelet senescence and phosphatidylserine exposure. Transfusion. 2010;**50**(10):2167-2175. DOI: 10.1111/j.1537-2995.2010.02676.x.Platelet

[125] Carbonara S et al. Response of severe HIV-associated thrombocytopenia to highly active antiretroviral therapy including protease inhibitors. The Journal of Infection. 2001;**42**(4):251-256. DOI: 10.1053/jinf.2001.0833

[126] Servais J et al. HIV-associated hematologic disorders are correlated with plasma viral load and improve under

highly active antiretroviral therapy. JAIDSs. 2001;**28**:221-225

[127] Lewis W. Mitochondrial toxicity of antiviral drugs. Nature Medicine. 1995;**1**(5):417-422

[128] Baum PD, Sullam PM, Stoddart CA, McCune JM. Abacavir increases platelet reactivity via competitive inhibition of soluble guanylyl cyclase. AIDS. 2011;**25**(18):2243-2248. DOI: 10.1097/QAD.0b013e32834d3cc3

[129] Khawaja AA et al. HIV antivirals affect endothelial activation and endothelial-platelet crosstalk. Circulation Research. 2020:1365-1380. DOI: 10.1161/CIRCRESAHA.119.316477

[130] Chini M et al. Effects of highly active antiretroviral therapy on platelet activating factor metabolism in naïve HIV-infected patients: II study of the abacavir/lamivudine/efavirenz haart regimen. International Journal of Immunopathology and Pharmacology. 2012;**25**(1):247-258. DOI: 10.1177/039463201202500127

[131] Jaschinski NJ, Greenberg L, Beesgaard B, et al. Recent abacavir use and incident cardiovascular disease in contemporary treated people living with HIV (PLWH) within the RESPOND cohort consortium. In: 18th European AIDS Conference. London, EACS 2021, October 27-30, 2021. Abstract BPD1/3

[132] Dorjee K, Baxi SM, Reingold AL, Hubbard A. Risk of cardiovascular events from current, recent, and cumulative exposure to abacavir among persons living with HIV who were receiving antiretroviral therapy in the United States: A cohort study. BMC Infectious Diseases. 2017;**17**(1):1-12. DOI: 10.1186/s12879-017-2808-8

[133] Baker JV, Hullsiek KH, Bradford RL, Prosser R, Tracy RP, Key NS. Circulating levels of tissue factor microparticle procoagulant activity are reduced with antiretroviral therapy and are associated with persistent inflammation and coagulation activation among HIV-positive patients. Journal of Acquired Immune Deficiency Syndromes. 2013;**63**(3):367-371. DOI: 10.1097/QAI.0b013e3182910121

[134] Funderburg NT et al. Shared monocyte subset phenotypes in HIV-1 infection and in uninfected subjects with acute coronary syndrome. Blood. 2012;**120**(23):4599-4608. DOI: 10.1182/blood-2012-05-433946

[135] Funderburg NT et al. Increased tissue factor expression on circulating monocytes in chronic HIV infection: Relationship to in vivo coagulation and immune activation. Blood. 2010;**115**(2):161-167. DOI: 10.1182/blood-2009-03-210179

[136] Østerud B. The role of platelets in decrypting monocyte tissue factor. Seminars in Hematology. 2001;**38**(Suppl 12):2-5. DOI: 10.1053/shem.2001.29508

[137] Scholz T, Temmler U, Krause S, Heptinstall S, Lösche W. Transfer of tissue factor from platelets to monocytes: Role of platelet-derived microvesicles and CD62P. Thrombosis and Haemostasis. 2002;**88**(6):1033-1038. DOI: 10.1055/s-0037-1613351

[138] Lösche W, Scholz T, Temmler U, Oberle V, Claus RA. Platelet-derived microvesicles transfer tissue factor to monocytes but not to neutrophils. Platelets. 2004;**15**(2):109-115. DOI: 10.1080/09537100310001649885

[139] De Pablo-Bernal RS et al. TNF-α levels in HIV-infected patients after long-term suppressive cART persist as high as in elderly, HIV-uninfected subjects. The Journal of Antimicrobial Chemotherapy.

2014;**69**(11):3041-3046. DOI: 10.1093/jac/dku263

[140] Laurence J, Elhadad S, Ahamed J. HIV-associated cardiovascular disease: Importance of platelet activation and cardiac fibrosis in the setting of specific antiretroviral therapies. Open Heart. 2018;**5**(2):1-13. DOI: 10.1136/openhrt-2018-000823

[141] Feinstein MJ et al. Characteristics, prevention, and Management of Cardiovascular Disease in people living with HIV: A scientific statement from the American Heart Association. Circulation. 2019;**140**(2):e98-e124. DOI: 10.1161/CIR.0000000000000695

[142] Currier JS et al. Coronary heart disease in HIV-infected individuals. JAIDS. 2003;**33**:506-512

[143] Boccara F et al. HIV and coronary heart disease: Time for a better understanding. Journal of the American College of Cardiology. 2013;**61**(5):511-523. DOI: 10.1016/j.jacc.2012.06.063

[144] Benjamin LA et al. HIV infection and stroke : Current perspectives and future directions. Lancet Neurology. 2012;**11**(10):878-890. DOI: 10.1016/S1474-4422(12)70205-3

[145] Lin HL, Muo CH, Lin CY, Chen HJ, Chen PC. Incidence of stroke in patients with HIV infection: A population-based study in Taiwan. PLoS One. 2019;**14**(5):1-14. DOI: 10.1371/journal.pone.0217147

[146] Currier JS et al. Epidemiological evidence for cardiovascular disease in HIV-infected patients and relationship to highly active antiretroviral therapy. Circulation. 2008;**118**(2):e29-e35. DOI: 10.1161/CIRCULATIONAHA.107.189624

[147] Obel N et al. Ischemic heart disease in HIV-infected and HIV-uninfected individuals: A population-based cohort study. Clinical Infectious Diseases. 2007;**44**(12):1625-1631. DOI: 10.1086/518285

[148] Archer O et al. Patients living with HIV and coronary disease: Are we using appropriate anti platelets as part of dual antiplatelet therapy? Cardiology & Vascular Research. 2021;**5**(1):1-5. DOI: 10.33425/2639-8486.1094

[149] Simpson SR, Singh MV, Dewhurst S, Schifitto G, Maggirwar SB. Platelets function as an acute viral reservoir during HIV-1 infection by harboring virus and T-cell complex formation. Blood Advances. 2020;**4**(18):4512-4521. DOI: 10.1182/bloodadvances.2020002420

Section 4

Care and Management

Chapter 7

Management Strategies in Perinatal HIV

Kayla Aleshire and Rima Bazzi

Abstract

Current management of perinatal HIV infections and exposures involves the administration of antiretroviral therapy to both the pregnant mother and to her child after delivery. Striving to achieve safe and effective medication management is key in preventing new pediatric HIV infections. Maternal HIV testing and subsequent monitoring can help to identify fetal HIV exposures during pregnancy, maternal nonadherence, insufficient treatment regimens, and otherwise undiscovered exposures during the delivery process. There are several well-constructed guidelines that offer expert references for healthcare providers. This chapter will summarize current recommendations from the United States, with a brief insight into select international guidelines. Although available guidelines provide a structured framework for the healthcare team, there has recently been a significant drive to advance current perinatal management and outcomes.

Keywords: pregnancy, perinatal, HIV, antiretrovirals, transmission

1. Introduction

Nearly 30 years ago, the Pediatric AIDS Clinical Trials Group (PACTG) Protocol 076 Study Group identified a reduction in the relative risk of perinatal transmission by almost 70 percent with the use of zidovudine monotherapy [1]. Zidovudine was administered to women starting in their second trimester and continued through the duration of the pregnancy [1]. Additionally, the medication was given to the mother during the intrapartum period, and postnatally to the infants [1]. A few decades later, triple antiretroviral therapy (ART) administered during pregnancy in the Promoting Maternal and Infant Survival Everywhere (PROMISE) trial proved more effective at reducing mother-to-child HIV transmission than with zidovudine monotherapy [2]. The PROMISE trial also demonstrated that there is a concern for transmission through breastfeeding, although this risk may be minimal with the use of ART [3]. Recent statistical evidence estimates that vertical transmission of HIV from mother to child is less than 1% in the United States [4], although it can exceed 10% in some countries [5]. Success in reducing perinatal transmission can presumably be attributed to the advancements in HIV care. Over the last three decades, prevention of mother-to-child transmission (MTCT) strategies have been continuously improving. There are several accepted guidelines that provide step-by-step recommendations for maternal HIV testing, management of acute HIV infection in the pregnant individual, use of antiretroviral (ARV) medications during pregnancy, the intrapartum period, and post-exposure prophylaxis to the newborn after delivery. The guideline recommendations provide slightly different options for treatment and prevention of perinatal HIV that are vital to controlling viremia in the pregnant mother and the developing child. Despite current information, therapeutic recommendations are more apt to utilize previously accepted regimens in the pregnant and neonatal populations. More recently, there is momentum directed toward conducting research trials with early pregnancies and neonates. Additional information regarding ARV safety and efficacy has the potential to further increase the therapeutic options in these respective populations.

2. Epidemiology

Nearly 5000 young women across the globe become infected with HIV each week, representing a profound population that warrants attention [6]. Centers for Disease Control and Prevention (CDC) data from the US population indicates that over 70% of new diagnoses in 2019 among females were those of childbearing age [4]. Of women who become pregnant, global estimates suggest that 80% have access to ART [6]. With many pregnant women having access to ARVs, it is important to consider implications in treatment management. Medications should be safe and effective in controlling maternal viremia to prevent newborn acquisition. In addition, HIV testing can help to identify new infections, thus enhancing earlier access to therapy. Over the last decade, new HIV diagnoses in children worldwide have dropped by half [6]. According to CDC statistics in the US population from 2015 to 2019, most children with perinatal HIV exposures in whom seroconversion did not occur were born to mothers who received HIV testing prior to the pregnancy [4]. Within the same period, the rates of acquired perinatal HIV were less than 1% in the United States [4]. Although testing prior to pregnancy is important, women can seroconvert later in the gestational period. Repeat testing should not be neglected as it has been demonstrated that a higher percentage of perinatal transmissions occur after 36 weeks' gestation [7]. In a US Epicenter for HIV, only about 80% of mothers were retested in their third trimester [8]. Furthermore, a study of pregnant women living with HIV in South Africa showed that only 11% of women were receiving all recommended tests throughout the perinatal period [9]. These examples highlight missed opportunities and the underutilization of HIV testing in some areas.

3. Future goals and challenges

In 2015, the United Nations endorsed a set of global goals to achieve a more promising future for all. One goal presented was to End AIDS by 2030 [10]. Subsequently, the United States advocated for Ending the Epidemic in the US—a plan for a 90% reduction in new HIV infections by 2030 [11]. More specifically, the CDC goal for HIV elimination is to reduce perinatal transmission to an incidence of <1 infection per 100,000 live births and a rate of <1% among infants exposed to HIV [12]. An essential component to achieving these goals is to understand the current approaches to the management of pregnant and pediatric populations and to identify barriers to treatment success. The optimization of medication therapy and performance of pertinent HIV tests are key strategies for preventing perinatal transmission [12–14]. Furthermore, the unique physiologies of neonates and pregnant women present challenges to enhancing medication therapy [15]. The paucity of data in these populations limits the recommended medication choices available for treatment and prophylaxis of HIV [12–14]. Currently, recommendations for medication dosing in pregnant women and neonates are often modeled after data obtained from non-pregnant adults or older pediatrics respectively. If efficacy and safety data were more comprehensive for the pregnant and neonatal populations, this would likely have a profound effect on achieving the elimination of MTCT. Additionally, opportunities exist for utilizing HIV testing during pregnancy and surrounding the time of delivery [8, 9]. Adhering to the current recommendations for HIV screening would shorten the time to treatment and potentially reduce viral exposure to the newborn [8].

4. Pharmacokinetic considerations for antiretroviral medications

The study of pharmacokinetics (PK) seeks to identify if an administered medication possesses the ability to reach therapeutic concentrations in the body, reach the proper site of action to exert its intended effect, and how long the intended effect will remain. Pharmacokinetic drug parameters include the absorption of drugs into the body, metabolism, and the excretion or removal of the drug and waste components from the body. Metabolism can create an active drug from a non-active one or change an active drug into non-active waste products. The products of a medication that result from a metabolic process in the body are termed metabolites. Drug metabolites can be eliminated by the liver or excreted by the kidneys. Another drug parameter to consider is drug distribution. Some medications readily exit the vascular system and distribute into neighboring tissues. Other medications predominantly remain within the vascular compartment. Many medications have a theoretical value, known as the volume of distribution (Vd), that describes this distribution property [16]. Pregnant women and neonates exhibit unique physiological properties that greatly alter medication PK [16, 17].

4.1 Pregnancy

Maternal physiology changes throughout the gestational period, thus PK parameters of a drug may be increasingly altered as the pregnancy progresses through each trimester. Most ARVs are administered orally and must be absorbed from the gastrointestinal tract. Consider a patient who is suffering from nausea and vomiting during pregnancy. If emesis occurs, then transit time in the stomach for an orally administered medication will be reduced and the medication may not be fully absorbed. If the patient requires antacids to alleviate symptoms, this, in turn, may increase the pH of the stomach. If the administered medication requires a low pH or acidic environment for absorption, an altered pH could affect therapeutic outcomes. Also, during pregnancy, there is a propensity for increased stomach pH, delayed gastric emptying, and slower intestinal motility altering the bioavailability of oral drugs. Enzymes, predominantly in the liver, are responsible for drug metabolism and are altered in the pregnant state. Some have increased activity (e.g., CYP3A4, CYP2D6, CYP2C9, UGT1A4, and UGT1A1/9), while others have decreased activity (e.g., CYP2C19, CYP1A2). This can have significant implications on how much active drug is available, and how fast or slow the administered medication is metabolized in the body. It changes the rate of conversion from active to inactive components or vice versa, depending on the properties of the drug. There is increased renal blood flow and glomerular filtration rate (GFR), resulting in increased elimination of renally-cleared medications, which may result in shorter half-lives and potential underdosing of those medications. During pregnancy, a woman's body fat, plasma volume, and water volume also significantly increase. In theory, this may create a larger Vd for both lipophilic and hydrophilic medications, requiring higher doses to maintain therapeutic drug concentrations. Albumin concentrations are markedly reduced when pregnancy progresses, and this affects the binding and transport of medications throughout the body. Medications that typically bind well to albumin may be found to have higher free or unbound concentrations, leading to greater efficacy, or an increase of unintended adverse effects. The placenta acts as a membrane where small, lipophilic medications are free to cross, thus medications with these properties may have more influence on the fetus [16].

Medications in the integrase strand transfer inhibitor (INSTI) and protease inhibitor (PI) classes have displayed altered PK in pregnancy. A small sample size of pregnant women living with HIV taking the combination of INSTI, elvitegravir, boosted with cobicistat at the approved doses, showed low concentrations of each drug in the third trimester. In most of these women, elvitegravir did not achieve the minimum effective concentration. Additionally, the boosting agent cobicistat was shown to have reduced AUC by about 50% [18]. Similar PK profiles were also observed in an earlier trial by Momper et al. [19]. Of the PI class, both darunavir and atazanavir, boosted with cobicistat have exhibited approximately 50% reductions in plasma concentrations in the third trimester [20]. Treatment regimens utilizing cobicistat as a boosting agent are not recommended in pregnancy by the United States Department of Health and Human Services (DHHS), the European AIDS Clinical Society (EACS), and the British HIV Association (BHIVA) guidelines [12–14]. The PK of nucleoside/nucleotide reverse transcriptase inhibitors (NRTIs) and non-nucleoside reverse transcriptase inhibitors (NNRTIs) are not expected to be altered during pregnancy [12].

4.2 Neonatal

Neonatal physiologic considerations are important when selecting safe and effective medications. Once clamping of the umbilical cord occurs, a newborn's body must compensate for life outside the womb. Neonatal development occurs rapidly within the first weeks of life. Throughout this period, the PK of medications can be varied as they are dependent on the maturity of the infant. Gestational age at birth and age after birth both influence pharmacokinetics and the sum of the two ages can be expressed as the postmenstrual age (PMA). Current neonatal dosing recommendations are commonly extrapolated from older pediatric populations and even sometimes from the adult population. Medications are often dosed by PMA and weight; however, this weight-based dosing strategy does not always account for the underexpression of liver enzymes required for drug metabolism and clearance. Full enzyme expression ranges from several days to years (e.g., CYP3A4, CYP2D6, CYP2C9, CYP2C19, and CYP1A1). A few enzymes are expressed in the womb but are eventually suppressed after birth (e.g., CYP3A7, FMO1). Medications that require adult enzyme expression for elimination may be overdosed in a newborn still expressing fetal enzymes. Hepatic blood flow rates increase as the newborn develops, so in the early stages of life, medications that are predominantly removed by the liver, exist in the body for a much longer period regardless of enzymatic expression. Weight-based dosing is not a perfect indicator of renal drug clearance either. Although larger infant body weight can be reflective of greater renal function, there is often slower renal development for premature neonates born at less than 34 weeks' gestation. Neonates have lower albumin concentrations which can lead to higher free drug concentrations that usually have a high binding affinity to albumin. Neonates have larger water volume, but they have low fat and muscle content. This can be further exaggerated in premature neonates. Lipophilic drugs with a propensity to enter adipose tissue could remain in the vasculature much longer, while hydrophilic drugs may exit the vasculature to a higher degree. Premature infants may also have slightly impaired gastrointestinal absorption [17].

Nevirapine is a medication often used in neonatal prevention of HIV and is largely dependent on CYP liver enzymes for elimination [12–14, 21]. DHHS guideline recommendations for gestational age of greater than 34 weeks up to 1 month are investigational and based on results from the IMPAACT P1115 trial [12, 22, 23]. The PACTG 1043 trial included a two-drug regimen for prophylaxis in infants with a high risk of perinatal exposure. This regimen was composed of standard zidovudine doses and additional fixed-dose nevirapine administered at 0, 2, and 6 days of life, for infants of at least 32 weeks gestational age [24]. The DHHS guidelines categorize this regimen as an option for high-risk exposure in infants born at 32 weeks' gestation or older [23]. A more recent study of premature infants used weight-based nevirapine dosing for post-exposure prophylaxis at a dose of 2 mg/kg/dose on days 0, 2, and 6 of life. This strategy resulted in no clinically significant adverse events. Infants with a gestational age of 28 weeks at birth who received this regimen achieved effective concentrations for prophylaxis and concentrations continued to remain above target concentrations at 2 weeks old. However, for infants greater than 28 weeks' gestational age at birth, plasma concentrations were shown to decline at day 12 [21]. Dosing under the age of 1 month has not been yet approved by the FDA due to insufficient data [23]. Though there is limited evidence for drug approval in the US, these trials illustrate the variability of pharmacokinetics in the neonate and highlight the necessity for additional studies for neonatal ARV dosing recommendations.

4.3 Drug-drug interactions

People living with HIV should be exposed to adequate concentrations of ARVs to achieve and maintain virological suppression. After considering the PK and pharmacodynamics (PD) of pregnancy, attention must be directed to important potential drug-drug interactions (DDIs) involved with HIV management in pregnancy. DDIs can occur at any step of the pharmacokinetic process where drug parameters are affected. As mentioned earlier, this may include absorption, distribution, metabolism, and elimination. DDIs can result in an increased concentration of ARV or concomitant drug, leading to potentially adverse effects. Alternatively, DDIs can lead to decreased ARV concentrations resulting in subtherapeutic concentrations and potential development of resistance.

Drug absorption can be affected by transit time in the stomach, chelation, or changes in pH. As discussed earlier, transit time can be reduced due to nausea and vomiting during pregnancy, slower intestinal motility, and delayed gastric emptying. Chelation occurs when components of an INSTI's chemical structure bind to polyvalent cations present in other medications such as calcium supplements, multivitamins, iron products, or antacids. The resultant chelated compounds are less likely to be absorbed and thus exhibit potential for reduced efficacy of the INSTI. As medications containing polyvalent cations are commonly used during pregnancy, mindful separation of these products from an INSTI-containing regimen is critical. As administration directions for each INSTI and polyvalent cations vary, in general, the recommendation is to give the INSTI about 2 h prior to any of the aforementioned medications to allow absorption to occur. If the supplement is administered first, then the INSTI is advised to be administered 4–6 h afterward. Some ARVs require an acidic environment for complete absorption. Acid-reducing agents such as proton pump inhibitors (PPIs), H2 receptor antagonists (H2RAs), or antacids will influence the absorption of these drugs. Ritonavir-boosted atazanavir is a PI recommended to be given during pregnancy. If a PPI or H2RA medication is utilized, it should be given about 12 h apart from ART. Rilpivirine, an NNRTI, should be given with food and separated from the H2RA. However, PPIs are specifically contraindicated with rilpivirine [12].

Hepatic metabolism can be influenced, not only by the pregnant state but also by select ARVs that are administered. PIs and their boosters inhibit many metabolizing enzymes, resulting in reduced elimination and increased plasma levels of other medications. Ondansetron is used to alleviate nausea and is a substrate of hepatic enzymes. Administration with PIs and their boosters can increase the side effects of ondansetron, notably cardiac prolongation of the QT interval. Clinical monitoring including electrocardiogram (ECG) assessments is recommended for prolonged concomitant drug therapy. Fentanyl plasma concentrations can be significantly increased by ritonavir, however, intrapartum epidural administration of fentanyl over a short period of 24 h has been suggested to be safe [12].

Although boosted atazanavir is expected to increase the concentrations of the NRTI tenofovir disoproxil fumarate (TDF), it is also apparent that TDF causes lower plasma concentrations of atazanavir (ATV) in the third trimester if the agents are combined in a regimen [12–14]. The BHIVA guidelines recommend that if this combination is used then therapeutic drug monitoring may be considered. They inform that it is not necessary to adjust the dose of ATV, when used in combination with TDF, but that dosage adjustments may be made on a case-by-case basis [14]. Furthermore, the combination of ATV and TDF is not recommended with additional use of an H2RA. If these three agents are still utilized concomitantly, then it is further recommended adjust the ATV dose from 300 to 400 mg daily [14]. The DHHS guidelines also do not recommend ATV in combination with TDF and an H2RA in a treatment experienced pregnant patient. They also do not instruct providers to adjust the dose if it is utilized. Instead, they inform that the increased dose reaches adequate plasma concentrations, and they provide recommendations from the FDA package insert for atazanavir. The Federal Drug Administration (FDA) label recommendation is that increased atazanavir dosing may be utilized if used in combination with both TDF and an H2RA [12]. All guidelines recommend that ATV is to be boosted with ritonavir during pregnancy [12–14].

Health care providers should consider that concentrations of methylergonovine, a medication used for post-partum hemorrhage, can be altered by ART. PIs and their boosters can increase the effect of methylergonovine resulting in increased uterine smooth muscle tone, posing risk for uterine tetany. Patients on ART containing PIs or boosting agents should not be prescribed methylergonovine unless oxytocin or misoprostol are not available. In contrast, methylergonovine can be reduced by medications in the NNRTI class, such as rilpivirine or efavirenz as they induce liver enzymes and increase the elimination of methylergonovine [12]. Due to the complexities of DDIs and ARVs, and the dire consequences of subtherapeutic ARV concentrations leading to potential resistance, health care prescribers are encouraged to refer to the product insert, treatment guidelines, online DDI websites or to consult with an HIV pharmacist for further assistance.

DOI: http://dx.doi.org/10.5772/intechopen.105451

5. Antiretroviral selection and initiation in the treatment naïve pregnant person living with HIV

One of the major goals of therapy in HIV treatment during pregnancy is to reduce the risk of transmission to the fetus. Since the initial use of zidovudine as monotherapy throughout pregnancy and intrapartum, it has been well established that the risk of perinatal transmission can be decreased when viral suppression is achieved [1]. When choosing a new regimen for a treatment naïve pregnant patient living with HIV, it is important to consider DDIs, PK, and side effects that may influence treatment efficacy or incur harm to the fetus.

Recommendations for the treatment of HIV during pregnancy vary slightly between the European AIDS Clinical Society (EACS), British HIV Association (BHIVA), and United States Department of Health and Human Services (DHHS) guidelines and preferred agents are summarized below (e.g., **Table 1**). ART is recommended for all pregnant women with HIV. The timeframe in which to initiate treatment in a pregnant woman living with HIV who is not currently on therapy is debated. If a pregnant woman is newly diagnosed with HIV, treatment should not be delayed according to DHHS and EACS, regardless of the patient's viral load, CD4 count, or pending resistance genotype results. In contrast, BHIVA recommends that treatment be started preferably during the second trimester, although it is permitted to start earlier if the patient's viral load exceeds 100,000 copies/ml or CD4 is less than 200 cells/mm^3. BHIVA also recommends that treatment not be initiated before HIV resistance genotype results are reviewed, except for women who present to care in the third trimester.

Collectively, the guidelines recommend a dual NRTI backbone in combination with a third agent as the choice treatment. The selected agents preferred in each of the dual NRTI backbones, and the third agent differ slightly among the guidelines. The guidelines share recommendations for an NRTI dual backbone of abacavir/lamivudine (ABC/3TC) and tenofovir disoproxil fumarate/emtricitabine (TDF/FTC) with the exclusion of any NRTI combination that includes zidovudine (ZDV). Zidovudine- based therapy is no longer preferred in the adult population due to concerns about toxicity, so aside from its short-term use in intrapartum care and infant prophylaxis, it has become an alternative agent. HLA-B*5701 testing

	Backbone	Third Agent		
	Dual NRTI	**INSTI**	**PI**	**NNRTI**
DHHS	ABC/3TC TDF/FTC TAF/FTC	DTG RAL*	DVR/r* ATV/r	
EACS	ABC/3TC TDF/FTC TAF/FTC⁺	DTG RAL*	DVR/r*	
BHIVA	ABC/3TC TDF/FTC		ATV/r	Efavirenz

**RAL 400 mg and DVR/r 600 mg/100 mg are recommended to be dosed twice daily.*
⁺TAF should only be initiated after 14 weeks' gestation according to EACS guidance.

Table 1.
Preferred ARV agents in the pregnant person living with HIV.

should be done prior to initiation of any regimen containing abacavir (ABC) to rule out hypersensitivity to the drug.

Regarding the tenofovir formulation, DHHS recommends that either tenofovir alafenamide (TAF) or tenofovir disoproxil fumarate (TDF) may be used as a preferred agent. EACS includes TAF among their preferred NRTI backbone options as well, but TAF is an alternative agent according to the BHIVA guidelines. BHIVA and EACS indicate that if TAF is to be included in a regimen, it should be used after 14 weeks of gestational age, due to its unevaluated safety and efficacy within the first trimester of pregnancy. Contrastingly, the DHHS panel does not place gestational age limits on the drug as the guidelines suggest the two agents have similar efficacy and safety profiles when used in pregnancy [12–14].

INSTIs have the ability to suppress viral load quickly and efficiently. As for the third agent comprising a complete regimen, INSTIs are preferred as indicated in both EACS and DHHS guidelines [12, 13]. In contrast, BHIVA suggests that INSTI regimens are to be reserved for pregnant patients presenting with high baseline viral loads of greater than 100,000 copies/ml or those with current ART that have failed to achieve adequate viral suppression [14]. Dolutegravir (DTG) is the INSTI of choice across the guidelines, though DHHS and EACS additionally include raltegravir (RAL) [12, 14]. It is important to note, however, that if raltegravir is used, it must be dosed twice daily in pregnancy, as there is insufficient information regarding the use of daily dosing of raltegravir during pregnancy [12]. In contrast to the US guidelines, both European guidelines state for dolutegravir to be included in a regimen, it should be started preferably after 6 weeks of gestation [13, 14]. This restriction is due to the previously proposed association of infant neural tube defects with dolutegravir use in pregnancy [25]. The guidelines further express that those pregnant women living with HIV should be fully informed prior to making the decision to initiate or switch therapy to dolutegravir [13, 14].

Although INSTIs are preferred agents to be included in a three-drug regimen within the EACS and DHHS guidelines, all three guidelines additionally recommend the use of a PI as the third ARV in a regimen [14]. Within the DHHS and BHIVA guidelines, ritonavir-boosted atazanavir (ATV/r) is recommended as a first-line agent from the PI class [12, 14]. Along with boosted atazanavir, DHHS also includes ritonavir-boosted darunavir (DTV/r) with twice-daily dosing as an appropriate third agent in a first-line treatment regimen [12]. In contrast, EACS lists DRV/r as a preferred agent only when used with a tenofovir-based NRTI backbone, not with ABC/3TC. Boosted atazanavir is not included in the EACS preferred regimens for pregnant patients initiating therapy [13]. The preferred boosting agent is ritonavir as regimens boosted with cobicistat have resulted in treatment failure during pregnancy, as mentioned previously [12–14].

Notably, the BHIVA guidelines also recommend efavirenz, an NNRTI, as an additional preferred agent to be used in combination with a dual NRTI backbone. This is due to its historically extensive use during pregnancy, thereby possessing the most data for its efficacy and safety [14]. In opposition to this BHIVA recommendation, DHHS and EACS both indicate that efavirenz is an alternative option for use in an ARV drug regimen during pregnancy [12, 13]. It should be carefully considered that NNRTI agents are not active against HIV-2 and so should be avoided in this population [12–14].

6. Testing and monitoring HIV clinical status in pregnancy

The DHHS guidelines recommend that all women be tested for HIV with each pregnancy at their earliest visit with their Obstetrician (OB). They further

DOI: http://dx.doi.org/10.5772/intechopen.105451

recommend repeat testing during the third trimester, even if the initial test was negative for mothers who may have a heightened risk of acquiring HIV. These women are identified as those who receive care in facilities or jurisdictions that have an increased incidence of HIV, women with behaviors that impose a high risk of HIV acquisition, or who present at any time during the pregnancy with another sexually transmitted infection (STI). Additionally, there are select states within the US that require a third trimester HIV test to be performed. If a mother presents in labor and her HIV status is unknown, HIV testing should be expedited with results available within the hour, to help determine if additional measures should be taken to prevent transmission to the child. If there was no HIV test conducted at any time during the pregnancy or during labor, it is advised that a mother is tested immediately postpartum to further determine any risk to the child. The HIV test that is recommended is a combination antibody/antigen test. Since it takes time for complete antibody development in response to an infection, this test could produce a false negative during the first 14 days of an acute HIV infection. Therefore, if an acute HIV infection is suspected, an HIV-1 RNA PCR test (viral load) is recommended as it can detect maternal viremia as early as 10 days post-exposure [12].

Several studies have demonstrated that maternal HIV testing may be underutilized [8, 9]. In a study conducted in a US epicenter for HIV, about 20% of women did not receive a second HIV test during their 3rd trimester. This is very unfortunate, as it could lead to delays in detection of previously unknown maternal HIV, thus resulting in delays to ARV access to the mother and to her child after birth.

One focus for improvement could be increasing provider awareness. Providers should be aware of the local prevalence of HIV infections and recommendations for HIV screening during all trimesters. Furthermore, conducting nonbiased social and sexual health histories during pregnancy would be useful to identify high-risk women who may benefit from a repeat HIV screening test in the third trimester [8].

If a pregnant mother has been living with HIV or is newly diagnosed during the pregnancy, there are additional testing recommendations for monitoring the clinical status of HIV, as well as the risk of transmission to the child. An HIV-1 RNA test should be conducted at the initial OB visit for any woman living with HIV. This helps to assess baseline viremia and establish immediate goals of care. The viral load is recommended to be repeated after 2–4 weeks if therapy is initiated or adjusted. Furthermore, once stabilized on an antiretroviral regimen, the viral load should be performed every month until viral suppression is achieved, then performed every 3 months thereafter. There should be an additional viral load conducted between 34 and 36 weeks' gestation in anticipation of delivery. This viral load will help to determine treatment measures that need to take place during the intrapartum and postpartum periods to prevent transmission. The CD4 count is not as critical to monitor throughout pregnancy if a mother has been previously stable on a regimen for at least 2 years. In this scenario, an initial CD4 collected at the first visit will suffice. However, if a mother was not virally suppressed on her ARV regimen, or has newly switched or initiated a ARVs during pregnancy, then CD4 testing should be conducted every 3 months until delivery. Antiretroviral resistance testing recommendations are similar to those in non-pregnant adult patients. As such, it is recommended that resistance testing be performed prior to initiation of ART, upon modification of a regimen, or if there is inadequate control of the viral load [12]. Resistance testing should not cause delays in care; thus, a clinician does not need to wait for the results of the genotype in order to start therapy. The therapy can be adjusted when the genotype results are available.

Based on monitoring during pregnancy, the child's risk for HIV acquisition can be categorized. The maternal viral load is the most important criterion for defining risk. Perinatal transmission can occur in utero at any time during the gestational period. It is especially important to assess the viral load late in the pregnancy, nearest to the time of delivery, as it is presumed that this time period is where most transmissions occur [7]. If a viral load is undetectable just prior to delivery, it is suggested that the infant is at low risk for the acquisition of HIV [12]. However, if the viral load is high during the late gestational period, the infant's risk is heightened [7, 12]. Other factors to consider in determining MTCT risk are the timing of the mother's antiretroviral treatment initiation, adherence to ARV medication throughout the pregnancy, and acute HIV infection during the pregnancy or during the breastfeeding period [12].

7. Antiretroviral selection for the intrapartum period

The PACTG 076 trial led to the recommendation of IV zidovudine during labor [1]. This initial recommendation preceded the current recommendations for women living with HIV to be on triple ART throughout pregnancy and as close to their normal schedule as possible even during the labor and delivery period [2, 12–14]. Thus, if the viral load is less than 50 copies/ml, the DHHS, BHIVA, and EACS guidelines agree that a pregnant mother on effective ART may proceed with a spontaneous vaginal delivery and the addition of IV zidovudine is not warranted [12–14]. However, if the viral load is not suppressed, the guidelines all support the use of IV zidovudine at the time of delivery. Zidovudine is administered as an initial loading dose of 2 mg/kg/h over the first hour of treatment, followed by a continuous infusion of 1 mg/kg/h until clamping of the umbilical cord has been performed [1, 12–14]. In the EACS guidelines, the threshold for when IV zidovudine is required is a viral load above 50 copies/ml or an unknown HIV status [13]. Contrastingly, BHIVA and DHHS provide that viral loads within the range of 50–1000 copies/ml do not necessitate IV zidovudine, although other factors, such as adherence, are to be considered when making the decision whether to initiate zidovudine [12–14]. Any time that a pregnant patient's HIV status is unknown or newly diagnosed during delivery, the guidelines agree that IV zidovudine should be initiated [12–14]. BHIVA furthermore recommends that the mother receive a single oral dose of nevirapine followed by oral zidovudine, lamivudine, raltegravir dosed twice daily, and IV zidovudine administered during delivery. BHIVA also indicates that if the infant is unlikely to take oral medications due to prematurity or other reasons, consider the addition of an oral double dose of TDF to the maternal oral regimen received prior to delivery [14]. The maternal viral load also influences the mode of delivery. Scheduled cesarean section (c-section) is strongly recommended by DHHS guidelines if the mother's viral load near delivery is >1000 copies/ml or unknown [12]. The urge for scheduled c-section is expressed by BHIVA guidelines with >400 copies/ml [14]. This threshold is further reduced in the EACS recommendations, at a viral load of 50 copies/ml or greater [13]. All c-sections are recommended to be scheduled at 38 weeks' gestation in hopes that the mother will not yet go into active labor [12–14].

8. Antiretroviral selection in the infant exposed to HIV

In order to determine the appropriate ARVs to initiate in the newborn who is born to a mother living with HIV, a clinical assessment of transmission risk needs to be performed. Risk stratification dictates whether a newborn will receive post-exposure prophylaxis (PEP) or an empiric initial ART. This stratification of risk is based on several factors. As discussed previously, it is important to appreciate the mother's viral load at or near the time of delivery. As a reflection of the viral load, it should be determined if the mother received the appropriate intrapartum antiretroviral medication(s). The mode of delivery should be noted. If the mother delivers via a spontaneous vaginal delivery, an assessment of the timing of placental rupture of membranes (PROM) is also an important consideration [12]. A duration of membrane rupture of greater than 4 h prior to delivery increases the chance of perinatal HIV transmission [26].

The recommendations for PEP of infants born to mothers with HIV are similar among both BHIVA and DHHS guidelines and are summarized below (e.g., **Table 2**) [12, 14]. BHIVA guidelines divide perinatal exposures into very low risk, low risk, and high risk [14]. The DHHS guidelines divide exposures into three groups as well, defined as low-risk, high-risk, and presumed newborn HIV infection [12]. In contrast, EACS defers PEP recommendations to local guidelines and only offers treatment recommendations for infants diagnosed with HIV [13].

According to the BHIVA panel, ARVs should be started within 4 h of delivery [14]. The DHHS broadens this window slightly to within 6 h of delivery [12]. The first risk category in the BHIVA guidelines is very low-risk and an infant is assigned this category when all the following criteria are met: the mother has been on appropriate antiretroviral therapy for greater than 10 weeks, had two documented HIV-1 RNA <50 copies/ml during pregnancy which were at least 4 weeks apart, and HIV-1 RNA <50 copies/ml at or after 36 weeks. Only 2 weeks of zidovudine monotherapy is indicated for such an infant [14]. The lowest risk category listed in the DHHS guidelines is the low-risk category, where the infant's mother received appropriate ART during pregnancy, and achieved viral suppression within 4 weeks, with no adherence concerns. In this scenario, a low-risk infant should receive 4 weeks of zidovudine monotherapy [12]. The BHIVA panel also recommends 4 weeks of zidovudine monotherapy for an infant in their low-risk category. An infant is considered low risk if the previous criteria are not met for very low risk, but maternal viral suppression is achieved at or after 36 weeks for a term baby, or near the delivery of a premature

DHHS		**BHIVA**	
Risk category	**ART**	**Risk category**	**ART**
Low risk	ZDV for 4 weeks	Very low risk	ZDV for 2 weeks
High risk	ZDV for 6 weeks+ 3TC/NVP* or 3TC/RAL for 2–6 weeks	Low risk	ZDV for 4 weeks
Presumed HIV Infection	ZDV for 6 weeks+ 3TC/NVP* or 3TC/RAL for 2–6 weeks	High risk	ZDV/3TC/NVP* for 4 weeks

**RAL should be considered for infants at high risk of perinatal HIV-2 transmission because HIV-2 is not susceptible to NVP [12]. In infants exposed to HIV-2, ZDV/3TC/RAL should be initiated until expert advice is available [14].*
+Duration of therapy depends on patient-specific risks and expert advice is recommended [12].
Note: EACS defers PEP recommendations to local guidelines [13].

Table 2.
Antiretroviral post-exposure prophylaxis in the infant exposed to HIV.

baby [14]. According to the DHHS guidelines, if a mother did not receive antepartum therapy, only received intrapartum ARVs, viral suppression was not achieved within 4 weeks of delivery on a regimen, or an acute or primary HIV infection was discovered during pregnancy, the infant would fall within the high-risk category [12]. For those in this DHHS high-risk category, presumptive HIV therapy should be initiated with at least 6 weeks of zidovudine and 2–6 weeks of lamivudine and nevirapine. One may also alternatively administer zidovudine, lamivudine, and raltegravir [12]. The BHIVA panel recommends that if maternal viral suppression was not achieved by the day of birth, viral load is unknown, or there is adherence uncertainty, this is considered high-risk and a 4-week course of combination PEP is indicated consisting of zidovudine, lamivudine, and nevirapine [14]. The DHHS panel recommends presumptive therapy for those newborns who are clinically suspected to have acquired HIV infection. This is when mothers with unconfirmed HIV status have at least one positive HIV test at delivery or postpartum or there is a positive HIV antibody test for the newborn [12]. The three-drug ART recommendations are similar in the DHHS high-risk category and the presumptive treatment category. The doses prescribed may change slightly with confirmed HIV infection [12]. For confirmed newborn HIV infection, EACS recommends that the infant be started on a three-drug combination regimen consisting of the dual NRTI-backbone zidovudine and lamivudine with the third agent options of lopinavir/ritonavir, nevirapine, or raltegravir [13].

9. Testing in the infant exposed to HIV

Once a child is known to have perinatal exposure, seroconversion must be ruled out or identified with HIV testing. In the neonate, antibody/antigen tests cannot be recommended. The general concept of passive immunity ensures that a mother protects her newborn infant from infections, by passing along her own antibodies through the placenta until the baby's own immune system can develop. The 4th generation antibody/antigen combination test is often performed for the adult population; however, this test could provide false results in an infant born to a mother living with HIV due to the presence of maternal antibodies in the infant's blood. Due to the underdeveloped immune system of the infant, the antigen test would not be as sensitive as virologic testing, thus it is important to test for HIV using virologic HIV RNA or HIV DNA Nucleic Acid Amplification Testing (NAAT). If a non-breastfeeding infant was exposed intrauterine or during the labor process, then either NAAT is recommended at birth and should be repeated 2–6 weeks after the cessation of PEP medications [12, 23]. According to DHHS protocol, infants born at high-risk for perinatal transmission should be tested as soon as possible and before initiation of ART so as not to skew test results. Despite this recommendation, however, ART should never be delayed [12]. A positive test within the first 2 days likely reflects an early intrauterine exposure. In non-breastfeeding infants who test negative during their first week of life, but test positive upon repeat testing, it can generally be assumed that they were exposed intrapartum, or later during the pregnancy [7].

10. Breastfeeding considerations

Perinatal transmission of HIV can occur in utero, labor, and delivery, or during the breastfeeding period. There are concerns about transmission risk to the infant

DHHS	EACS	BHIVA
Breastfeeding is not recommended for individuals with HIV in the US	The panel advises against breastfeeding for those living with HIV	The panel recommends that women living with HIV feed their infants with formula milk
Those that desire to breastfeed should receive patient-centered, evidence-based counseling on infant feeding options. Those that choose to breastfeed should be supported in risk-reduction measures to minimize risk of HIV transmission to their infants	If they choose to breastfeed, the panel recommends discussion from an interdisciplinary team of HIV specialist, pediatrician and OBGYN. The panel provides guidance on what to monitor and how often to monitor maternal and infant viral load	Those that choose to breastfeed in the UK, who are virologically suppressed on ART with good adherence should be supported and informed of the low risk of vertical transmission. These patients may need additional maternal/child monitoring

Table 3.
Summary of guideline recommendations for persons living with HIV who are breastfeeding.

through breastmilk versus the benefits that breastmilk can provide. These concerns differ between high-income (HIC) and low-middle income countries (LMIC). It can be estimated that postnatal vertical transmission rates during breastfeeding range from 5 to 20% without intervention [27]. HIV viral load is collected from plasma samples for monitoring, however, there is less information on viral load in breastmilk. The Undetectable = Untransmittable (U = U) concept derived from the PARTNER study provides that people living with HIV who are on ARV and are undetectable cannot sexually transmit the virus to their partners [28]. There is interest in expanding the U = U concept to breastfeeding mothers on ART. Part of the PROMISE study compared postpartum ARV prophylaxis in mother-baby pairs where breastfeeding occurred. The pairs were randomized to one of two ARV prophylaxis arms where either maternal ART versus daily infant NVP was administered [3]. In the primary analysis, the same number of infants were infected with HIV-1 from each arm. Thus, there was no difference between arms with vertical transmission and infant HIV-free survival at 24 months of age was high in both arms [3]. Importantly, the trial was not able to demonstrate a difference between arms due to the low degree of acquired infections. This demonstrates that both regimens were very effective in preventing transmission [3]. However, a secondary analysis of the trial did result in two infants in the maternal ART arm acquiring HIV despite maternal viral loads of less than 40 copies/ml [12]. Although U = U in the setting of breastfeeding is still undetermined, data from women in LMIC and emerging data from HIC show the transmission risk is low in the setting of strict adherence to ART and being virally suppressed [29, 30]. Although transmission risk is low, it is still possible. A summary of the breastfeeding recommendations by each guideline is provided in **Table 3** [12–14].

11. Modern considerations for ethics and research

In 2018, clinical alarm spread across the globe after results from the Tsepamo surveillance study in Botswana suggested a relationship between dolutegravir exposure at conception and infant neural tube defects [25]. At the time, Botswana had switched from efavirenz-based to dolutegravir-based first-line therapy for the adult treatment of HIV [25]. Dolutegravir is a vivid example of how newly approved medications become available to the majority of women of child-bearing age, despite having never been tested in the pregnant population. Fortunately, by 2020, additional data collection on the prevalence of neural tube defects in infants exposed to dolutegravir at the time of conception stabilized the previously alarming numbers to less than 0.2%. This was comparable to the 0.11% prevalence rate of neural tube defects in infants of mothers who were not on dolutegravir at conception [31]. As discussed earlier, dolutegravir is now recommended as a preferred agent by the DHHS guidelines for women of childbearing potential [12]. However, it is not recommended until after the first trimester by other panels [13, 14]. The dolutegravir-scare sparked an international momentum for modifying the ethical considerations surrounding drug research and pregnancy [32]. The Tsepamo study highlights the importance of conducting earlier and more frequent trials including large study populations of pregnant women.

The intricate nature of balancing maternal benefit versus fetal harm has been a long-standing phenomenon in the field of drug research. This balancing act teeters between providing effective therapy for a pregnant mother while preventing harm to her developing child. For a long time, the scales tilted in favor of omitting useful medications, thus avoiding potential harm to the fetus. This one-sided sway reflects the perception that the fetus is so vulnerable to harm that providing appropriate maternal treatment for an array of maternal medical conditions does not provide sufficient benefit [15, 32]. This view also assumes that what may be safe for the fetus is also most appropriate for the mother [33]. First, this idea is an underrepresentation of how effective maternal medication management, directly improving maternal health, can indirectly result in improved pregnancy outcomes for the child-in-utero [33]. Second, this concept neglects a pregnant mother's ability to make decisions for herself and for her own child [33, 34]. Instead, it leaves both providers and their pregnant patients to make less informed decisions from the limited academic information available to them [33–35]. Third, it results in more off-label use in the post-marketing pregnant population rather than use in carefully conducted and monitored trials [33, 34]. Fortunately, HIV is one chronic medical condition for which there have been considerable efforts through the years to obtain pregnancy data [32, 33]. This can be largely attributed to organizations such as the Pharmacokinetics of newly developed ANtiretroviral agents in HIV-infected pregNAnt women (PANNA) and the International Maternal Pediatric Adolescent AIDS Clinical Trials (IMPAACT) Network [36, 37]. The IMPAACT network was originally established 16 years ago as the Pediatric AIDS Clinical Trials Group (PACTG) and the Perinatal Scientific Working Group of the HIV Prevention Trials Network (HPTN) joined forces to end the HIV epidemic with a special focus on pediatric and pregnant populations. The IMPAACT Network is a global collaborative effort based in the United States to conduct quality research [37]. The PANNA study is a European Network that collects pharmacokinetic data in pregnant women and aims to obtain information on new antiretroviral medications with little to no information on this population [36]. Although there is some clinical research information available for antiretrovirals in pregnancy, it is a research area with a great opportunity [15, 32–34]. Generally, pregnancy data for ARVs are obtained when women living with HIV become pregnant on a stable ART, and the decision is made to continue the regimen throughout the pregnancy. Aside from the limited pregnancy data available, guideline recommendations are often based on extrapolations from the non-pregnant adult population. Most research today does not present separate PK data for men and women, therefore extrapolation can be difficult to draw from women of childbearing potential to women who become pregnant when it often includes male data [16].

The agencies that influence drug approval in the United States are the Federal Drug Association (FDA) and DHHS. There are drug research regulations that were originally designed to protect human rights in drug trials, including the protection of women of child-bearing potential, pregnant women, and their children [38, 39]. Additionally, there are provisions for these populations in DHHS protocols [38]. Although adherence to these DHHS protocols is not mandated in FDA-conducted drug trials, the FDA still has recommended the DHHS guidance to be followed [38]. Historically, regulations have emphasized much effort in protecting the fetus, and pregnant women are often excluded from drug research trials [39]. If there was a shift in focus from protecting women and their unborn children by omitting them from drug trials to including them, there could be great potential. This could provide more available treatment options and identify early in the gestational period if medications are not effective. There would be information on how to adjust medication doses during pregnancy [33, 34]. This shift in focus can also be applied to the neonatal population. If there were additional information on the PK and PD of ARVs in the neonatal population, there could be more successful outcomes. Luckily, there has recently been a turning point in history. In 2017, the Third Conference on Antiretroviral Drug Optimization (CADO 3) was held to discuss the implications of newer antiretroviral agents to current standards of care, and the re-sequencing of first-, second-and third-line therapies for the future [40]. Shortly following this, the statistical results of neural tube defects discovered by the Tsepamo study raised a global alert [25] and the FDA issued draft guidance for reconsidering the ethics and science behind drug research regulations for the pregnant population [38]. The World Health Organization (WHO) also held a pediatric antiretroviral drug optimization (PADO) meeting in which the regulatory framework for research in pregnancy was determined to be outdated [32]. The CADO and PADO experts, among many others, proposed adjusting the drug approval timeline to shorten the delay of access to new antiretroviral medications for pregnant women [32, 40]. A WHO-IMPAACT-led workshop was held to address evidence gaps and identify opportunities for change. The workshop included experts from the fields of research and pharmacokinetic studies, regulatory agencies, public organizations, and stakeholders. Their consensus statement was published in 2019 which proposes earlier conducted research trials and the barriers that need to be addressed to conduct these trials [15]. In July 2020, The PHASES Working Group - Pregnancy and HIV/AIDS: Seeking Equitable Study issued a 12-step recommendation pathway for the industry [33, 34]. It stressed evidence gaps in dosing, fetal safety, and maternal outcomes and identified that in order to close these gaps changes needed to be made to the concept of ethics in pregnant women. Their call-to-action plan sought to address the inequities presented to pregnant women in access to first-line therapies, respecting pregnant women by allowing them to choose a therapy that would enhance their own health outcomes, and protection from drug-related risks when using medications "off-label" because there is no pregnancy data [33, 34]. At the end of 2021, the World Health Organization (WHO), the IMPAACT Network, and the International AIDS Society launched another "Call-to-Action" campaign [35]. This was a call for the inclusion of the female voices of women living with HIV and to change from viewing pregnant women as a vulnerable population to a population with many intricacies that should be addressed. This call to action speaks to stop protecting patients by excluding them and to instead protect them by including them [35].

12. Conclusion

The ethical considerations for pregnancy and neonatal populations are beginning to change. The focus is shifting in the direction of protecting these populations by conducting medication research trials that are inclusive. There are many advancements in HIV management, however, the field continues to evolve with more research and practical world experience. As more data unfolds, this may lead to more drug therapy options for the management of perinatal HIV. In turn, it may result in the use of safer and more effective ARVs in the pregnant and neonatal populations. With the availability of more reliable ARV options, utilization of these medications, and adherence to recommended HIV screening guidelines, there is more potential to reduce the transmission of HIV from mother to child, moving the HIV field toward achieving ending the HIV epidemic globally.

Acknowledgements

We would like to acknowledge our dear friend and colleague in the field of HIV Jean C. Lee, PharmD, AAHIVP for her invaluable support and feedback for our chapter.

Conflict of interest

The authors declare no conflict of interest.

Author details

Kayla Aleshire and Rima Bazzi*
PharmD AAHIVP, Beaumont Health, Dearborn, USA

*Address all correspondence to: rima.bazzi@beaumont.org

References

[1] Connor EM, Sperling RS, Gelber R, et al. Reduction of maternal-infant transmission of human immunodeficiency virus type 1 with zidovudine treatment. Pediatric AIDS Clinical Trials Group Protocol 076 Study Group. The New England Journal of Medicine. 1994;**331**(18):1173-1180. DOI: 10.1056/NEJM199411033311801

[2] Fowler MG, Qin M, Fiscus SA, et al. Benefits and risks of antiretroviral therapy for perinatal HIV prevention. The New England Journal of Medicine. 2016;**375**(18):1726-1737. DOI: 10.1056/NEJMoa1511691

[3] Flynn PM, Taha TE, Cababasay M, et al. Prevention of HIV-1 transmission through breastfeeding: Efficacy and safety of maternal antiretroviral therapy versus infant nevirapine prophylaxis for duration of breastfeeding in HIV-1-infected women with high CD4 cell count (IMPAACT PROMISE): A randomized, open-label, clinical trial. Journal of Acquired Immune Deficiency Syndromes. 2018;**77**(4):383-392. DOI: 10.1097/QAI.0000000000001612

[4] Centers for Disease Control and Prevention. HIV Surveillance Report, 2019. Vol. 32 [Internet]. 2021. Available from: http://www.cdc.gov/hiv/library/reports/hiv-surveillance.html. [Accessed: April 18, 2022]

[5] World Health Organization. Global Health Sector Strategy on HIV: 2016-2021 Towards Ending AIDS: Prevention of HIV Infection in Infants [Internet] 2016. Available from: https://apps.who.int/iris/bitstream/handle/10665/246178/WHO-HIV-2016.05-eng.pdf. [Accessed: April 18, 2022]

[6] Unaids.org. Global HIV & AIDS Statistics Fact Sheet [Internet]. 2021. Available from: https://www.unaids.org/en/resources/fact-sheet. [Accessed: April 18, 2022]

[7] Kourtis AP, Bulterys M, Nesheim SR, Lee FK. Understanding the timing of HIV transmission from mother to infant. Journal of the American Medical Association. 2001;**285**(6):709-712. DOI: 10.1001/jama.285.6.709

[8] Szlachta-McGinn A, Aserlind A, Duthely L, et al. HIV screening during pregnancy in a U.S. HIV Epicenter. Infectious Diseases in Obstetrics and Gynecology. 2020;**2020**:8196342. DOI: 10.1155/2020/8196342

[9] de Beer S, Kalk E, Kroon M, et al. A longitudinal analysis of the completeness of maternal HIV testing, including repeat testing in Cape Town, South Africa. Journal of the International AIDS Society. 2020;**23**(1):e25441. DOI: 10.1002/jia2.25441

[10] United Nations: Office on Drugs and Crime. Sustainable Development [Internet]. 2022. Available from: https://www.unodc.org/unodc/en/hiv-aids/new/Sustainable_development.html. [Accessed: April 18, 2022]

[11] HIV.gov. Ending the HIV Epidemic: About Ending the HIV Epidemic in the U.S.: Overview [Internet]. 2021. Available from: https://www.hiv.gov/federal-response/ending-the-hiv-epidemic/overview. [Accessed: April 18, 2022]

[12] Department of Health and Human Services Panel on Treatment of HIV during Pregnancy and Prevention of Perinatal Transmission. Recommendations for the Use of Antiretroviral Drugs during Pregnancy and Interventions to Reduce Perinatal

HIV Transmission in the United States [Internet]. 2022. Available from: https://clinicalinfo.hiv.gov/en/guidelines/perinatal. [Accessed: April 18, 2022]

[13] European AIDS Clinical Society (EACS) Treatment Guidelines Panel. EACS Guidelines Version 11.0 [Internet]. 2021. Available from: https://www.eacsociety.org/guidelines/eacs-guidelines/. [Accessed: April 18, 2022]

[14] Gilleece Y, Tariq S, Bamford A, et al. British HIV Association guidelines for the management of HIV in pregnancy and postpartum 2018: 2020 third interim update. HIV Medicine. 2019;**20**(Suppl 3):s2-s85. Available from: bhiva.org/pregnancy-guidelines. [Accessed: April 18, 2022]

[15] Eke AC, Olagunju A, Momper J, et al. Optimizing pharmacology studies in pregnant and lactating women using lessons from HIV: A consensus statement. Clinical Pharmacology and Therapeutics. 2021;**110**(1):36-48. DOI: 10.1002/cpt.2048

[16] Feghali M, Venkataramanan R, Caritis S. Pharmacokinetics of drugs in pregnancy. Seminars in Perinatology. 2015;**39**(7):512-519. DOI: 10.1053/j.semperi.2015.08.003

[17] Ku LC, Smith PB. Dosing in neonates: Special considerations in physiology and trial design. Pediatric Research. 2015;**77**(1-1):2-9. DOI: 10.1038/pr.2014.143

[18] Bukkems V, Necsoi C, Tenorio CH, et al. Clinically significant lower elvitegravir exposure during the third trimester of pregnant patients living with human immunodeficiency virus: Data from the pharmacokinetics of ANtiretroviral agents in HIV-infected pregNAnt women (PANNA) network. Clinical Infectious Diseases. 2020;**71**(10):e714-e717. DOI: 10.1093/cid/ciaa488

[19] Momper JD, Best BM, Wang J, et al. Elvitegravir/cobicistat pharmacokinetics in pregnant and postpartum women with HIV. AIDS. 2018;**32**(17):2507-2516. DOI: 10.1097/QAD.0000000000001992

[20] Momper JD, Wang J, Stek A, et al. Pharmacokinetics of darunavir and cobicistat in pregnant and postpartum women with HIV. AIDS. 2021;**35**(8):1191-1199. DOI: 10.1097/QAD.0000000000002857

[21] Hirt D, Kubota Kilengelela J, Jarreau PH, Tréluyer JM, Marcou V. Nevirapine pharmacokinetics in neonates between 25 and 32 weeks gestational age for the prevention of mother-to-child transmission of HIV. The Pediatric Infectious Disease Journal. 2021;**40**(4):344-346. DOI: 10.1097/INF.0000000000002994

[22] Ruel TD, Capparelli EV, Tierney C, et al. Pharmacokinetics and safety of early nevirapine-based antiretroviral therapy for neonates at high risk for perinatal HIV infection: A phase 1/2 proof of concept study. Lancet HIV. 2021;**8**(3):e149-e157. DOI: 10.1016/S2352-3018(20)30274-5

[23] Department of Health and Human Services Panel on Antiretroviral Therapy and Medical Management of Children Living with HIV. Guidelines for the Use of Antiretroviral Agents in Pediatric HIV Infection Pages C1-6, L75-L78, G12 [Internet]. 2022. Available from: https://clinicalinfo.hiv.gov/en/guidelines/pediatric-arv. [Accessed: April 18, 2022]

[24] Nielsen-Saines K, Watts DH, Veloso VG, et al. Three postpartum antiretroviral regimens to prevent intrapartum HIV infection. The New England Journal of Medicine.

2012;**366**(25):2368-2379. DOI: 10.1056/NEJMoa1108275

[25] Zash R, Holmes L, Diseko M, et al. Neural-tube defects and antiretroviral treatment regimens in Botswana. The New England Journal of Medicine. 2019;**381**(9):827-840. DOI: 10.1056/NEJMoa1905230

[26] Landesman SH, Kalish LA, Burns DN, et al. Obstetrical factors and the transmission of human immunodeficiency virus type 1 from mother to child. The Women and Infants Transmission Study. The New England Journal of Medicine. 1996;**334**(25):1617-1623. DOI: 10.1056/NEJM199606203342501

[27] World Health Organization. HIV Transmission through Breastfeeding: A Review of Available Evidence 2007 Update, Table 1 [Internet]. 2008. Available from: https://apps.who.int/iris/handle/10665/43879. [Accessed: May 10, 2022]

[28] Rodger AJ, Cambiano V, Bruun T, et al. Sexual activity without condoms and risk of HIV transmission in serodifferent couples when the HIV-positive partner is using suppressive antiretroviral therapy [published correction appears in JAMA. 2016 Aug 9;316(6):667] [published correction appears in JAMA. 2016 Nov 15;316(19):2048]. Journal of the American Medical Association. 2016;**316**(2):171-181. DOI: 10.1001/jama.2016.5148

[29] Yusuf HE, Knott-Grasso MA, Anderson J, et al. Experience and outcomes of breastfed infants of women living with HIV in the United States: Findings from a single-center breastfeeding support initiative [published correction appears in J Pediatric Infect Dis Soc. 2022 Mar 14]. Journal of the Pediatric Infectious Diseases Society. 2022;**11**(1):24-27. DOI: 10.1093/jpids/piab116

[30] Nashid N, Khan S, Loutfy M, et al. Breastfeeding by women living with human immunodeficiency virus in a resource-rich setting: A case series of maternal and infant management and outcomes. Journal of the Pediatric Infectious Diseases Society. 2020;**9**(2):228-231. DOI: 10.1093/jpids/piz003

[31] Zash R, Holmes L, Diseko M, et al. Update on neural tube defects with antiretroviral exposure in the Tsepamo Study, Botswana. AIDS 2020: 23rd International AIDS Conference Virtual. July 6-10, 2020. Abstract OAXLB0102

[32] Abrams EJ, Mofenson LM, Pozniak A, et al. Enhanced and timely investigation of ARVs for use in pregnant women. Journal of Acquired Immune Deficiency Syndromes. 2021;**86**(5):607-615. DOI: 10.1097/QAI.0000000000002597

[33] The PHASES Working Group. Executive Summary- Ending the Evidence Gap for Pregnant Women around HIV & Co-infections: A Call to Action [Internet]. 2020. Available from: https://static1.squarespace.com/static/53f27090e4b0dbe1ff72f27c/t/5f07a4610d10336a0a5f852a/1594336355653/PHASES_Guidance_Executive_Summary_%28July_2020%29.pdf. [Accessed: April 18, 2022]

[34] Lyerly AD, Beigi R, Bekker LG, et al. Ending the evidence gap for pregnancy, HIV and co-infections: Ethics guidance from the PHASES project. Journal of the International AIDS Society. 2021;**24**(12):e25846. DOI: 10.1002/jia2.25846

[35] World Health Organization. Research for Informed Choices—Accelerating the

Study of New ARVs in Pregnancy: Call to Action [Internet]. 2021. Available from: https://www.who.int/news/item/01-12-2021-call-to-accelerate-the-study-of-new-drugs-for-hiv-in-pregnant-and-breastfeeding-women. [Accessed: April 18, 2022]

[36] Pannastudy.com. PANNA Study Home Page [Internet]. 2022. Available from: https://www.pannastudy.com/home.html. [Accessed: April 18, 2022]

[37] Impaactnetwork.org. About IMPAACT [Internet] 2020. Available from: https://www.impaactnetwork.org/about. [Accessed: April 18, 2022]

[38] U.S. Food and Drug Administration. Pregnant Women: Scientific and Ethical Considerations for Inclusion in Clinical Trials [Internet]. 2018. Available from: https://www.fda.gov/regulatory-information/search-fda-guidance-documents/pregnant-women-scientific-and-ethical-considerations-inclusion-clinical-trials. [Accessed: April 28, 2022]

[39] U.S. Food and Drug Administration. General Considerations for the Clinical Evaluation of Drugs [Internet]. 1997. Available from: https://www.fda.gov/regulatory-information/search-fda-guidance-documents/general-considerations-clinical-evaluation-drugs. [Accessed: April 28, 2022]

[40] World Health Organization. Third Conference on Antiretroviral Drug Optimization (CADO 3): Summary Meeting Report, 29 Nov-1 Dec 2017, Rosebank Crowne Plaza, Johannesburg, South Africa [Internet]. World Health Organization; 2018. Available from: https://apps.who.int/iris/handle/10665/272291. [Accessed: April 18, 2022]

Chapter 8

HIV Infection and Oral Manifestations: An Update

Ricardo Roberto de Souza Fonseca, Rogério Valois Laurentino, Luiz Fernando Almeida Machado, Carlos Eduardo Vieira da Silva Gomes, Tatiany Oliveira de Alencar Menezes, Oscar Faciola Pessoa, Aldemir Branco Oliveira-Filho, Tábata Resque Beckmann Carvalho, Paula Gabriela Faciola Pessoa de Oliveira, Erich Brito Tanaka, Jorge Sá Elias Nogueira, Douglas Magno Guimarães, Marcelo Newton Carneiro, Paula Mendes Acatauassú Carneiro, Aluísio Ferreira Celestino Junior, Patricia de Almeida Rodrigues and Silvio Augusto Fernandes de Menezes

Abstract

Human immunodeficiency virus (HIV) causes a complete depletion of the immune system; it has been a major health issue around the world since the 1980s, and due to the reduction of CD4+ T lymphocytes levels, it can trigger various opportunistic infections. Oral lesions are usually accurate indicators of immunosuppression because these oral manifestations may occur as a result of the compromised immune system caused by HIV infection; therefore, oral lesions might be initial and common clinical features in people living with HIV. So, it is necessary to evaluate and understand the mechanism, prevalence, and risk factors of oral lesions to avoid the increase morbidity among those with oral diseases.

Keywords: HIV, acquired immunodeficiency syndrome, immune deficiency disease, oral cavity, oral manifestations, periodontal disease

1. Introduction

Since the twentieth century, the human immunodeficiency virus (HIV) has been a global public health problem, and for about 40 years, the structural aspects, pathogenic mechanisms, forms of transmission, and cycle of infection have continued to be studied in order to reach a detailed understanding of the infection of this virus in its carriers [1–3], especially in key populations such as men who have sex with men, transgender people, sex workers, people who inject drugs, indigenous people, and prisoners [4–11], in order to seek to develop solutions for immunosuppression caused by HIV, such as antiretroviral therapies and even effective vaccines [12–14].

HIV is a member of the order *Ortervirales*, family *Retroviridae*, subfamily *Orthoretrovirinae*, and genus *Lentivirus*, which are currently grouped into two types, HIV-type 1 (HIV-1) and HIV-type 2 (HIV-2) and infections caused by HIV. Lentiviruses generally have a chronic aspect of development, with a long period of clinical latency and persistent viral replication, and cause progressive immunosuppression in their hosts [2, 15–17]. Both HIV-1 and HIV-2 will infect specific cells of the immune system, such as CD4+ T lymphocytes, macrophages, dendritic cells, and mucosal lining cells such as vaginal, anorectal, and oral, which will later spread to regional lymph nodes and, consequently, into the bloodstream, which will cause changes in the development and function of the immune response [18–23]. Although certain differences can be seen between the two types, such as HIV-2 greater predilection for central nervous system infections and a lower virulent potential than HIV-1 [24–28].

In practice, HIV transmission requires direct exposure to blood or fluids, or secretions contaminated with areas such as skin or mucous membranes with mechanical trauma or discontinuity of integrity, either by punctures with needles or cuts with cutting instruments or abrasions of mucosal tissues during sexual relations or the vertical route [29, 30]. Furthermore, it should be understood that HIV transmission is directly dependent on the viral load, its concentration in the infected body fluid, and the susceptibility of the host [31, 32]. It is necessary to emphasize this because HIV cannot survive outside the bloodstream or lymph tissue and is easily inactivated by exposure to common detergents and disinfectants, so understanding the means of transmission is essential to reduce the stigma around people living with HIV (PLWH), mainly among health professionals [33].

Between the initial contamination and severe cases of immunosuppression such as the acquired immunodeficiency syndrome (AIDS), basically, the pathogenesis of HIV infection and the progression between its phases are related between the properties of the virus, risk factors, and the host's immune response. Patient adherence to antiretroviral therapy, that is, the balance between these items, will determine the development of the symptomatic and asymptomatic phase, AIDS, and even the medium- and long-term experience of the host [2, 32–34]. Among the main properties of HIV is the viral replication cycle that can be in the following steps: (1) binding in the cell receptor; (2) cell surface fusion; (3) uncoating; (4) reverse transcription; (5) integration of proviruses; (6) translation; (7) assembly of viral proteins; (8) budding; and (9) release [2, 35, 36].

In summary, HIV replication occurs when the heterodimer proteins gp120 and gp41 of the viral envelope bind to proteins in the cell membrane of target cells; that is, gp120 binds to CD4 monomeric glycoprotein on the cell surface of T lymphocytes or precursor T cells of lymphatic tissues such as bone marrow and thymus, macrophages, eosinophils, dendritic cells, and microglial cells [2, 21, 37–39] and after that, viral RNA is released inside the cells and tissues that will follow its cycle replication from the early stages of infection can be intensely active, as well as allowing the establishment of a latent infection, particularly known as permanent viral reservoirs promoting a major obstacle in the complete eradication of HIV infection and effectiveness in antiretroviral treatment [40–44].

It is estimated that between 10 and 12 days after the initial infection, the levels of viral RNA viremia in the blood plasma will increase slightly providing the anti-HIV antibody seroconversion phase that occurs in a variable period of 3–5 weeks, and this period of the infection is critical, as it indicates that the infected host is transmissible [45–48] and is also possible to detect viral RNA in blood plasma by amplification methods such as reverse transcription polymerase chain reaction (RT-PCR) [49–51]. However, prior to the seroconversion of anti-HIV antibodies, there is a period of time in which the infection is present, but the antibodies are still not detectable; this period is known as the serological window, which, according to the literature, varies from 3 months to a longer period [52–54].

In the acute phase, the CD4+ T cell count decreases dramatically, while the serum levels of viral particles rise proportionally, which is usually of short duration because the host begins to generate humoral and cellular immune responses that partially control viral replication [55, 56]. And as the specific immune response progresses, primarily mediated by cytotoxic CD8+ T cells that produce the initial control of viral replication at this stage of infection, viremia tends to decrease until it reaches stable or undetectable levels signaling the beginning of the chronic phase [57–59]. However, even with this immune response, it is possible to verify the qualitative functional impairment of the immune responses due to HIV, which can be described as a dysfunction of CD4+ T cells and other cells of the immune system, with the need to complement the host's defense lines with antiretroviral therapy [2].

Clinically, PLWH in most cases will present symptoms from a few days to weeks from exposure and contamination by HIV; usually, individuals have systemic symptoms similar to flu or mononucleosis, such as fever, weight loss, night sweats, constant diarrhea, malaise, lymphadenopathy, arthralgia, pharyngitis, and myalgia [60, 61]. These clinical characteristics mentioned above are heterogeneous and may vary between cases; however, something that is common and previously documented is that individuals who delay in starting antiretroviral therapy or maintain inconsistency in treatment and who present the above-mentioned symptoms for a longer duration, which may worsen the infection, leading to systemic and oral opportunistic infections, secondary malignancies, and neurologic manifestations [62, 63].

2. HIV and oral manifestations

2.1 HIV and oral cavity

Systemic and local opportunistic infections caused by HIV will directly impact the innate immune response, impact and trigger negative consequences on quality of life, and increase the morbidity of HIV infection; among the main local opportunistic infections, we cite oral lesions (OLs) [64, 65]. OLs are commonly among the first signs and symptoms of HIV infection, and certain lesions, such as necrotizing periodontitis (NP), Kaposi's sarcoma, or linear gingival erythema (LGE), as they are naturally found in PLWH, can serve as a means of diagnosis or indications for individuals with HIV infection status unknown [66–68].

In the past, when the individual was diagnosed with HIV or was undisciplined about antiviral treatment and oral hygiene, the occurrence of certain OLs could predict the progression of chronic infection to acute phases and even AIDS [68, 69]. The presence of OLs in PLWH using antiretroviral therapy (ART) can serve as a marker of viral resistance to medication and, consequently, reduce the effectiveness of ART, indicating the replacement of the current medication. According to Heron and Elahi [70], the prevalence of OL will vary with the use of ART, so specific lesions, such as candidiasis, hairy leukoplakia, and Kaposi's sarcoma, clinically, have shown a lower prevalence in patients who are regular users; however, evidence has shown that lesions, such as oral warts (OWs) and salivary gland diseases, are more prevalent resulting from the use of ART [71].

Oral health care is a vital component for maintaining a satisfactory general state of health and quality of life for PLWH, so it is interesting for health professionals to recognize and reinforce this care of adequate oral hygiene [72, 73], because when there is no such care and due to the immunosuppression conditions and systemic proinflammatory state of HIV-infected individuals and when we associate these systemic conditions with PLWH sites, they are simultaneously more prone to develop moderate and severe OLs such as oral candidiasis (OC), oral hairy leukoplakia (OHL), oral warts, oral aphthous ulcers, and oral herpes even in the presence of ART, demonstrating that the lack of oral hygiene or inadequate hygiene will have a high direct negative impact on the health of this population [74–76].

2.2 HIV and risk of oral transmission

Since HIV discovery, the means of transmission of HIV has been routinely studied aspects of infection, and until the present day, they are reasons for fear and stigma by the general population and even health professionals such as dentists [33]. Among the most controversial means of transmission is the oral cavity, and the presence of OLs that can serve as facilitators for transmission and contagion has been widely discussed [43]. Although it is known that HIV has periodontal tissues as reservoirs for its latency period, some studies that tried to detect the presence of viral particles in the cells of the oral epithelium demonstrated the absence of HIV in their results, making the transmission through the oral cavity as a somewhat questionable [77].

In theory, HIV infection *via* oral route would occur through oral sex; however, the data indicate low rates of oral HIV transmission. According to the literature studies, when there are cases of serodiscordant partners, the risk of contracting HIV by oral sex is estimated at between 0.04 and 0.06%, which has been shown to be well below the rates of anal sex, which is estimated at around 1.4%, and through sharing sharp instruments, which is estimated at between 0.63 and 2.4% [78–81]. To understand this low prevalence of oral transmission, we first need to understand that the oral epithelium is part of the innate immune system acting as a physical barrier that protects the underlying tissues from infection by pathogenic microorganisms such as HIV; that is, for oral contagion to occur by HIV, there must be a discontinuity in this oral tissue and, beyond this line of defense, the oral cavity [79]. In addition, the oral cavity has saliva and crevicular fluid as a means of defense, due to its low hypotonicity, which can act as antimicrobial factors, as well as macrophages, natural killer cells, and neutrophils, which will play important roles in the immune response of the oral mucosa [43, 70].

Although clinical and statistical data show that the oral transmission of HIV in adults is uncommon, it is understood that OL or mechanical trauma to the tissues of the oral mucosa causing ruptures or damage to the oral epithelium may be risk factors for the oral transmission of HIV, and key populations such as crack users, sex workers, and men who have sex with men may be more likely to be infected due to risky behaviors. As seen above, transmission in adults is rare, but postnatal vertical transmission seems to be a risky means of transmission to neonates, since in cases of HIV-infected postpartum women and neonates who were not contaminated via the uterus, they may contract HIV at ingesting infected vaginal secretions or amniotic fluids during childbirth or even while breastfeeding [82, 83].

2.3 HIV infection and oral mucosal

As discussed above, oral mucosal infections are commonly seen in HIV-infected individuals, suggesting that HIV infection is a risk factor for pathologies such as periodontal disease (PD), oral candidiasis, oral ulcers (OUs), angular cheilitis, and verrucous lesions [84, 85]. In fact, the literature indicates that ART-naïve PLWH users are more likely to have at least one OL during their lifetime, around 70–90% more likely when compared with PLWH ART users. Interestingly, this relationship may be proportional, because in the case of ART use, the appearance of these oral manifestations is still commonplace, but at a lower incidence, which is due to the fact that OLs, such as periodontitis, have multifactorial etiologies such as the presence of dental biofilm, and in cases of inadequate oral hygiene or absence of it, there will still be risks of oral manifestations [86, 87].

Therefore, it should be understood that the etiology of infections in the oral mucosa of ART-naïve PLWH has an intriguing combination because of systemic immunodeficiency due to the depletion of CD4+ T cells; local factors such as dental biofilm, environmental factors such as smoking, and compromise of oral defense cells producing interleukin-17 (IL-17) may be associated with increased susceptibility to opportunistic oral lesions. However, when ART is present, this incidence rate of OL tends to decrease; studies show that after the prescription and continuous use of ART, oral manifestations such as candidiasis, oral warts, hairy leukoplakia, and angular cheilitis will resolve as the immunosuppression is resolved by increasing the CD4+ T cell count and decreasing the viral load; however, it should be noted that each lesion will take a certain time to resolve due to the different associated causal factors as mentioned above, mainly factors related to impaction in the oral microbiota that undergo changes in the oral bacterial ecosystem [88–90].

2.4 HIV infection and oral microbiome

In the oral cavity, the role of the oral microbiota is extremely relevant to determine the health or disease of individuals; that is, when there is a process of oral dysbiosis, the diversity and composition of the oral microbiome changes overmuch. In PLWH cases, oral infections are commonly associated with significant proportions of highly pathogenic species such as *Fusobacterium nucleatum*, *Porphyromonas gingivalis*, *Prevotella denticola*, *Tannerella forsythia*, *Prevotella intermedia*, *Treponema denticola*, and *Aggregatibacter actinomycetemcomitans*. In the oral cavity of PLWH, microbial diversity was lower in individuals of this group than in individuals free of HIV infection and patients using ART; that is, in this HIV-infected population, the presence of aggressive bacteria was greater, and moreover, the presence of more virulent fungal communities can be identified. Therefore, the literature suggests that oral dysbiosis in PLWH promote greater chances of OL appearances due to the presence of more aggressive bacterial and fungal communities, even with a lower diversity of strains in the region [91–93].

2.5 Oral lesions caused by HIV infection

Several studies in the literature show the great harmful impact of HIV infection on the quality of life and oral health of this population [69, 94–104]. According to the Joint United Nations Program on HIV/AIDS (UNAIDS) in 2020, globally, there are about 37.7 million people living with HIV, with 1.5 million newly cases in 2020 alone, and according to studies, the prevalence of OL in PLWH has a range between 40 and 93%, and this variance will depend on geographic and socioeconomic issues, access to ART and health services, and factors influencing a good quality of life [105]. As seen, OLs are commonly among the first signs and symptoms of a possible HIV infection and can be used as a diagnostic method suggestive of HIV, and these lesions were classified as lesions strongly associated with HIV infection, lesions commonly associated with HIV infection, and lesions seen in HIV infection (**Table 1**) [106, 107]. As for the quality of life of PLWH, OL can be associated with acute pain, chewing and feeding difficulties, esthetic impairment, speech problems, and impaired social life; thus, the need for adequate care, management, and treatment, as well as the prevention of oral diseases, is the duty of health professionals [33].

2.6 Oral lesions and their relationship with CD4 count and viral load

In addition to their diagnostic importance, OLs are useful to base a prognosis on the stages of infection, as, according to the literature, they will serve as clinical parameters with CD4+ and CD8+ cell counts. Since the introduction of ART, there has been a vertiginous drop in the morbidity and mortality of PLWH, and the lower presence of OLs in HIV-infected patients is also associated with this. That is, the literature indicates that the amount and severity of OL is also directly associated with immunosuppression, so the tendency is to have a high prevalence of OL in patients with a low CD4+ cell count (<200 cells/mm^3) and high viral load (>55,000 copies/mL). In cases of ART-naïve or newly diagnosed individuals, the presence of moderate or severe OL and a CD4+ cell count below 200 cells/mm^3, it is necessary to start treatment with ART and dental treatment [75, 108–111].

3. Oral lesions clinical characteristics

3.1 Oral candidiasis

Oral candidiasis (OC) is among the most common opportunistic infections among PLWH, with an estimated prevalence of between 15% and 80% in adults living with HIV. The OC is a fungal infection caused by the proliferation of different strains such as *Candida albicans*, *Candida tropicalis*, *Candida parapsilosis*, *Candida glabrata*, *Candida krusei*, and *Candida dubliniensis* and is usually associated with low CD4+ cell counts and risk factors such as smoking, being an important marker for the individual's immunity status and among the clinical features of OC we cite [112–120]:

- White and pasty stains (removable during smear);
- Pain or burning during chewing and swallowing;
- Oral ulcers;
- Bleeding;
- Reddish lesions on the palate due to dental prostheses;
- Dysgeusia or ageusia;

DOI: http://dx.doi.org/10.5772/intechopen.105894

A- Lesions strongly associated with HIV infection	1. Oral candidiasis
	• Erythematous candidiasis
	• Pseudomembranous candidiasis
	2. Oral hairy leukoplakia
	3. Kaposi's sarcoma
	4. Non-Hodgkin's lymphoma
	5. Periodontal disease
	• Linear gingival erythema
	• Necrotizing gingivitis
	• Necrotizing periodontitis
	• Necrotizing stomatitis
B- Lesions less commonly associated with HIV infection	6. Bacterial infections
	• *Mycobacterium avium—intracellulare*
	• *Mycobacterium tuberculosis*
	7. Viral infections
	• Herpes simplex virus
	• Human papillomavirus (wart-like lesions)
	• Condyloma acuminatum
	• Focal epithelial hyperplasia
	• Verruca vulgaris
	• Varicella zoster virus
	• Herpes zoster
	• Varicella
	8. Melanotic hyperpigmentation
	9. Salivary gland disease
	• Xerostomia (decreased salivary flow rate)
	• Unilateral or bilateral swelling of salivary glands
	10. Thrombocytopenic purpura
	11. Various types of ulceration
C- Lesions seen in HIV infection	12. Bacterial infections
	• *Actinomyces israelii*
	• *Escherichia coli*
	• *Klebsiella pneumoniae*
	13. Fungal infections (different from candidiasis)
	• *Cryptococcus neoformans*
	• *Histoplasma capsulatum*
	• *Geotrichum candidum*
	• *Mucoraceae mucormycosis*

	• *Mucoraceae zygomycosis*
	• *Aspergillus flavus*
	14. Cat-scratch disease
	15. Drug reactions
	16. Epithelioid angiomatosis
	17. Viral infections
	• Cytomegalovirus
	• *Molluscum contagiosum*
	18. Neurologic disturbances
	• Facial palsy
	• Trigeminal neuralgia

Table 1.
EC-clearinghouse oral lesions associated with HIV infection classification.

- Edema.

Currently, three types of OC are observed: pseudomembranous candidiasis, erythematous candidiasis, and angular cheilitis [112–120].

3.1.1 Pseudomembraneous candidiasis

They appear as whitish plaques, pasty consistency, can be found on the buccal mucosa, lingual belly, periodontium, hard and soft palate, labial region, and oropharyngeal region. Such plaques are formed by a mixture of fungal hyphae, desquamated epithelium, and proinflammatory cells that, when removed, leave the underlying surface red or bleeding. As for the clinical diagnosis, it is made through clinical symptoms, and the histological diagnosis can be used through the direct smear [112–118].

3.1.2 Erythematous candidiasis

They appear as petechiae or reddish ecchymoses, commonly associated in the region of the hard palate (indiscriminate use of complete dentures), dorsum of the tongue (similar to areas of depapillation), and buccal mucosa. In most cases, these lesions present characteristic symptoms such as burning mouth and altered taste. As for the clinical diagnosis, it is made through clinical symptoms, and the histological diagnosis can be used through incisional biopsy [112–118].

3.1.3 Angular cheilitis

It presents as linear fissures or ulcers in the flaky labial commissures, which can be unilateral or bilateral, with a whitish color, sometimes blisters, and are usually associated with small white plaques. In cases of severe immunosuppression or AIDS, angular cheilitis may be related to erythematous candidiasis or pseudomembranous candidiasis. Clinically, the patient reports itching and burning in the labial commissure; the clinical diagnosis is made through clinical symptoms, and the histological diagnosis can be used through incisional biopsy [112–118].

3.1.4 Treatment

The treatment of OC can be topical and/or systemic, depending on the severity of candidiasis, immunosuppression, and risk factors.

- Topical therapy:
- Mouthwash:

  a. Chlorhexidine digluconate (0.12%): use two to three times a day for 10–14 days, dosage: 3 mL of oral solution.

  b. Amphotericin B (0.1 mg/mL): use three to five times a day for 14–42 days, dosage: 1.0–5.0 mg/kg/day of oral solution.

  c. Cleaning or replacing dental prosthesis.

- Dermatological cream:

  a. Clotrimazole (10 mg/g): use three times a day for up to 28 days.

- Systemic therapy:
- Oral suspension:

  a. Nystatin (100,000 IU/ml): use four times a day for 14 days, dosage: 1 to 6 ml of oral suspension.

- Oral pill:

  a. Fluconazole (150–200 mg): use once daily for 14 to 42 days.

  b. Ketoconazole (200 mg): use once daily for up to 14 days.

  c. Itraconazole (100 mg): use once daily for up to 7 days, dosage: 2 tablets (200 mg) daily.

3.2 Periodontal disease

Periodontal disease (PD) can be categorized simply as gingivitis and periodontitis; PD is an infectious inflammatory disease of multifactorial etiology [121, 122]. Its main etiology is the interaction among dental biofilm, host immune defense, and risk factors. Therefore, the association among pathological microorganisms, proinflammatory cytokines, oral dysbiosis, and cytotoxic factors causes an intense inflammatory response, which leads to the destruction of periodontal tissues and potentially resulting in tooth and bone loss [123–125].

Host habits, such as poor oral hygiene and smoking, and systemic diseases, such as AIDS, can predispose and worsen the progression of PD, as HIV infection alters the immune system, progressively impairing the immune response, favoring a more intense PD, such as acute and necrotizing. Necrotizing periodontal disease is the most severe form of PD due to rapid onset, severe pain, severe bone loss, suppuration, ulcerations, and areas of tissue necrosis. Among the clinical features of gingivitis and necrotizing periodontitis, we have the following [126, 127]:

- Intense pain;
- Spontaneous or provoked bleeding;
- Spontaneous or provoked suppuration;
- Areas of tissue necrosis;
- Ulcers in the periodontium (secondary aspects of the lesion);
- Presence of metallic taste in the mouth;
- Edema and gingival swelling;
- Presence of interproximal black space (interproximal bone loss);
- Increase in the degree of tooth mobility;
- Clinical attachment level loss;
- Halitosis;
- Periodontal pockets or gingival recessions (depending on tissue phenotype);
- Tooth loss.

3.2.1 Linear gingival erythema

Linear gingival erythema (LGE) is characterized by an erythematous band located on the free marginal gingiva; it can be generalized or localized and usually does not show signs of inflammation due to bacterial plaque accumulation. In other words, LGE can be considered a chronic non-plaque-induced gingivitis, a precursor of necrotizing diseases (**Figure 1**).

LGE is among the main oral signs and symptoms of HIV infection and possibly occurs due to the dysbiosis of the gingival sulcus microbiota and systemic immunosuppression. As a form of differential diagnosis between a common chronic gingivitis and LGE, in addition to the low presence and biofilm, the negative response to scaling and root planning treatment can be fundamental for the diagnosis [112–114, 128].

3.2.2 Necrotizing gingivitis

Necrotizing gingivitis (NG), also known as Vincent's disease or trench mouth, is the most severe form of PD and tends to be present in individuals with severe immunosuppression; it is characterized by rapid onset, ulcerations, tissue necrosis,

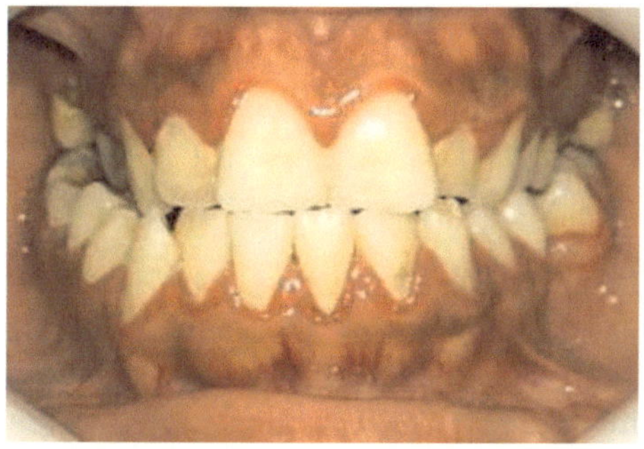

Figure 1.
Clinical linear gingival erythema.

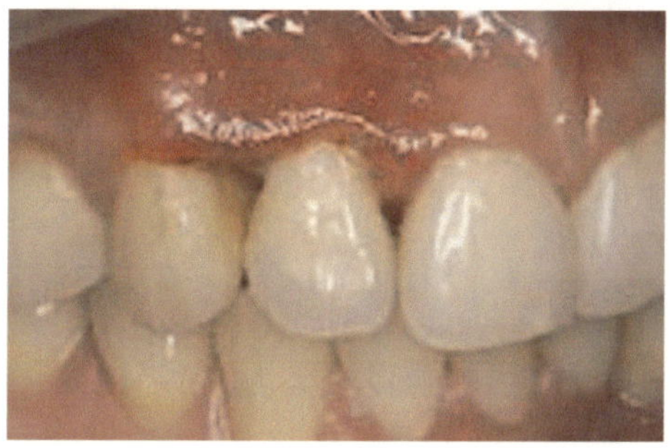

Figure 2.
Clinical necrotizing gingivitis.

suppuration, bleeding, foul odor, severe pain, and loss of interdental papillae (**Figure 2**) [127].

3.2.3 Necrotizing periodontitis

Necrotizing periodontitis (NP) is the natural evolution of NG; it is characterized by loss of soft tissue as a direct result of necrosis and acute ulceration arising from NG and presents a rapid bone destruction and extensive loss of the clinical level of bone attachment that can be generalized or located (**Figure 3**) [127].

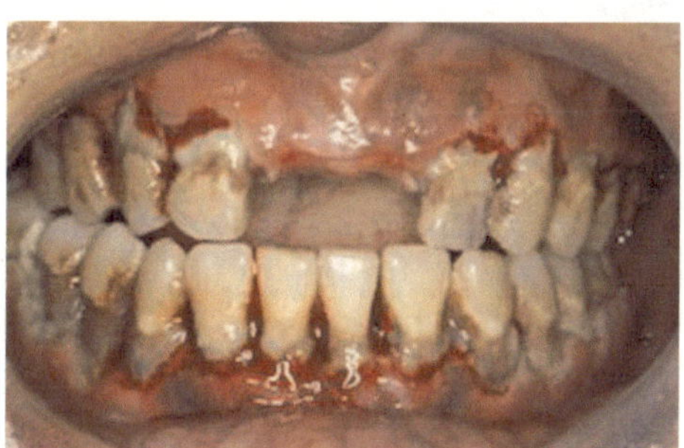

Figure 3.
Clinical necrotizing periodontitis.

3.2.4 Treatment

The treatment of periodontal diseases boils down to topical and systemic chemical-mechanical therapy [127].

- Topical therapy:
- Mouthwash:

    a. Chlorhexidine digluconate (0.12%: use two to three times a day for 10–14 days, dosage: 3 mL of oral solution.

- Scaling and root planing associated with tissue debridement.
- Oral hygiene instructions.
- Systemic therapy:
- Oral pill:

    a. Amoxicillin (500 mg): use three times a day for 7 days.

    b. Metronidazole (250 mg): use twice daily for up to 10 days.

    c. Amoxicillin and metronidazole can be combined to broaden the spectrum of action of antibiotic therapy.

3.3 Oral hairy leukoplakia: (OHL)

Oral hairy leukoplakia (OHL) is also among the most common oral signs and symptoms of HIV infection; it is usually caused by Epstein-Barr virus infections and is white asymptomatic plaques with a corrugated surface or a velvety hair-like appearance, which can be found on the lateral borders, unilaterally or bilaterally, of the tongue and in more severe cases also found on the dorsum or belly of the tongue, on the floor of the mouth, and on the buccal mucosa. If there is no removal of the plaque, the suggestive diagnosis is OHL, and if it comes out, it will be candidiasis. Among the histological features of OHL, we evidenced areas of hyperkeratosis, parakeratosis, acanthosis, papillomatosis, and the presence of layers of ballooned cells similar to koilocytes with nuclear alterations in the spinous layer, epithelial inflammatory infiltrate, and connective tissue [112–114, 129–132].

3.3.1 Treatment

The treatment of OHL is not just periodontal, and necrotizing diseases boils down to topical and systemic chemical-mechanical therapy [129–132].

- Topical therapy:
    - Podophyllin (25%): use three times a day for 7–14 days, use by applying the oral solution locally.

DOI: http://dx.doi.org/10.5772/intechopen.105894

- Systemic therapy:
    - Prevention of smoking and alcoholism.
    - Acyclovir (800 mg): use five times daily for 7–14 days.
    - Desciclovir (250 mg): use three times daily for 7–14 days.
    - Valacyclovir (1000 mg): use three times daily for 7–14 days.
    - Surgical excision of the lesion with an electric scalpel or laser.

3.4 Kaposi's sarcoma

Kaposi's sarcoma is a neoplasm commonly associated with individuals with AIDS; its etiology is usually linked to the oncovirus human herpes virus-8 (HHV-8) and originates from endothelial cells as a direct response to HHV-8 infection and immunosuppression caused by HIV. Clinically, the lesions are found in the form of asymptomatic macules or nodules, fast growing, reddish, bluish, or purple, and in some cases, in addition to the OL, lesions in the gastrointestinal and pulmonary tracts can be found. They are usually located in the palate or alveolar process and can lead to bone destruction, tooth mobility, and invariably tooth loss. Histologically, this neoplasm presents fusiform tumor cells, similar to smooth muscle, fibroblasts, and myofibroblasts [108, 112–114].

3.4.1 Treatment

The treatment of Kaposi's sarcoma consists of excisional biopsy, radiation therapy, or chemotherapy [108, 112–114].

3.5 Non-Hodgkin's lymphoma (NHL)

Non-Hodgkin's lymphoma (NHL) is the most uncommon OL associated with HIV infection; however, apart from Kaposi's sarcoma, it is the second most common malignancy among PLWH, with an average prevalence of 4%. NHL is a type of malignant neoplasm of origin in the cells of the lymphatic system and with an unordered diffusion and clinically appears as lymphadenopathy of the head and neck, armpits, and/or groin; among the most common signs and symptoms, the individual has nocturnal sweating, pyrexia or hyperpyrexia, itching, weight loss, and rapidly growing oral nodules in the alveolar process and tongue [112–114, 133–135].

3.5.1 Treatment

The treatment of NHL is based on excisional biopsy or puncture and with confirmation the individual should start with immunotherapy, radiotherapy, or chemotherapy [112–114, 133–135].

3.6 Oral ulcers

Oral ulcers (OUs) are erosive lesions that occur in the oral epithelium, and when the epithelium sloughs, the nerve endings of the oral epithelium will be exposed and trigger symptoms such as pain provoked and exudate, causing difficulty in swallowing and impaired speech and chewing. They can appear in all the areas of the oral mucosa, and among PLWH, it has a prevalence of about 50%; OUs can be classified into minor aphthous ulcers and major aphthous ulcers [112–114].

3.6.1 Minor aphthous ulcers

They are minor ulcerative lesions with about 2–5 mm in diameter and occur on nonkeratinized mucosa, have a predilection for areas of the buccal mucosa and lips, are clinically more superficial, covered by a whitish pseudomembrane, surrounded by an erythematous halo, and are extremely painful [112–114].

3.6.2 Major aphthous ulcers

They are larger ulcerative lesions measuring over 1 cm in diameter and can occur in both keratinized and nonkeratinized areas, generally affecting the lateral border of the tongue, soft palate, floor of the mouth, buccal mucosa, oropharynx, and alveolar process. Clinically, they have a crater-like appearance with raised edges and covered by a yellowish-white pseudomembrane and may be accompanied by regional lymphadenopathy [112–114].

3.6.3 Treatment

The treatment of OU is summarized in a topical therapy, in which the individual must maintain good oral hygiene, use 0.12% chlorhexidine digluconate mouthwash or dexamethasone mouthwash (0.5 mg/5 cc), rinse for 5 minutes before spitting, and use three to four times a day for up to 10 days. The use of topical ointments, such as triamcinolone acetonide, can be applied under the ulcer area two to three times daily for up to 7 days [112–114].

3.7 Salivary gland diseases

The enlargement of the major salivary glands affects the parotid, sublingual, and submandibular glands; clinically, xerostomia, unilateral or bilateral, and asymptomatic edema, in addition to esthetic embarrassment and social stigma, are observed. Histologically, the presence of focal sialoadenitis with an infiltrate of proinflammatory cells and CD8+ T lymphocytes can be observed [112–114].

3.7.1 Treatment

A specific treatment for the enlargement of the major salivary glands does not exist; to treat symptoms such as xerostomia, the use of artificial saliva or the habit of chewing gum to increase salivary volume is recommended, and some studies have shown that radiotherapy may be a viable treatment to reduce the size of the glands [112–114].

3.8 Melanotic hyperpigmentation

Oral melanotic hyperpigmentation is another common lesion in PLWH, and once the differential diagnosis of ethnic melanic pigmentation is removed, it can be indicated that, once present in the oral cavity, it is a possible factor of HIV infection. Clinically, there is a black, brownish, or brown spot or macula, typically asymptomatic and may occur due to increased release and dysregulation of alpha melanocytes caused by certain types of ART, such as zidovudine and antifungal drugs, especially to treat and *Mycobacterium avium* intracellulare [112–114].

3.9 Human papillomavirus

Human papillomavirus (HPV) can infect the oral mucosa, resulting in the development of oral verrucous lesions. Oral warts (OWs) usually present nodular or pedunculated lesions with a sessile base, with a firm consistency; they can be solitary or multiple lesions, white or pink in color, and can have smooth or irregular surfaces, similar to a cauliflower. The OWs caused by HPV are among the most prevalent lesions of PLWH with a reported prevalence of about 0.5–6.9%, and HPV can be classified into subtypes according to its oncogenic level, and in the oral cavity, subtypes 6 and 11 are the most prevalent; about 90%, in OWs such as condylomas and laryngeal papillomas, have lower oncogenic potential. HPV is highly sexually transmitted; being frequent in the genital and anal region, its incidence in the oral mucosa is due to acts of self-inoculation or oral sexual contact [112–114, 136–139].

3.9.1 Treatment

The basic treatment of OW is summarized in the excisional biopsy of the nodule, either by removal with a surgical laser or by electric scalpel or cryosurgery. Topically, a cream called imiquimod (50 mg/g) serves as an immunomodulatory cream that must be applied to the wart site once a day, three times a week for up to 28 days. Systemically, the use of antivirals such as cidofovir (5 mg/kg) is recommended, which should be administered once a week for up to 14 days [112–114, 136–139].

4. Conclusion

Host's immune, oral hygiene, and HIV infection course could be considered a directly key determinant for oral mucosal infection linked to HIV. Therefore, to understand the immunological key elements in the oral health of PLWH is essential to alerted healthcare workers regarding HIV infection severity, because compromised oral barrier integrity will facilitate HIV infection, oral dysbiosis, microbial translocation along different types of mucosal tissue, and the spread of microorganism products into the oral epithelial tissue, which may predispose to opportunistic infections and systemic inflammation, such as various oral lesions and neoplasms. This chapter presented various studies and discussed the newly knowledge about HIV infection and its importance to oral mucosa infections, so this review might be helpful to the diagnosis and treatment of various oral lesions in PLWH.

Acknowledgements

The authors would like to acknowledge the help from Coordenação de Aperfeiçoamento de Pessoal de Nível Superior (CAPES), Ministry of Education - Brazil– Grant code 001. LFAM is a CNPq Grantee (#314209/2021-2). Publication of the article was supported by Public Notice PAPQ, PROPESP/FADESP of the Federal University of Pará.

Conflict of interest

The authors declare no conflict of interest.

Appendices and nomenclature

Human Immunodeficiency Virus (HIV);
HIV-type 1 (HIV-1);
HIV-type 2 (HIV-2);
People Living with HIV (PLWH);
Acquired Immunodeficiency Syndrome (AIDS);
Reverse Transcription Polymerase Chain Reaction (RT-PCR);
Oral lesions (OL);
Antiretroviral therapy (ART);
Joint United Nations Programme on HIV/AIDS (UNAIDS);
Oral candidiasis (OC);
Periodontal disease (PD);
Linear gingival erythema (LEG);
Necrotizing gingivitis (NG);
Necrotizing periodontitis (NP);
Oral hairy leukoplakia (OHL);
Human Herpes Virus-8 (HHV-8);
Non-Hodgkin's lymphoma (NHL);
Human papillomavirus (HPV);
Oral warts (OW).

Author details

Ricardo Roberto de Souza Fonseca[1,2*], Rogério Valois Laurentino[1,2], Luiz Fernando Almeida Machado[1,2], Carlos Eduardo Vieira da Silva Gomes[3], Tatiany Oliveira de Alencar Menezes[3], Oscar Faciola Pessoa[3], Aldemir Branco Oliveira-Filho[4], Tábata Resque Beckmann Carvalho[5], Paula Gabriela Faciola Pessoa de Oliveira[5], Erich Brito Tanaka[5], Jorge Sá Elias Nogueira[5], Douglas Magno Guimarães[5], Marcelo Newton Carneiro[5], Paula Mendes Acatauassú Carneiro[5], Aluísio Ferreira Celestino Junior[5], Patricia de Almeida Rodrigues[5] and Silvio Augusto Fernandes de Menezes[5]

1 Biology of Infectious and Parasitic Agents Post-Graduate Program, Federal University of Pará, Belém, Brazil

2 Virology Laboratory, Institute of Biological Sciences, Federal University of Pará, Belém, Brazil

3 Dentistry Post-Graduate Program, School of Dentistry, Federal University of Pará, Belém, Brazil

4 Study of Research Group on Vulnerable Populations, Institute of Coastal Studies, Bragança, Brazil

5 School of Dentistry, University Center of State of Pará, Belém, Brazil

*Address all correspondence to: ricardofonseca285@gmail.com

References

[1] Lucas S, Nelson AM. HIV and the spectrum of human disease. The Journal of Pathology. 2015;**235**(2):229-241. DOI: 10.1002/path.4449

[2] Fanales-Belasio E, Raimondo M, Suligoi B, Buttò S. HIV virology and pathogenetic mechanisms of infection: A brief overview. Annali dell'Istituto Superiore di Sanità. 2010;**46**(1):5-14. DOI: 10.4415/ANN_10_01_02

[3] U.S. Department of Health & Human Services. A Timeline of HIV and AIDS. 2020. Available from: https://www.hiv.gov/hiv-basics/overview/history/hiv-and-aids-timeline

[4] Joint United Nations Programme on HIV/AIDS (UNAIDS). Update. 2020. Available from: https://www.unaids.org/en/resources/presscentre/featurestories/2020/september/20200928_new-hiv-infections-increasingly-among-key-populations

[5] Crispim MAE, Reis MNDG, Abrahim C, Kiesslich D, Fraiji N, Bello G, et al. Homogenous HIV-1 subtype B from the Brazilian Amazon with infrequent diverse BF1 recombinants, subtypes F1 and C among blood donors. PLoS One. 2019; **14**(9):e0221151. DOI: 10.1371/journal.pone.0221151

[6] Oliveira-Filho AB, Silva FQ, Santos FJA, Cardoso YMN, Di Miceli JFF, Resque RL, et al. Prevalence and risk factors for HIV-1 infection in people who use illicit drugs in northern Brazil. Transactions of the Royal Society of Tropical Medicine and Hygiene. 2020; **114**(3):213-221. DOI: 10.1093/trstmh/trz106

[7] Zhang J, Fan Q, Luo M, Yao J, Pan X, Li X. Phylogenetic evidence of HIV-1 transmission linkage between two men who have sex with men. Virology Journal. 2021;**18**(1):106. DOI: 10.1186/s12985-021-01573-5

[8] de Souza RL, Pereira MVS, da Silva RM, Sales JBL, Gardunho DCL, Monteiro JC, et al. Molecular epidemiology of HIV-1 and HTLV-1/2 among female sex workers in four cities in the state of para, northern Brazil. Frontiers in Microbiology. 2020;**11**: 602664. DOI: 10.3389/fmicb.2020.602664

[9] Machado LF, Vallinoto AC, Souza MI, Azevedo VN, Ishak MO, Ishak R. Serological and molecular typing of HIV type 1 infection in the Tiriyo tribe, a native Indian community of the Amazon region of Brazil. AIDS Research and Human Retroviruses. 2006;**22**(12):1267-1270. DOI: 10.1089/aid.2006.22.1267

[10] Rubenstein LS, Amon JJ, McLemore M, Eba P, Dolan K, Lines R. HIV, prisoners, and human rights. Lancet. 2016;**388**(10050):1202-1214. DOI: 10.1016/S0140-6736(16)30663-8

[11] Baral SD, Poteat T, Strömdahl S, Wirtz AL, Guadamuz TE, Beyrer C. Worldwide burden of HIV in transgender women: A systematic review and meta-analysis. The Lancet Infectious Diseases. 2013;**13**(3):214-222. DOI: 10.1016/S1473-3099(12)70315-8

[12] Machado LF, Costa IB, Folha MN, da Luz AL, Vallinoto AC, Ishak R, et al. Lower genetic variability of HIV-1 and antiretroviral drug resistance in pregnant women from the state of Pará, Brazil. BMC Infectious Diseases. 2017;**17**(1):270. DOI: 10.1186/s12879-017-2392-y

[13] Burton DR. Advancing an HIV vaccine; advancing vaccinology. Nature Reviews. Immunology. 2019;**19**(2):77-78. DOI: 10.1038/s41577-018-0103-6

[14] Bandera A, Gori A, Clerici M, Sironi M. Phylogenies in ART: HIV reservoirs, HIV latency and drug resistance. Current Opinion in Pharmacology. 2019;**48**:24-32. DOI: 10.1016/j.coph.2019.03.003

[15] World Health Organization (WHO). HIV/AIDS. 2020. Available from: https://www.who.int/news-room/fact-sheets/detail/hiv-aids

[16] International Committee on Taxonomy of Viruses (ICTV). 2020. Available from: http://www.ictvonline.org/virusTaxonomy.asp

[17] Gelderblom HR, Ozel M, Pauli G. Morphogenesis and morphology of HIV. Structure-function relations. Archives of Virology. 1989;**106**(1–2):1-13. DOI: 10.1007/BF01311033

[18] Hemelaar J, Elangovan R, Yun J, Dickson-Tetteh L, Kirtley S, Gouws-Williams E, et al. Global and regional epidemiology of HIV-1 recombinants in 1990-2015: A systematic review and global survey. Lancet HIV. 2020;7(11):e772-e781. DOI: 10.1016/S2352-3018(20)30252-6

[19] Sabin CA, Lundgren JD. The natural history of HIV infection. Current Opinion in HIV and AIDS. 2013;**8**(4): 311-317. DOI: 10.1097/COH.0b013e328361fa66

[20] Kedzierska K, Crowe SM. The role of monocytes and macrophages in the pathogenesis of HIV-1 infection. Current Medicinal Chemistry. 2002;**9**(21): 1893-1903. DOI: 10.2174/0929867023368935

[21] Fauci AS, Pantaleo G, Stanley S, Weissman D. Immunopathogenic mechanisms of HIV infection. Annals of Internal Medicine. 1996;**124**(7):654-663. DOI: 10.7326/0003-4819-124-7-199604010-00006

[22] Nittayananta W, Tao R, Jiang L, Peng Y, Huang Y. Oral innate immunity in HIV infection in HAART era. Journal of Oral Pathology & Medicine. 2016; **45**(1):3-8. DOI: 10.1111/jop.12304

[23] Challacombe SJ, Naglik JR. The effects of HIV infection on oral mucosal immunity. Advances in Dental Research. 2006;**19**(1):29-35. DOI: 10.1177/154407370601900107

[24] Gallo RC, Garzino-Demo A, DeVico AL. HIV infection and pathogenesis: What about chemokines? Journal of Clinical Immunology. 1999; **19**(5):293-299. DOI: 10.1023/a:1020539524373

[25] Broder CC, Berger EA. Fusogenic selectivity of the envelope glycoprotein is a major determinant of human immunodeficiency virus type 1 tropism for CD4+ T-cell lines vs. primary macrophages. Proceedings of the National Academy of Sciences of the United States of America. 1995;**92**(19):9004-9008. DOI: 10.1073/pnas.92.19.9004

[26] Dupont M, Sattentau QJ. Macrophage cell-cell interactions promoting HIV-1 Infection. Viruses. 2020;**12**(5):492. DOI: 10.3390/v12050492

[27] Zoeteweij JP, Blauvelt A. HIV-Dendritic cell interactions promote efficient viral infection of T cells. Journal of Biomedical Science. 1998;**5**(4): 253-259. DOI: 10.1007/BF02255856

[28] Nyamweya S, Hegedus A, Jaye A, Rowland-Jones S, Flanagan KL, Macallan DC. Comparing HIV-1 and HIV-2 infection: Lessons for viral immunopathogenesis. Reviews in Medical Virology. 2013;**23**(4):221-240. DOI: 10.1002/rmv.1739

[29] Hassan AS, Pybus OG, Sanders EJ, Albert J, Esbjörnsson J. Defining HIV-1

transmission clusters based on sequence data. AIDS. 2017;**31**(9):1211-1222. DOI: 10.1097/QAD.0000000000001470

[30] Goldman G, Budhram S. A retrospective cohort study comparing pregnancy outcomes and neonatal characteristics between HIV-infected and HIV-non-infected mothers. South African Medical Journal. 2020;**110**(6): 502-504. DOI: 10.7196/SAMJ.2020.v110i6.14357

[31] Hemelaar J. The origin and diversity of the HIV-1 pandemic. Trends in Molecular Medicine. 2012;**18**(3):182-192. DOI: 10.1016/j.molmed.2011.12.001

[32] Goodsell DS. Illustrations of the HIV life cycle. Current Topics in Microbiology and Immunology. 2015; **389**:243-252. DOI: 10.1007/82_2015_437

[33] Fonseca RRS, Laurentino RV, Menezes SAF, Oliveira-Filho AB, Alves AC, Frade PCR, et al. digital form for assessing dentists' knowledge about oral care of people living with HIV. International Journal of Environmental Research and Public Health. 2022;**19**: 5055. DOI: 10.3390/ijerph19095055

[34] Henrard DR, Daar E, Farzadegan H, Clark SJ, Phillips J, Shaw GM, et al. Virologic and immunologic characterization of symptomatic and asymptomatic primary HIV-1 infection. Journal of Acquired Immune Deficiency Syndromes and Human Retrovirology. 1995;**9**(3):305-310

[35] Ferguson MR, Rojo DR, von Lindern JJ, O'Brien WA. HIV-1 replication cycle. Clinics in Laboratory Medicine. 2002;**22**(3):611-635. DOI: 10.1016/s0272-2712(02)00015-x

[36] Christensen DE, Ganser-Pornillos BK, Johnson JS, Pornillos O, Sundquist WI. Reconstitution and visualization of HIV-1 capsid-dependent replication and integration in vitro. Science. 2020;**370**(6513):eabc8420. DOI: 10.1126/science.abc8420

[37] Price DA, Goulder PJ, Klenerman P, Sewell AK, Easterbrook PJ, Troop M, et al. Positive selection of HIV-1 cytotoxic T lymphocyte escape variants during primary infection. Proceedings of the National Academy of Sciences of the United States of America. 1997;**94**(5): 1890-1895. DOI: 10.1073/pnas.94.5.1890

[38] Falcinelli SD, Ceriani C, Margolis DM, Archin NM. New frontiers in measuring and characterizing the HIV reservoir. Frontiers in Microbiology. 2019;**10**:2878. DOI: 10.3389/fmicb.2019.02878

[39] Garzino-Demo A. Chemokines and defensins as HIV suppressive factors: An evolving story. Current Pharmaceutical Design. 2007;**13**(2):163-172. DOI: 10.2174/138161207779313696

[40] Castro-Gonzalez S, Colomer-Lluch M, Serra-Moreno R. Barriers for HIV cure: The latent reservoir. AIDS Research and Human Retroviruses. 2018;**34**(9): 739-759. DOI: 10.1089/AID.2018.0118

[41] Pedro KD, Henderson AJ, Agosto LM. Mechanisms of HIV-1 cell-to-cell transmission and the establishment of the latent reservoir. Virus Research. 2019;**265**:115-121. DOI: 10.1016/j.virusres.2019.03.014

[42] Wallet C, De Rovere M, Van Assche J, Daouad F, De Wit S, Gautier V, et al. Microglial cells: The main HIV-1 reservoir in the brain. Frontiers in Cellular and Infection Microbiology. 2019;**9**:362. DOI: 10.3389/fcimb.2019.00362

[43] Moyes DL, Islam A, Kohli A, Naglik JR. Oral epithelial cells and their

interactions with HIV-1. Oral Diseases. 2016;**22**(Suppl. 1):66-72. DOI: 10.1111/odi.12410

[44] George J, Wagner W, Lewis MG, Mattapallil JJ. Significant depletion of CD4(+) T cells occurs in the oral mucosa during simian immunodeficiency virus infection with the infected CD4(+) T cell reservoir continuing to persist in the oral mucosa during antiretroviral therapy. Journal of Immunology Research. 2015; **2015**:673815. DOI: 10.1155/2015/673815

[45] Schechter MT, Craib KJ, Le TN, Montaner JS, Douglas B, Sestak P, et al. Susceptibility to AIDS progression appears early in HIV infection. AIDS. 1990;**4**(3):185-190. DOI: 10.1097/00002030-199003000-00002

[46] Keet IP, Krijnen P, Koot M, Lange JM, Miedema F, Goudsmit J, et al. Predictors of rapid progression to AIDS in HIV-1 seroconverters. AIDS. 1993; 7(1):51-57. DOI: 10.1097/00002030-199301000-00008

[47] Busch MP, Satten GA. Time course of viremia and antibody seroconversion following human immunodeficiency virus exposure. The American Journal of Medicine. 1997;**102**(5B):117-124; 125-6. DOI: 10.1016/s0002-9343(97)00077-6

[48] Xavier Ruiz F, Arnold E. Evolving understanding of HIV-1 reverse transcriptase structure, function, inhibition, and resistance. Current Opinion in Structural Biology. 2020;**61**: 113-123. DOI: 10.1016/j.sbi.2019.11.011

[49] Sarafianos SG, Marchand B, Das K, Himmel DM, Parniak MA, Hughes SH, et al. Structure and function of HIV-1 reverse transcriptase: Molecular mechanisms of polymerization and inhibition. Journal of Molecular Biology. 2009;**385**(3):693-713. DOI: 10.1016/j.jmb.2008.10.071

[50] Yilmaz G. Diagnosis of HIV infection and laboratory monitoring of its therapy. Journal of Clinical Virology. 2001;**21**(3):187-196. DOI: 10.1016/s1386-6532(01)00165-2

[51] Alexander TS. Human Immunodeficiency virus diagnostic testing: 30 years of evolution. Clinical and Vaccine Immunology. 2016;**23**(4): 249-253. DOI: 10.1128/CVI.00053-16

[52] Kucirka LM, Sarathy H, Govindan P, Wolf JH, Ellison TA, Hart LJ, et al. Risk of window period HIV infection in high infectious risk donors: Systematic review and meta-analysis. American Journal of Transplantation. 2011;**11**(6):1176-1187. DOI: 10.1111/j.1600-6143.2010.03329.x

[53] Salles NA, Nishiya AS, Ferreira SC, Rocha VG, Mendrone-Junior A. Detection of HIV-1 infections in blood donors during the pre-seroconversion window period in São Paulo Brazil. Revista da Sociedade Brasileira de Medicina Tropical. 2019;**52**:e20180432. DOI: 10.1590/0037-8682-0432-2018

[54] Whitlock G, Nwokolo N, Dean Street Collaborative Group. Does qualitative viral load testing shorten the window period for diagnosing HIV in individuals attending for post-exposure prophylaxis? International Journal of STD & AIDS. 2020;**31**(9):816-819. DOI: 10.1177/0956462420923883

[55] Gomes STM, Gomes ÉR, Dos Santos MB, Lima SS, Queiroz MAF, Machado LFA, et al. Immunological and virological characterization of HIV-1 viremia controllers in the North Region of Brazil. BMC Infectious Diseases. 2017; **17**(1):381. DOI: 10.1186/s12879-017-2491-9

[56] Gomes STM, da Silva Graça Amoras E, Gomes ÉR, MAF Q, ECS J, de Vasconcelos Massafra JM, et al. Immune

escape mutations in HIV-1 controllers in the Brazilian Amazon region. BMC Infectious Diseases. 2020;**20**(1):546. DOI: 10.1186/s12879-020-05268-0

[57] Gulzar N, Copeland KF. CD8+ T-cells: Function and response to HIV infection. Current HIV Research. 2004; **2**(1):23-37. DOI: 10.2174/1570162043485077

[58] Wilson SS, Wiens ME, Smith JG. Antiviral mechanisms of human defensins. Journal of Molecular Biology. 2013;**425**(24):4965-4980. DOI: 10.1016/j.jmb.2013.09.038

[59] Tumwesigye E. Telling signs and symptoms. African Women Health. 1994;**2**(3):31-37

[60] Vanhems P, Dassa C, Lambert J, Cooper DA, Perrin L, Vizzard J, et al. Comprehensive classification of symptoms and signs reported among 218 patients with acute HIV-1 infection. Journal of Acquired Immune Deficiency Syndromes. 1999;**21**(2):99-106

[61] Hoenigl M, Green N, Camacho M, Gianella S, Mehta SR, Smith DM, et al. Signs or symptoms of acute HIV infection in a cohort undergoing community-based screening. Emerging Infectious Diseases. 2016;**22**(3):532-534. DOI: 10.3201/eid2203.151607

[62] Pamplona MCDCA, Chaves EC, Carvalho AC, Pamplona RDCA, Vallinoto ACR, Queiroz MAF, et al. Influence of exposure and vertical transmission of HIV-1 on the neuropsychomotor development in children. Revista da Sociedade Brasileira de Medicina Tropical. 2019;**52**: e20180263. DOI: 10.1590/0037-8682-0263-2018

[63] Munishi OM, McCormack V, Mchome B, Mangi G, Zullig LL, Bartlett J, et al. Awareness of cancer risk factors and its signs and symptoms in Northern Tanzania: A cross-sectional survey in the general population and in people living with HIV. Journal of Cancer Education. 2020;**35**(4):696-704. DOI: 10.1007/s13187-019-01513-6

[64] John CN, Stephen LX, Joyce Africa CW. Is human immunodeficiency virus (HIV) stage an independent risk factor for altering the periodontal status of HIV-positive patients? A South African study. BMC Oral Health. 2013; **13**:69. DOI: 10.1186/1472-6831-13-69

[65] Weinberg A, Tugizov S, Pandiyan P, Jin G, Rakshit S, Vyakarnam A, et al. Innate immune mechanisms to oral pathogens in oral mucosa of HIV-infected individuals. Oral Diseases. 2020;**26**(Suppl. 1):69-79. DOI: 10.1111/odi.13470

[66] Greenspan D, Greenspan JS. HIV-related oral disease. Lancet. 1996; **348**(9029):729-733. DOI: 10.1016/S0140-6736(96)02308-2

[67] Hodgson TA, Greenspan D, Greenspan JS. Oral lesions of HIV disease and HAART in industrialized countries. Advances in Dental Research. 2006; **19**(1):57-62. DOI: 10.1177/154407370601900112

[68] Petersen PE, Bourgeois D, Ogawa H, Estupinan-Day S, Ndiaye C. The global burden of oral diseases and risks to oral health. Bulletin of the World Health Organization. 2005;**83**(9):661-669

[69] Patton L. Progress in understanding oral health and HIV/AIDS. Oral Diseases. 2014;**20**(3):223-225. DOI: 10.1111/odi.12220

[70] Heron SE, Elahi S. HIV infection and compromised mucosal immunity: Oral manifestations and systemic

inflammation. Frontiers in Immunology. 2017;**8**:241. DOI: 10.3389/fimmu.2017.00241

[71] Khoury ZH, Meeks V. The influence of antiretroviral therapy on HIV-related oral manifestations. Journal of the National Medical Association. 2021; **113**(4):449-456. DOI: 10.1016/j.jnma.2021.02.008

[72] Phanuphak N, Gulick RM. HIV treatment and prevention 2019: Current standards of care. Current Opinion in HIV and AIDS. 2020;**15**(1):4-12. DOI: 10.1097/COH.0000000000000588

[73] Shirlaw PJ, Chikte U, MacPhail L, Schmidt-Westhausen A, Croser D, Reichart P. Oral and dental care and treatment protocols for the management of HIV-infected patients. Oral Diseases. 2002;**8**(Suppl. 2):136-143. DOI: 10.1034/j.1601-0825.2002.00025.x

[74] Aškinytė D, Matulionytė R, Rimkevičius A. Oral manifestations of HIV disease: A review. Stomatologija. 2015;**17**(1):21-28

[75] Rocha GCT, Fonseca RRS, Oliveira-Filho AB, Ribeiro ALR, de Menezes SAF, Laurentino RV, et al. Evaluation of sociodemographic factors and prevalence of oral lesions in people living with HIV from Cacoal, Rondônia, Amazon region of Brazil. International Journal of Environmental Research and Public Health. 2022;**19**(5):2614. DOI: 10.3390/ijerph19052614

[76] Menezes TO, Rodrigues MC, Nogueira BM, Menezes SA, Silva SH, Vallinoto AC. Oral and systemic manifestations in HIV-1 patients. Revista da Sociedade Brasileira de Medicina Tropical. 2015;**48**(1):83-86. DOI: 10.1590/0037-8682-0179-2014

[77] Pólvora TLS, Nobre ÁVV, Tirapelli C, Taba M Jr, Macedo LD, Santana RC, et al. Relationship between human immunodeficiency virus (HIV-1) infection and chronic periodontitis. Expert Review of Clinical Immunology. 2018;**14**(4):315-327. DOI: 10.1080/1744666X.2018.1459571

[78] Shugars DC, Sweet SP, Malamud D, Kazmi SH, Page-Shafer K, Challacombe SJ. Saliva and inhibition of HIV-1 infection: Molecular mechanisms. Oral Diseases. 2002;**8** (Suppl. 2):169-175. DOI: 10.1034/j.1601-0825.8.s2.7.x

[79] Baggaley RF, White RG, Boily MC. Systematic review of orogenital HIV-1 transmission probabilities. International Journal of Epidemiology. 2008;**37**(6): 1255-1265. DOI: 10.1093/ije/dyn151

[80] Boily MC, Buvé A, Baggaley RF. HIV transmission in serodiscordant heterosexual couples. BMJ. 2010;**340**: c2449. DOI: 10.1136/bmj.c2449

[81] Baggaley RF, White RG, Boily MC. HIV transmission risk through anal intercourse: Systematic review, meta-analysis and implications for HIV prevention. International Journal of Epidemiology. 2010;**39**(4):1048-1063. DOI: 10.1093/ije/dyq057

[82] Guo Y, Huang X, Sun X, Yu Y, Wang Y, Zhang B, et al. The underrated salivary virome of men who have sex with men infected with HIV. Frontiers in Immunology. 2021;**12**:759253. DOI: 10.3389/fimmu.2021.759253

[83] Cresswell FV, Ellis J, Hartley J, Sabin CA, Orkin C, Churchill DR. A systematic review of risk of HIV transmission through biting or spitting: Implications for policy. HIV Medicine. 2018;**19**(8):532-540. DOI: 10.1111/hiv.12625

[84] Lopez R, Fernandez O, Jara G, Baelum V. Epidemiology of necrotizing ulcerative gingival lesions in adolescents. Journal of Periodontal Research. 2002; **37**(6):439-444. DOI: 10.1034/j.1600-0765.2002.01377.x

[85] Patton LL, Phelan JA, Ramos-Gomez FJ, Nittayananta W, Shiboski CH, Mbuguye TL. Prevalence and classification of HIV-associated oral lesions. Oral Diseases. 2002;**8**(Suppl 2): 98-109. DOI: 10.1034/j.1601-0825.2002.00020.x

[86] Kamiru HN, Naidoo S. Oral HIV lesions and oral health behaviour of HIV-positive patients attending the Queen Elizabeth II Hospital, Maseru, Lesotho. Journal of the South African Dental Association. 2002;**57**(11):479-482

[87] Agbelusi GA, Wright AA. Oral lesions as indicators of HIV infection among routine dental patients in Lagos Nigeria. Oral Diseases. 2005;**11**(6): 370-373. DOI: 10.1111/j.1601-0825.2005.01132.x

[88] Moodley A, Wood NH. HIV-associated oral lesions as an indicator for HAART failure: A review. Journal of the South African Dental Association. 2012; **67**(7):348-352

[89] Aquino-García SI, Rivas MA, Ceballos-Salobreña A, Acosta-Gio AE, Gaitán-Cepeda LA. Oral lesions in HIV/AIDS patients undergoing HAART including efavirenz. AIDS Research and Human Retroviruses. 2008;**24**(6): 815-820. DOI: 10.1089/aid.2007.0159

[90] Vohra P, Jamatia K, Subhada B, Tiwari RVC, Althaf MN, Jain C. Correlation of CD4 counts with oral and systemic manifestations in HIV patients. Journal of Family Medicine and Primary Care. 2019;**8**(10):3247-3252. DOI: 10.4103/jfmpc.jfmpc_767_19

[91] Li S, Su B, He QS, Wu H, Zhang T. Alterations in the oral microbiome in HIV infection: Causes, effects and potential interventions. Chinese Medical Journal. 2021;**134**(23):2788-2798. DOI: 10.1097/CM9.0000000000001825

[92] Fidel PL Jr, Moyes D, Samaranayake L, Hagensee ME. Interplay between oral immunity in HIV and the microbiome. Oral Diseases. 2020;**26**(Suppl. 1):59-68. DOI: 10.1111/odi.13515

[93] Perez Rosero E, Heron S, Jovel J, O'Neil CR, Turvey SL, Parashar P, et al. Differential signature of the microbiome and neutrophils in the oral cavity of HIV-infected individuals. Frontiers in Immunology. 2021;**12**:780910, 2021. DOI: 10.3389/fimmu.2021.780910. eCollection

[94] Patton LL, van der Horst C. Oral infections and other manifestations of HIV disease. Infectious Disease Clinics of North America. 1999;**13**(4):879-900. DOI: 10.1016/s08

[95] Gennaro S, Naidoo S, Berthold P. Oral health & HIV/AIDS. MCN: American Journal of Maternal Child Nursing. 2008;**33**(1):50-57. DOI: 10.1097/01.NMC.0000305658.32237.7d

[96] de Aguiar RA, Portela MB, de Souza IP. The oral health of HIV-infected Brazilian children. International Journal of Paediatric Dentistry. 2013;**23**(5):359-365. DOI: 10.1111/ipd.12008

[97] Kumar S, Mishra P, Warhekar S, Airen B, Jain D, Godha S. Oral health status and oromucosal lesions in patients living with HIV/AIDS in India: A comparative study. AIDS Research and Treatment. 2014;**2014**:480247. DOI: 10.1155/2014/480247

[98] Nouaman MN, Meless DG, Coffie PA, Arrivé E, Tchounga BK, Ekouévi DK, et al. Oral health and HIV infection among female sex workers in Abidjan, Côte d'Ivoire. BMC Oral Health. 2015;**15**(1):154. DOI: 10.1186/s12903-015-0129-0

[99] Oyedeji OA, Gbolahan OO, Abe EO, Agelebe E. Oral and dental lesions in HIV infected Nigerian children. The Pan African Medical Journal. 2015;**20**: 287. DOI: 10.11604/pamj.2015.20.287.5273

[100] Shiboski CH, Webster-Cyriaque JY, Ghannoum M, Dittmer DP, Greenspan JS. Oral HIV/AIDS research alliance, subcommittee of the aids clinical trial group. The Oral HIV/AIDS research alliance program: Lessons learned and future directions. Oral Diseases. 2016;**22**(Suppl 1):128-134. DOI: 10.1111/odi.12409

[101] Ottria L, Lauritano D, Oberti L, Candotto V, Cura F, Tagliabue A, et al. Prevalence of HIV-related oral manifestations and their association with HAART and CD4+ T cell count: A review. Journal of Biological Regulators and Homeostatic Agents. 2018;**32**(2 Suppl. 1):51-59

[102] Chaudhary P, Manral K, Gupta R, Bengani AKS, Chauhan BI, Arora D. Oral health status and treatment needs among HIV/AIDS patients attending antiretroviral therapy center in Western India: A cross-sectional study. Journal of Family Medicine and Primary Care. 2020;**9**(7):3722-3728. DOI: 10.4103/jfmpc.jfmpc_411_20

[103] Muralidharan S, Mahendrakar S, Talekar A, Nara A, Kanitkar AA, Kanitkar A, et al. Oral health-related quality of life in HIV: A systematic review. The Journal of Contemporary Dental Practice. 2020;**21**(5):585-592

[104] Barbi W, Shalini K, Kumari A, Raaj V, Gupta H, Gauniyal P, et al. Assessment of oral health and prevalence of oral conditions in human immunodeficiency virus-infected subjects visiting antiretroviral therapy centers. Journal of Pharmacy & Bioallied Sciences. 2021;**13**(Suppl. 2):S1470-S1473. DOI: 10.4103/jpbs.jpbs_256_21

[105] Joint United Nations Programme on HIV/AIDS (UNAIDS). Global HIV & AIDS statistics — Fact sheet. 2021. Available from: https://www.unaids.org/en/resources/fact-sheet.

[106] Greenspan JS, Barr CE, Sciubba JJ, Winkler JR. Oral manifestations of HIV infection. Definitions, diagnostic criteria, and principles of therapy. Oral Surgery, Oral Medicine, and Oral Pathology. 1992;**73**(2):142-144. DOI: 10.1016/0030-4220(92)90185-s

[107] EC-Clearinghouse on Oral Problems Related to HIV Infection and WHO Collaborating Centre on Oral Manifestations of the Immunodeficiency Virus. Classification and diagnostic criteria for oral lesions in HIV infection. Journal of Oral Pathology & Medicine. 1993;**22**:289-291

[108] Sousa RH, Souza LL, Guedes PT, Prado-Ribeiro AC, Rodrigues-Oliveira L, Brandão TB, et al. Oral Kaposi sarcoma development is associated with HIV viral load, CD4+ count and CD4+/CD8+ ratio. Medicina Oral, Patología Oral y Cirugía Bucal. 2021;**26**(6):e748-e753. DOI: 10.4317/medoral.24708

[109] Baba MM, Buba F, Talle MA, Umar H, Garbati M, Abdul H. Relationship between CD4 cell count, viral load and left ventricular function among HIV-1 infected patients asymptomatic for cardiac disease on HAART. West African Journal of Medicine. 2021;**38**(6):571-577

[110] Shu W, Li C, Du F, Bai J, Duan K. A real-world, cross sectional study of oral lesions and their association with CD4 cell counts and HIV viral load in Yunnan, China. Medicine (Baltimore). 2020;**99**(40):e22416. DOI: 10.1097/MD.0000000000022416

[111] Memish ZA, Al-Tawfiq JA, Filemban SM, Qutb S, Fodail A, Ali B, et al. Antiretroviral therapy, CD4, viral load, and disease stage in HIV patients in Saudi Arabia: A 2001-2013 cross-sectional study. Journal of Infection in Developing Countries. 2015;**9**(7): 765-769. DOI: 10.3855/jidc.6588

[112] Patton LL, Ramirez-Amador V, Anaya-Saavedra G, Nittayananta W, Carrozzo M, Ranganathan K. Urban legends series: Oral manifestations of HIV infection. Oral Diseases. 2013;**19**(6): 533-550. DOI: 10.1111/odi.12103

[113] Berberi A, Aoun G. Oral lesions associated with human immunodeficiency virus in 75 adult patients: A clinical study. Journal of the Korean Association of Oral and Maxillofacial Surgeons. 2017;**43**(6): 388-394. DOI: 10.5125/jkaoms.2017.43.6.388

[114] Ranganathan K, Umadevi KMR. Common oral opportunistic infections in human immunodeficiency virus infection/acquired immunodeficiency syndrome: Changing epidemiology; diagnostic criteria and methods; management protocols. Periodontology. 2000. 2019;**80**(1):177-188. DOI: 10.1111/prd.12274

[115] Orlandini RK, Bepu DAN, Saraiva MDCP, Bollela VR, Motta ACF, Lourenço AG. Are Candida albicans isolates from the oral cavity of HIV-infected patients more virulent than from non-HIV-infected patients? Systematic review and meta-analysis. Microbial Pathogenesis. 2020;**149**: 104477. DOI: 10.1016/j.micpath.2020.104477

[116] Spalanzani RN, Mattos K, Marques LI, Barros PFD, Pereira PIP, Paniago AMM, et al. Clinical and laboratorial features of oral candidiasis in HIV-positive patients. Revista da Sociedade Brasileira de Medicina Tropical. 2018;**51**(3):352-356. DOI: 10.1590/0037-8682-0241-2017

[117] Ribeiro Ribeiro AL, de Alencar Menezes TO, de Melo A-JS, de Menezes SA, Marques-da-Silva SH, Rosário Vallinoto AC. Oral carriage of Candida species in HIV-infected patients during highly active antiretroviral therapy (HAART) in Belém, Brazil. Oral Surgery, Oral Medicine, Oral Pathology, Oral Radiology. 2015;**120**(1):29-33. DOI: 10.1016/j.oooo.2015.03.008

[118] Paula SB, Morey AT, Santos JP, Santos PM, Gameiro DG, Kerbauy G, et al. Oral Candida colonization in HIV-infected patients in Londrina-PR, Brazil: Antifungal susceptibility and virulence factors. Journal of Infection in Developing Countries. 2015;**9**(12): 1350-1359. DOI: 10.3855/jidc.6970

[119] Greenspan D. Treatment of oral candidiasis in HIV infection. Oral Surgery, Oral Medicine, and Oral Pathology. 1994;**78**(2):211-215. DOI: 10.1016/0030-4220(94)90149-x

[120] Menon T, Umamaheswari K, Kumarasamy N, Solomon S, Thyagarajan SP. Efficacy of fluconazole and itraconazole in the treatment of oral candidiasis in HIV patients. Acta Tropica. 2001;**80**(2):151-154. DOI: 10.1016/s0001-706x(01)00170-x

[121] Caton JG, Armitage G, Berglundh T, Chapple ILC, Jepsen S, Kornman KS, et al. A new classification scheme for

periodontal and peri-implant diseases and conditions - Introduction and key changes from the 1999 classification. Journal of Clinical Periodontology. 2018; **45**(Suppl 20):S1-S8. DOI: 10.1111/jcpe.12935

[122] Jakubovics NS, Goodman SD, Mashburn-Warren L, Stafford GP, Cieplik F. The dental plaque biofilm matrix. Periodontology 2000. 2021;**86**(1):32-56. DOI: 10.1111/prd.12361

[123] Socransky SS, Haffajee AD, Cugini MA, Smith C, Kent RL Jr. Microbial complexes in subgingival plaque. Journal of Clinical Periodontology. 1998;**25**(2):134-144. DOI: 10.1111/j.1600-051x.1998.tb02419.x

[124] de Menezes S, Menezes T, Rodrigues T, Nogueira B, Fonseca R. Analysis of IL-10 in HIV-1 patients with chronic periodontitis in northern Brazil. Brazilian Journal of Oral Sciences. 2017; **16**:17072-17081

[125] Shaikh HFM, Patil SH, Pangam TS, Rathod KV. Polymicrobial synergy and dysbiosis: An overview. Journal of Indian Society of Periodontology. 2018;**22**(2): 101-106. DOI: 10.4103/jisp.jisp_385_17

[126] Herrera D, Retamal-Valdes B, Alonso B, Feres M. Acute periodontal lesions (periodontal abscesses and necrotizing periodontal diseases) and endo-periodontal lesions. Journal of Periodontology. 2018;**89**(Suppl. 1):S85-S102. DOI: 10.1002/JPER.16-0642

[127] Fonseca RRS, Carvalho CA, Rodrigues TMS, Cavaleiro RMS, Menezes SAF, Machado LFA. Severe necrotizing periodontitis in an HIV-infected patient: Case report and non-surgical treatment. Clinical Advances in Periodontics. 2021;**11**(2):59-63. DOI: 10.1002/cap.10105

[128] Gomez RS, da Costa JE, Loyola AM, de Araújo NS, de Araújo VC. Immunohistochemical study of linear gingival erythema from HIV-positive patients. Journal of Periodontal Research. 1995;**30**(5):355-359. DOI: 10.1111/j.1600-0765.1995.tb01287.x

[129] Mete O, Keskin Y, Hafiz G, Kayhan KB, Unur M. Oral proliferative verrucous leukoplakia: Underdiagnosed oral precursor lesion that requires retrospective clinicopathological correlation. Dermatology Online Journal. 2010;**16**(5):6

[130] Carrard VC, van der Waal I. A clinical diagnosis of oral leukoplakia; A guide for dentists. Medicina Oral, Patología Oral y Cirugía Bucal. 2018; **23**(1):e59-e64. DOI: 10.4317/medoral.22292

[131] van der Waal I. Oral leukoplakia; A proposal for simplification and consistency of the clinical classification and terminology. Medicina Oral, Patología Oral y Cirugía Bucal. 2019;**24**(6):e799-e803. DOI: 10.4317/medoral.23372

[132] Ghosh S, Rao RS, Upadhyay MK, Kumari K, Sanketh DS, Raj AT, et al. Proliferative verrucous leukoplakia revisited: A retrospective clinicopathological study. Clinics and Practice. 2021;**11**(2):337-346. DOI: 10.3390/clinpract11020048

[133] Sandler AS, Kaplan LD. Diagnosis and management of systemic non-Hodgkin's lymphoma in HIV disease. Hematology/Oncology Clinics of North America. 1996;**10**(5):1111-1124. DOI: 10.1016/s0889-8588(05)70387-7

[134] Ji Y, Lu H. Malignancies in HIV-infected and AIDS patients. Advances in Experimental Medicine and Biology. 2017;**1018**:167-179. DOI: 10.1007/978-981-10-5765-6_10

[135] Thandra KC, Barsouk A, Saginala K, Padala SA, Barsouk A, Rawla P. Epidemiology of non-hodgkin's lymphoma. Medical Sciences. 2021;**9**(1): 5. DOI: 10.3390/medsci9010005

[136] Muller K, Kazimiroff J, Fatahzadeh M, Smith RV, Wiltz M, Polanco J, et al. Oral human papillomavirus infection and oral lesions in HIV-positive and HIV-negative dental patients. The Journal of Infectious Diseases. 2015;**212**(5):760-768. DOI: 10.1093/infdis/jiv080

[137] Vianna LMS, Carneiro FP, Amorim R, Guerra ENDS, Cavalcanti Neto FF, Tiziani V, et al. Oropharynx HPV status and its relation to HIV infection. PeerJ. 2018;**6**:e4407. DOI: 10.7717/peerj.4407

[138] Johnson NW, Anaya-Saavedra G, Webster-Cyriaque J. Viruses and oral diseases in HIV-infected individuals on long-term antiretroviral therapy: What are the risks and what are the mechanisms? Oral Diseases. 2020;**26** (Suppl. 1):80-90. DOI: 10.1111/odi.13471

[139] Cavallari EN, Ceccarelli G, Santinelli L, Innocenti GP, De Girolamo G, Borrazzo C, et al. Clinical effects of oral bacteriotherapy on anal HPV infection and related dysplasia in HIV-positive MSM: Results from the "HPVinHIV" trial. Biomedicine. 2021; **9**(11):1738. DOI: 10.3390/biomedicines9111738

Chapter 9

Psychiatric Problems in HIV Care

Seggane Musisi and Noeline Nakasujja

Abstract

Psychiatric problems associated with HIV/AIDS are many, varied and often bidirectional and they are often neglected. Their presence compromises HIV care and prevention efforts. Unaddressed, they compromise treatment outcomes, increase HIV virus–resistant strains, leave pockets of potential HIV spread in the community and lead to poor quality of life and early death of Persons Living With HIV/AIDS. This chapter focuses on specific HIV-associated mental disorders and their management. However, the mental health problems of HIV/AIDS go beyond disorders to include social, family and community problems such as the problems faced by AIDS orphans, widowhood, family disruptions, multiple deaths, bereavements, poverty, stigma, caregiver burden, education and occupational difficulties etc. All these need to be addressed in holistic HIV care. This calls for more research and integration of mental healthcare in all HIV/AIDS treatment and prevention programs.

Keywords: HIV/AIDS, anxiety, depression, mania, psychosis, dementia

1. Introduction

HIV/AIDS is an intimately sexually embedded disease and as such connected to human reproduction and hence human perpetuation [1]. Sexuality, itself, is a bio-psycho-social phenomenon, the regulation of which has fascinated humans from time immemorial. It is a subject of religious, cultural and ultimately government concern especially as it impacts human health and hence healthcare provision. Secondly, HIV/AIDS is a fatal condition and mainly a disease of those in the reproductive age. However, it now spans all ages as it can be transmitted perinatally from mother to fetus and, can be managed with modern drugs up to old age. This makes HIV/AIDS a chronic disease for which one has to adjust and take medications for life hence inherently laden with problems associated with medication compliance and adherence. Being predominantly sexually transmitted and fatal makes HIV/AIDS highly stigmatized. HIV is an infectious disease which is predominantly sexually transmitted [2]. Prevention of HIV infection is a prolog of public health, but in the domain of human behavioral change, calling for measures to regulate human behavior to curb HIV infection risk. Thus, mental health problems impacting HIV infection risk become of utmost concern in HIV care [3]. The HIV virus is neuropathic invading brain tissue soon after infection and giving rise to a host of psychiatric disorders which call for treatment [2]. The secondary infections associated with HIV/AIDS and the drugs to treat them as well as the antiretroviral (ARVs) drugs themselves may also cause psychiatric complications [1]. Lastly, the high numbers of HIV/AIDS deaths have caused much family disruptions due to the orphans left behind as well as widowhood with significant socio-economic, educational and occupational ramifications [4–6]. For all these reasons and many more as will be seen, the psychiatric, social and behavioral mental health problems associated with HIV/AIDS are many and call for their management in HIV care [5–7]. This chapter will give an overview of the mental health problems which are frequently encountered in HIV care, their effects and how to manage them. It will also discuss the need to integrate mental health care in HIV/AIDS management and how this impacts outcomes of treatment.

1.1 Classification of the mental health problems encountered in HIV care

Significant research has shown that the relationship between mental illness and HIV/AIDS is bidirectional. First, mental illness and other premorbid psycho-behavioral patterns are risk factors to contracting HIV infection [2, 5, 7]. On the other hand HIV/AIDS predisposes to getting psychiatric disorder. Both have to be addressed in HIV care efforts and infection spread prevention. Unaddressed, they leave pockets in the population which hinder effective control of the HIV pandemic.

2. Premorbid behavioral psychopathology in HIV/AIDS

In HIV-related mental health problems and illness, it is important to discuss premorbid psychopathology and psychosocial risk behaviors in HIV/AIDS as these factors complicate the post-infection clinical picture and impact treatment outcomes including treatment adherence and HIV infection risk [5]. Premorbid behavioral psychopathology in HIV/AIDS includes the following:

1. Personality Disorders

2. High HIV-infection risk groups

3. Pre-existing psychiatric illness

4. Substance Abuse

5. Vulnerable populations

    a. Orphans and other vulnerable children (OVCs)

    b. Marginalized poor communities

    c. Conflict communities—Refugees, Displaced Persons, war & disaster affected

    d. The elderly

    e. Women

Personality disorders represent enduring maladaptive ways of behaving and coping with life's challenges often with non-conformity to society's expectations, adjusting to stresses, or relating to others [8]. Examples include Antisocial Personality

Disorder, Borderline Personality Disorder, Dependent Personality Disorder or Avoidant Personality Disorder. Individuals with Personality disorders are more likely to not comply with treatment recommendations, to break rules, to abuse substances, not to practice safe sex and to present as difficult patients including being manipulative, dependent or avoidant. They present problems of treatment non-compliance and high HIV-infection risk behaviors. Management consists of long-term psychotherapy geared to behavior change, setting boundaries and instituting firm limitations.

In Western countries, high HIV-infection risk groups were classified as Homosexual men, Hemophiliacs, Intravenous drug users (Heroin) and Blacks (Haitians) [5]. In Africa, HIV-transmission is by and large heterosexual followed by mother-to-child (vertical) transmission [5]. The determinants to HIV infection here are related to socio-economic and power dynamics [2]. Thus high rates of HIV have been found in post-conflict communities, fishing villages and overcrowded urban centers with high rates of poverty and loosely connected family ties such as slums, casual workers, recreation and bar attenders [5, 7]. Mother-to-child transmission remains a big problem because of the unbalanced power dynamics in matters pertaining to negotiating sex and money which makes women more subordinate and thus more susceptible to HIV infection. These social determinants also operate for the common mental disorders of depression, anxiety, post-traumatic disorder associated with family violence and substance abuse.

Individuals with pre-existing Severe Mental Illness (SMI), such as Schizophrenia, Bipolar Disorder and Major Depression, have been found to have a higher prevalence of HIV infection compared to those without SMI [9, 10] . In a study of SMI patients at a psychiatric hospital in Uganda, Maling et al. [9] found a prevalence of HIV infection of 18% compared to 7% in the general population. Lundberg et al. [10] found an HIV prevalence of 11.3% in hospitalized SMI patients. Thus SMI predisposes to HIV infection risk. Lastly, Nakimuli et al. [11, 12] found a high prevalence of HIV-infection in individuals with alcohol dependence and depression in Uganda. These groups of individuals with pre-existing mental disorders are usually less likely to be compliant with ARV medication adherence and they are also less likely to practice safe sex such as condom use [13]. Moreover, often HIV prevention efforts have not targeted the population of the mentally ill for their messaging thus leaving a pocket of potential HIV infection spread in the community. Management calls for definitive treatment of the SMI with appropriate psychotropic medications and psychotherapy and follow up as these conditions tend to be life-long [14]. All this points to the need to integrate mental healthcare in efforts of HIV care and prevention.

Vulnerable populations comprise of those groups of people or communities within a country that have characteristics putting them at risk of being excluded from social, economic, political or environmental resources hence needing humanitarian assistance due to the barriers they face [15]. In HIV/AIDS care, these groups often comprise of, but are not limited to, orphans and other vulnerable children (OVCs), marginalized poor communities,, the elderly, and conflict/post-conflict communities including refugees, immigrants and displaced persons, as well as the war and disaster affected. These groups tend to have poor access to health services and have higher rates of mental illness, especially depression and Post-traumatic Stress disorder and are at increased risk of HIV-infection [16]. They are also less likely to be targeted in HIV care and prevention messaging. Specific measures need to be taken to ensure their access to psychosocial care. Group Support Psychotherapy (GSP) has been found to be especially effective in addressing their care needs [16, 17].

3. Acute psychological problems and reactions following the HIV/AIDS diagnosis

Despite effective pharmacotherapies in HIV care, a positive HIV test still invokes stressful psychological reactions, which are not the result of HIV neuronal involvement [5]. The reasons for these reactions are many including the following:

1. *STD*: HIV infection is to a large extent a Sexually Transmitted Disease, STD. Because of this, it remains secretive and associated with social, cultural, religious and moral judgments including sexual looseness, sexual orientation and character integrity.

2. *Stigma*: Because of the sexual nature of the disease it attracts both internalized (self) and externalized (others) stigma. Stigma in society, including among health-workers, compromises access to care by the affected person.

3. *Infectious*: HIV is highly infectious and concerns of contagion still loom high in society e.g. school children at play or other potentially bruising physical contacts.

4. *Chronic and Fatal*: HIV/AIDS is still a fatal disease despite advanced and effective pharmacotherapies but which only make it a chronic diseases for which one has to take medications and attend clinics for life. HIV Chronicity and fatality invokes fear.

5. *Disfiguring*: Dermatological, body image and tumor disfigurements may still occur in HIV/AIDS including hair changes despite taking ARVs.

6. *CNS Involvement*: HIV infection invades the brain early and may cause transient changes in thinking, cognition and perception.

7. *The Medications*: ARV medications have serious side effects which may make it difficult to take them. Moreover, one has to adjust to taking them daily for life without fail for them to work well.

8. *Opportunistic Infections*: These occur frequently in HIV/AIDS due to immunosuppression. These opportunistic infections may be associated with stigma e.g. fungal dermatoses and nail infections, pulmonary tuberculosis, Kaposi's Sarcoma, GIT upsets, GU candidiasis etc.

The observed psychological reactions do not connote brain pathology but a psychological, emotional and behavioral reaction to the news that indeed one is now infected with HIV hence challenging the individual's ego defense and coping mechanisms. The frequently encountered psychological reactions to the HIV diagnosis include Adjustment Disorders, Acute Stress Disorder, Post-traumatic Stress Disorder and Suicidal ideations [5]. They occur early on learning of the diagnosis and often present as psychiatric emergences demanding immediate intervention e.g. suicidal attempts, panic attacks etc.

3.1 Adjustment disorders

News of a positive HIV-infection diagnosis is traumatic and the recipient has to adjust to the new reality. Adjustment disorders occur as emotional or behavioral symptoms occurring within 3 months following the psychologically traumatic stressor of the HIV-positive news causing clinically significant marked distress and causing impairment in social, occupational, academic or other performance [8]. Adjustment disorders occur within 3 months of the diagnosis and do not persist for longer than 6 months. They may take any of the following six forms [8]:

i. *Adjustment Disorder with Depressed Mood.* Symptoms include: depressed mood, sleeplessness, tearfulness, hopelessness, and suicidal ideation.

ii. *Adjustment Disorder with Anxiety.* Symptoms include nervousness, panic, worry, jitteriness and fear.

iii. *Adjustment Disorder with Anxiety and Depressed Mood.* This involves a combination *of symptoms of both anxiety and depression.*

iv. *Adjustment Disorder with Disturbance of Conduct.* Symptoms include: aggressiveness, violence, destruction of property, recklessness, reckless sex, fighting, substance abuse, or other antisocial behavior.

v. *Adjustment Disorder with Mixed Disturbance of Emotions and Conduct*. This involves a combination of symptoms of anxiety, depression and disturbance of conduct.

vi. *Adjustment Disorder Unspecified.* Symptoms do not fit any of the above. They include behaviors like social withdrawal/inhibitions or dis-inhibitions not normally exhibited by the person.

3.2 Acute stress disorder and post-traumatic stress disorder (PTSD)

Acute Stress Disorder (ASD) has also called Acute Stress Reaction is a transient mental disorder that develops following the traumatic mental stressor, e.g. news of HIV diagnosis [8]. Individual vulnerability and coping capacity play a role in the occurrence and severity of the ASD. The symptoms appear within minutes to 30 days of the impact of the stressful traumatic news of the HIV diagnosis but may disappear within 30 days. If the symptoms persist longer than this, the diagnosis is then changed to Post-traumatic Stress Disorder, PTSD, otherwise the DSM-5 diagnostic criteria for ASD and PTSD are similar and they include [8]:

- Experiencing or learning of the traumatic event (news of the HIV diagnosis)

- Re-experiencing intrusive symptoms—recurrent, involuntary thoughts, dreams (nightmares) and flashbacks causing intense psychological or physiological distress with reminders of the traumatic event (news of the HIV diagnosis).

- Dissociative symptoms—altered sense of reality with depersonalization and derealization and inability to recall details of events with selective dissociative amnesia.

- Avoidance symptoms—patient avoids reminders of the trauma of the news of the HIV diagnosis including avoiding memories, thoughts, feelings, people, places, events, conversations, activities, things or situations.

- Arousal symptoms—sleep disturbances, irritability, anger outbursts, verbal or physical aggression, poor concentration, hyper- vigilance or exaggerated startle response.

- Negative mood—inability to experience positive emotions: happiness, satisfaction, love. Also there are stress emotions of increased autonomic activity which include anger outbursts, hyper-vigilance, startle response, or, verbal or physical aggression, recklessness, poor concentration, feelings of tension, fear and anxiety (panic).

- For PTSD, the duration of symptoms must be for more than 1 month and causing significant distress to the ones affected with impairment of social and occupational/school functioning. The PTSD symptom constellations evolve in a timely fashion which constitutes the sub-types of PTSD as follows:

    1. *ASD*: The symptoms occur within 30 days of the trauma (of the HIV diagnosis)

    2. *Acute PTSD*: The duration of PTSD symptoms is 30 to 90 days.

    3. *Chronic PTSD*: The duration of PTSD symptoms is 90 or more days.

    4. *Delayed Onset PTSD*: The PTSD symptoms occur within 6 months or more of the trauma (of the HIV diagnosis).

The risk factors for developing the acute psychological disorders to the HIV diagnosis include [5, 7]:

- A previous history of psychiatric illness,
- Lack of social, occupational and family support
- Financial and logistical uncertainty
- Poor access to healthcare
- Unavailability of adequate pre- and post-test counseling

The management of the acute psychological reactions includes [5]:

- Adequate pre- and post-test counseling and follow-up.
- Psychosocial and family support.
- Psychotherapy: CBT, Supportive individual, family and group support psychotherapy (GSP).
- Medications: benzodiazepines (alprazolam, clonazepam), antidepressants (tricyclics—imipramine, amitriptyline and SSRIs—fluoxetine, paroxetine, sertraline).
- Hospitalization is indicated for the severely affected or those with suicidal ideation.

4. The specific HIV-associated mental disorders

These are classified as [5, 7]:

1. Anxiety Disorders
2. Mood Disorders
3. Psychotic Disorders
4. HIV-Associated Neurocognitive Disorders, HAND.
5. Substance Use Disorders

4.1 Anxiety disorders

Anxiety is defined as an emotional response of excessive fear to a real, imagined or perceived threat or anticipation of a future threat. Affected individuals may experience one or more anxiety states comprising of physiological activation, increased behavioral response, restlessness and cognitive dissonance [8]. Anxiety disorders differ from normative anxiety by being excessive, persistent, typically lasting 6 months or more, and causing impairment in one's life functioning [8]. The prevalence of Anxiety disorders in the general population is about 18% [18] but is higher occurring in about 20–35% of individuals with HIV/AIDS and may evolve from Adjustment Disorders or occur on their own [5, 7, 19]. They take the form of generalized anxiety, panic attacks or obsessional fears. The affected individuals have difficulty controlling apprehension and worry coupled with increased muscular tension, and autonomic hyper-arousal resulting in fear symptoms which include shaking or tremulousness, choking feelings, hyperventilation, increased heart rate, sweating, goose flesh, sleeplessness, increased urinary frequency and gastrointestinal upset with frequent loose stools or even frank diarrhea [8]. Cognitively, one becomes restless, hyper-vigilant, irritable, tense and has difficulty in concentration accompanied by fears of dying, loss of control or something dreadful happening

Anxiety disorder	Characteristic symptoms	Prevalence (%)
Generalized anxiety disorder (GAD)	Excessive anxiety and worry about a number of events or activities. Difficulty controlling worry.	0.4–3.6
Panic disorder	Recurrent unexpected panic attacks. At least one panic attack followed by worry of future attacks accompanied with changes in behavior to avoid future attacks.	2–3
Social anxiety disorder	Marked fear or anxiety about one or more social situations in which the individual is exposed or for possible scrutiny by others. Fear of negative evaluation e.g. in audiences.	2–7
Agoraphobia	Marked fear or anxiety about situations in which one may have a panic attack, such as being in open crowds, being outside of the home alone etc. Avoidance of such situations where escape or exit may not be easily available.	1.7
Specific phobia	Marked fear or anxiety about a specific object or situation	7–9

Table 1.
Symptoms and prevalence of anxiety disorders found in HIV/AIDS.

to them. Some patients develop hypochondriacally fixated with excessive concerns about bodily functions and exaggerating any bodily discomforts or pains. The specific DSM-5 Anxiety disorders found in HIV/AIDS are Generalized Anxiety Disorder (GAD), Panic Disorder, Social Anxiety Disorder, Agoraphobia and Specific phobias [8]. Brandt et al. [19] summarized their symptom characteristics and prevalence as indicated in **Table 1**.

Symptomatic anxiety is arguably the most prevalent psychiatric disorder in HIV/AIDS. It may occur as Adjustment disorder with Anxious Mood, be persistent as GAD and panic attacks, arise sporadically with reminders of the HIV infection (e.g. news of HIV/AIDS deaths, development of new symptoms such as TB or skin changes including Herpes Zoster rashes etc.) or become a chronic condition with preoccupation with physical symptoms or with illness progression. Anxiety Disorders in HIV/AIDS must be treated as they often impair daily functioning interfering with Quality of Life. Psychotherapy with Supportive Counseling and Behavioral Activation techniques should be tried first. Long-term psychotherapy is often useful individually or in groups employing Interpersonal Psychotherapy, IPT [20]; Interpersonal Group Psychotherapy, IGPT [21]; Group Support Psychotherapy, GSP [16]; or Cognitive Behavioral Psychotherapy, CBT [22]. Psychopharmacotherapy is indicated when symptoms persist, are debilitating or present as panic emergences with patients running to hospitals or clinics repeatedly [23]. Short acting benzodiazepines such as Alprazolam or Lorazepam are useful in controlling the acute symptoms of panic attacks. The persistent tension and sleeplessness can be controlled using longer acting benzodiazepines such as Clonazepam. Use of benzodiazepines should be brief, not lasting more than 2 to 3 weeks to avoid dependence to these medications. Antidepressants are indicated for persistent or recurrent symptoms or when depression sets in. The antidepressants of choice include tricyclic antidepressants (imipramine or amitriptyline), SSRIs (fluoxetine, paroxetine, sertraline) or SNRIs such as venlafaxine. These antidepressants must be given in clinically therapeutic dosages and for sufficient duration of at least 6-months, but may stretch to 1–2 years in some patients. Concomitant use of non-prescription medications and substance abuse (alcohol and or illicit drugs) must be looked out for and addressed.

4.2 Mood disorders

Mood disorders of major concern in HIV/AIDS comprise of Depression and Bipolar Affective Disorder. HIV-associated mood disorders must be distinguished from Primary mood disorders. However, it is important to effectively treat and, if possible, prevent Primary Affective Disorders as these are risk factors for HIV infection as composite SMIs. If not properly addressed, both HIV-associated mood disorders and Primary mood disorders compromise HIV/AIDS care outcomes, increase risk of HIV infection spread and impact the Quality of Life of individuals living with HIV/AIDS.

4.2.1 Depression

Depression is common in people living with HIV/AIDS (PLWH) with a lifetime prevalence of about 40% [24] compared to 4–8% in the general population [25] and also about 41% of HIV-affected children and adolescents [26]. DSM-5 gives diagnostic criteria for depression as comprising of two or more weeks of depressed mood most of the day, nearly every day and/or diminished interest/pleasure in activities previously enjoyed [8]. These two are accompanied by at least 4 of the following: loss of appetite and weight, sleep disturbance (usually poor sleep), psychomotor agitation or retardation, fatigue or loss of energy, feelings of worthlessness and/or hopelessness, poor concentration and memory, indecisiveness, suicidal ideation or attempts or pre-occupation with death. These depressive symptoms cause clinically significant distress and impairment of functioning and must not be due to effects of substances, other medical conditions or bereavement. Akena et al. [27] described the clinical and associated features of HIV- associated depression in adults as distinct from Depression in HIV-negative individuals. They found that the Depression of HIV/AIDS tended to occur earlier on in the HIV disease (WHO stages I & II) and was not associated with increased immunosuppression (as measured with CD4 counts) but was associated with cognitive decline as measured by the Mini Mental Status Examination, MMSE. Its onset was in older patients, (>30 years), who were more likely to be widowed or never married and had a negative a family history of affective disorder compared to HIV-negative depressed patients. On the Beck Depression Inventory, BDI, depressed PLWH were more likely to have more loss of appetite and weight, had poorer sleep, felt more fatigue, and were more self-critical and indecisive. Studies of Depression in HIV/AIDS have found poorer treatment outcomes and a poorer quality of life in untreated depressive PLWH [28]. They have poorer adherence to treatment recommendations including poor adherence to ARVs [29, 30] and are more likely to engage in risky sexual behaviors including non-condom use [31] and substance abuse [11] as well as domestic violence, child abuse and suicide [5].

Treatment of depression in PLWH includes Social treatments, Psychotherapy and antidepressant medications [30]. Antidepressant medications are almost always indicated in the management of HIV-associated depression because of the biological nature of its etiology being linked to early CNS HIV viral involvement [5]. Commonly used antidepressants include tricyclic antidepressants—imipramine, amitriptyline or their breakdown products of desipramine and nortriptyline respectively; and the SSRI group of antidepressants as quite effective and associated with fewer side effects [32]. These medications include fluoxetine, sertraline, citalopram, escitalopram, paroxetine as well as other types of antidepressants including SNRIs like Venlafaxine. Individual and group psychotherapy has been found to be effective and should always be combined with the pharmacotherapy. Of particular effectiveness has been IPT and IGPT [20, 21]. More recently GSP as developed by Nakimuli et al. [17] has been found to be especially effective in LMIC in Africa as it addresses commonly associated family and social issues such as stigma, poverty, neighborhood wrangles, poor community welfare including insecurity, water and food shortages in especially post-conflict communities where PTSD, substance abuse and domestic as well as other violence is also common.

4.2.2 Bipolar affective disorder

Bipolar affective disorder frequently occurs in HIV/AIDS with a prevalence of up to 4.3% compared to 1% in the general population [33]. The DSM-5 diagnostic criteria for Bipolar Affective Disorder, Manic Phase, include at least 1 week of a distinctively elevated, expansive or irritable mood with persistently increased goal-directed activity or energy present most of the day, nearly every day and calling for a need for intervention [8]. This is then accompanied with at least 4 of the following symptoms: inflated self-esteem or grandiosity, decreased need for sleep, increased talkativeness, racing thoughts with flight of ideas, distractibility, over-activity including risky behaviors such buying sprees, high libido with sexual indiscretions, unrealistic business deals, argumentativeness with sometimes aggressiveness and violence. In one study, Nakimuli et al. [34] described the clinical features of HIV-associated secondary mania as distinct compared to Primary Bipolar mania. HIV-related secondary mania is characterized by older age of onset, higher prevalence in females, more likely to occur in widowed, separated or divorced PLWH. Symptomatically, it has more manic symptoms as measured on the Young Mania Rating Scale (YMRS), has more irritable/elated mood, is more aggressive and disruptive with more decreased need for sleep, paranoid delusions, visual and auditory hallucinations and showing more cognitive impairment on the Mini Mental Status Examination (MMSE). The causes of secondary mania of HIV/AIDS include HIV being the sole organic brain insult to the brain as the virus invades the brain early on, HIV-related opportunistic infections, medication-induced mania e.g. psychotropic medications such as antidepressants, steroids, or even ARVs themselves such as zidovudine or didanosine [5]. An individual with a primary bipolar affective disorder can also be infected with HIV, in which case the Bipolar disorder is considered as comorbid with of HIV/AIDS.

A manic episode in PLWH is disruptive of care and leads to poor treatment compliance, non-adherence to ARVs, risky and unsafe sex as well as substance abuse [7, 35]. Untreated, bipolar affective disorder is associated with job losses, marital breakups and poor quality of life. There is also an increased risk of suicide in Bipolar Affective Disorders compared to the general population. The treatment of HIV-related mania follows the same principles as primary mania [36]. Often, a manic episode demands hospitalization including involuntary commitment and or use of restraints or isolation on a secure ward due to the presenting aggression, violence or its disruptive nature. It is important to achieve quick control of the disruptive manic symptoms as they pause a psychiatric emergence with possible harm to others or property. Quick acting parenteral antipsychotics and benzodiazepines are administered and the patient is placed in a quiet isolated room, secure ward or psychiatric intensive care unit. Rapid neuroleptization using intramuscular injections of Haloperidol Hcl or zuclopenthixol acetate combined with injectable promethazine or lorazepam achieve quick control of the patient's symptoms with the required sedation. These are followed by regular 8 or 12 hourly oral doses of atypical antipsychotics such as olanzapine, quetiapine, ziprasidone or risperidone and a longer acting benzodiazepine such as Clonazepam at bedtime for about 1–2 weeks. These are then be tapered down as the symptoms become controlled and mood stabilizers are added to the regimen, such as Lithium Carbonate or anticonvulsants such as sodium valproate, carbamazepine or lamotrigine. Blood levels of these drugs must be checked after 2 weeks of equilibration, to avoid toxicity and maintain therapeutic levels. When all symptoms are controlled medications are tapered down to minimal maintenance doses, to avoid relapses and preferably administered at bedtime only. Bipolar disorders in HIV/AIDS respond very quickly to medications but it needs maintenance therapy to avoid relapses which may become more frequent with cognitive decline. Psychotherapy is commenced as more of a supportive and psycho-educative nature initially and should involve the family as a trialogue involving the patient, supporting family caretaker and the clinician. Family Psychosocial Involvement Interventions have been found to be effective in SMI including Bipolar Affective Disorders [36].

4.3 Psychotic disorders

Similar to mood disorders in PLWH, psychotic disorders can be either primary predating HIV infection and considered as comorbid to HIV/AIDS or as secondary to HIV infection as new onset psychotic illnesses associated with the HIV/AIDS disease [7, 33, 37]. Severe mental illness (SMI), a category to which psychotic disorders belong, has been associated with high rates of HIV-infection [9, 10]. In a study of individuals with first episode psychosis in Uganda, Maling et al. [9] found an HIV infection prevalence of 18.3% in patients with newly onset psychosis in a psychiatric hospital in Uganda. Lundberg et al. [10] found 11.3% of persons hospitalized with SMI in Uganda to have a HIV infection which prevalence was greater in women. The prevalence of psychosis in PLWH has been reported to be in range of 5–15% [37] . Psychotic disorder is characterized by the presence of delusions, hallucinations, disordered thinking, speech and behavior as well as deterioration in social, occupational and daily functioning due to distorted reality testing [8]. The mechanism of causation of new onset psychotic disorders in HIV/AIDS is complex and multifactorial. Viral invasion of the brain, opportunistic infections and the multiple medications used as well as general debilitation and progression of the disease with cognitive impairment all contribute to causing new onset psychosis of HIV/AIDS [5, 37]. The HIV virus invades sub-cortical structures of the brain including the limbic system. The presence of psychosis in PLWH heralds poor prognosis as untreated or poorly treated psychosis compromises treatment adherence with non-attendance of follow ups and a consequent poor quality of life as well as high HIV infection risk sexual behavior. Early death is common.

The clinical presentation of new onset HIV-related psychosis includes late onset psychosis (>30 years), presence of auditory, visual and tactile hallucinations, paranoid and bizarre delusions, affective symptoms, cognitive impairment and behavioral disturbances [5, 37]. HIV associated psychosis is more common in the late stages of the diseases, especially in untreated or poorly treated PLWH. The symptoms are often of a mixed bag and not well formed unlike those of the classical SMIs. There is usually a negative family history of mental illness.

Management of HIV-related psychosis follows the same principles as the non-HIV related psychoses but with concomitant treatment of the HIV/AIDS itself using ARVs and any associated opportunistic infections [5, 37]. Antipsychotic medications are always indicated and are quite effective, starting with small doses and watching out for side effects which are then also treated. The medications include the typical antipsychotics like haloperidol, trifluoperazine, flupenthixol, fluphenazine or with atypical antipsychotics which usually have less extrapyramidal side effects but more metabolic dyslipidemias. The atypical antipsychotics include Olanzapine, Risperidone, Quetiapine, Ziprasidone, Aripiprazole etc. Often PLWH who have psychosis have poor medication compliance, in which case long acting depot preparations are useful such as monthly Risperidone Consta, Abilify Maintena (Depot Aripirazole), Haloperidol Decanoate, Fluphenazine decanoate, Flupenthixol decanoate or even three monthly depot preparations such as Paliperidone Palmitate. Extrapyramidal side effects are managed with anticholinergic medications such as benzhexhol, benztropine or procyclidine. Unlike classical SMIs, new onset HIV-related psychoses respond quickly to medications and which may then be tapered off after 3–6 months of effective treatment. However, in some cases long-term maintenance treatment with low antipsychotic doses is necessary. Psychotherapy of a supportive and psycho-educative nature must always be added to the pharmacotherapy and should involve the family as a trialogue involving the patient, supporting family caretaker and the clinician as Family Psychosocial Involvement Intervention [38].

4.4 HIV-associated neurocognitive disorders (HAND)

HIV-associated cognitive disorder has had considerable research attention in the past 20 years, especially HIV-associated dementia [39]. Neurocognitive disorders or dementias are characterized by difficulties in *attention* (sustenance, selectiveness & processing), *executive function* (planning, habits, decision making, responses, flexibility & error correction), *learning* (memory—immediate, short and long term), *language* (receptive-comprehension, expressive, fluency, grammar, syntax), *perceptiveness* (visual, constructional, motor integration and knowing-gnosis) *social cognition* (recognition of situations/circumstances, emotions and consideration of others) and *motoric praxis* (integrity of learned movements, gesturing, understanding of commands & intentions) [5, 8]. Neurocognitive disorders can be acute, chronic, mild, moderate or severe and debilitating/terminal. DSM 5 classifies dementia as either Mild or Major Neurocognitive Disorder, then specify what it is due to and state whether with or without behavioral disturbance [8].

4.5 HIV dementia

Dementia of HIV infection has gone by many names including HIV-associated dementia (HAD), HIV encephalopathy, AIDS dementia complex, or HIV- associated neurocognitive disorder [40]. DSM 5 classifies it as Mild or Major Neurocognitive Disorder Due To HIV Infection [8]. The Frascati criteria described three cognitive sub-types based on 5 cognitive domains to establish the classification of the neurocognitive effects of the HIV virus on the brain as the HIV-Associated Neurocognitive Disorder (HAND) criteria [41]. The HAND criteria are useful in the identification of cases, monitoring of treatment and instituting caregiving especially in the severe form of the illness. The three HAND categories are Asymptomatic Neurocognitive Impairment (ANI), Mild Neurocognitive Disorder (MND) and HIV-Associated Dementia, HAD as shown in **Table 2**.

In Africa, the prevalence of HAND, with or without ARV treatment was found to be 31% [42]. The prevalence was higher in females and with advanced immunosuppression as measured by low CD4 counts. Adherence to ARV treatment with immune

HAND Category	Asymptomatic Neurocognitive Impairment, ANI	Mild Neurocognitive Disorder, MND	HIV-Associated Dementia, HAD
Activities of Daily Living, ADL	No interference	Mild interference	Marked interference
Cognitive Level	At least 1.0 SD below mean of normative population in one cognitive domain	At least 1.0 SD below mean of normative population in two cognitive domains	At least 2.0 SD below mean of normative population in two cognitive domains

Table 2.
Classification of HIV-associated neurocognitive disorder (HAND).

HAND subtype	Pre ART prevalence (%)	Post ART prevalence (%)
HAD	17	2
MND	10	12
ANI	20	32
No Impairment	53	54

Table 3.
HAND subtypes prevalence in the pre and post ART era.

reconstruction reduces the severity of HAND but does not eliminate it. Nevertheless, this is of utmost importance for PLWH in HIV care as advanced HAND impairs function and QoL. **Table 3** below shows the HAND subtypes prevalence in the pre and post ART era [37].

Screening for HAND is therefore of great importance in HIV care in PLWH. However the cognitive test performances and the tools used are often influenced by educational, cultural and socioeconomic factors. Sacktor et al. [42] reported on the IHDS as a culturally and educationally sensitive instrument for assessing HAD.

The mainstay of treatment for HAND is combination Highly Active Anti-retroviral Therapy, HAART requiring a more than 90% adherence to the ARVs to ensure a very low or undetectable viral load, VL, in order to achieve the necessary immunosuppression. Individual and family psychosocial support is crucial in this exercise. This underscores the importance of integrating mental health care in any HIV care and prevention programs.

4.6 HIV associated delirium

The American DSM-5 diagnostic criteria for delirium are a an acute disturbance in attention and awareness that develops over a short period of time (hours to days) and representing a change from baseline, fluctuating in severity during the course of the day, with disturbances in cognition (memory, disorientation, language, perception) as a direct consequence of a medical condition, substance intoxication or its withdrawal, toxins or due to multiple etiologies [8]. Delirium in HIV/AIDS manifests clinically in the context of high viremia, advanced HIV disease, other infections, drug toxicities and substance abuse or metabolic disturbances [5]. The prevalence of delirium in of hospitalized HIV+ people may be as high as 30–40% [43] especially in those with advanced disease. Untreated delirium often leads to stupor, coma or death.

The mortality rate of delirium can be as high as 20–40% [5, 43]. It is considered a medical emergency and diagnosing it and finding the cause(s) can be lifesaving.

A delirious person has disturbances in sleep continuity and presents as confused in relationship to time, the environment (location) and others, and the confusion waxes and wanes throughout the day, going in and out of a disoriented state, seeing things as they clearly are not, experiencing hallucinations and illusions and often paranoid thinking with behaviors of agitation, fear, anxiety, irritability, restlessness, anger and aggression. They cannot comprehend instructions. The delirium subtypes reflect psychomotor activity and include hyperactive delirium (agitated, hyperalert), hypoactive delirium (lethargic, hypoalert) and mixed states (combination of the two). Seizures are not uncommon in delirium. Dementia and depression must be excluded especially for hypoactive delirium.

Delirium is a medical emergency with a case fatality of 40% and thus calling for immediate hospitalization, sometimes to an intensive care unit [43]. Because of the ever-changing condition of the patient and to reduce external stimuli, delirious patients are managed in the hospital, in a quiet room with clear lighting, constant observation, regular monitoring of vital signs and psychiatric NOBS (Nursing Observation Sheet). The first priority in treating delirium is to ascertain patient safety as they are confused and often fall and injure themselves. They can be aggressive and cannot look after themselves in terms of steadiness, feeding, hygiene, toilet or even dressing. The second priority is to treat the underlying cause (hypoxemia, septicemia, anemia, metabolic and electrolyte imbalances, intoxications, medications, alcohol and illicit drug intoxications or their withdrawal etc.). Disorientation, aggression, paranoia, hallucinations, delusions and anxiety (fear) are treated with parenteral antipsychotic medications (haloperidol, risperidone, olanzapine) often combined with a benzodiazepine (Lorazepam, clonazepam), as tolerated by the patient [43]. Parenteral Thiamine is always administered in alcohol-related delirium. Delirium is frightening to the patient, family and friends. Repeated reassurance and re-orienting of the patient, explaining procedures and establishing a calm and constant environment and nurse/attendant are crucial. Providing a wall clock and calendar that the patient sees easily, and keeping the patient's room well-lighted during the day with dimmed lights at night are useful for patient orientation. For psychotherapy, on recovery, the patient and family are educated about the apparent cause of the delirium to avoid future risk e.g. substance abuse, non-compliance to ARVs and causing worsening of the HIV disease etc. [5, 43]. Psychotherapy helps alleviate the anxiety, guilt, anger, depression, or other emotional states and family dynamics. Prognosis of delirium is usually poor depending on its underlying cause with a fatality rate of 40% within a year of the delirium diagnosis.

4.7 Substance abuse

Substance abuse is defined as the use of illicit drugs and alcohol as well as misuse of prescription and over-the-counter medications [5]. Substances of common abuse in Africa include alcohol, marijuana, cathenone (khat), stimulants (amphetamines) and recently opiates (pain medications) and anxiolytics (benzodiazepines). Drug and alcohol abuse usually increases the indulgence into HIV infection risk behaviors including unsafe sex (multiple partners, unprotected sex), non-disclosure of HIV status to sex partners, sharing needles (in IV drug use) and passing HIV onto others [11]. Substance use leads to reduced judgment and compromises adherence to ART medications and increases chances of engaging in risky sexual behavior. Drugs and alcohol also weaken the immune system, may interact with ARVs reducing efficacy or causing toxic side effects. Alcohol and drugs damage body organs including the liver which is responsible for drug metabolism. They may also lead to other mental disorders including delirium, seizures, depression and even dementia. They are also associated with family, social, educational, occupational and economic problems.

Treatment of drug and alcohol abuse begins with clinician suspicion and detection by direct inquiry and collateral information from family, friends and caretakers [5]. Drug screens and Liver Function tests such as GGT and pancreatic enzymes are helpful in pinpointing end organ (liver, pancreas) damage. Heavy substance dependence often needs hospitalization for medical detoxification followed by referral to Residential Rehabilitation programs for 3, 6, or 12 months and thereafter follow up aftercare for 1–2 years. Self-help support groups are helpful such as Alcoholics Anonymous, AA or Narcotics Anonymous, NA. Detoxification involves prophylactic treatment for withdrawal symptoms including tremors, sweats, rebound insomnia and anxiety and even psychotic symptoms and seizures. Any associated substance-induced mental disorder such as anxiety, depression, psychosis or seizures is specifically treated. Family support is necessary to help the individual to stay totally abstinent from the substance of abuse.

5. Conclusion

Psychiatric problems associated with HIV/AIDS are many, varied and often bidirectional and they are often neglected. Their presence compromises HIV care and prevention efforts. Unaddressed, they compromise treatment outcomes, increase HIV virus resistant strains, leave pockets of potential HIV spread in the community and lead to poor quality of life and early death of PLWH. This calls for integration of mental healthcare in all HIV/AIDS treatment and prevention programs [44]. This chapter has focused on specific HIV-associated mental disorders. However, the mental health problems of HIV/AIDS go beyond disorders to include social, family and community problems such as the problems faced by AIDS orphans, widowhood, family disruptions, multiple deaths, bereavements, poverty, stigma, caregiver burden, education and occupational difficulties etc. All these need to be addressed in holistic HIV care. There is need for more research to address brain impairment in HIV/AIDS and its sequels and ways for total integration of mental health care in HIV care and prevention.

Author details

Seggane Musisi[1,2*] and Noeline Nakasujja[1]

1 Makerere University College of Health Sciences, Kampala, Uganda

2 Entebbe Lakeside Hospital, Entebbe, Uganda

*Address all correspondence to: segganemusisi@yahoo.ca

References

[1] Sewankambo N. Forward. In: Musisi S, Kinyanda E, editors. Psychiatric Problems of HIV/AIDS and Their Management in Africa. Kampala, Uganda: Fountain Publishers; 2009

[2] Breuer E, Myer L, Struthers H, Joska JA. HIV/AIDS and mental Health Research in sub-Saharan Africa: A systematic review. African Journal of AIDS Research. 2011;**10**(2):101-122

[3] Musisi S, Wagner GJ, Ghosh-Dastidar B, Nakasujja N, et al. Depression and sexual risk behavior among clients about to start HIV antiretroviral therapy in Uganda. International Journal of STDs & AIDS. 2013;**25**(2):130-137. DOI: 10.1177/0956462413495186

[4] Heggenhougen K, Sabin L, Laurence K, (Eds), (2004): Comparative Studies of Orphans and Non-Orphans in Uganda. A Monograph of International Health and Development, Center for International Health and Development. Boston University School of Public Health. Boston, MA

[5] Musisi S, Kinyanda E, editors. Psychiatric Problems of HIV/AIDS and Their Management in Africa. Kampala, Uganda: Fountain Publishers; 2009

[6] Musisi S, Kinyanda E, Nakasujja N, et al. A comparison of the behavioral and emotional problems of orphans vs non-orphans in Uganda. African Health Sciences Journal. 2007;**7**(4):202-213

[7] Owe-Larsson B, Säll L, Salamon E, Allgulander C. HIV infection and psychiatric illness. African Journal of Psychiatry. 2009;**12**:115-128

[8] DSM 5. Diagnostic and Statistical Manual of Mental Disorders. 5th ed. Arlington, VA, USA: American Psychiatric Association, APA; 2013

[9] Maling S, Todd J, Van der Paal L, Grosskurth H, Kinyanda E. HIV-1 Seroprevalence and risk factors for HIV infection among first-time psychiatric admissions in Uganda. AIDS Care. 2011;**23**(2):171-178. DOI: 10.1080/09540121.2010.498939

[10] Lundberg P, Nakasujja N, Musisi S, Thorson AE. Cantor-Graae E and Allebeck P (2013): HIV prevalence in persons with severe mental illness in Uganda: A cross-sectional hospital-based study. International Journal of Mental Health Systems. 2013;**7**:20

[11] Nakimuli-Mpungu E, Bass JK, Musisi S, et al. Depression, alcohol use and adherence to antiretroviral therapy in Sub-Saharan Africa: A systematic review. AIDS Behavior. 2011;**16**:2101-2118. DOI: 10.1007/s10461-011-0087-8

[12] Nakimuli-Mpungu E, Musisi S, Katabira E, et al. Prevalence and factors associated with depressive disorders in an HIV–positive population in southern Uganda. Journal of Affective Disorders. 2011;**135**(1-3):160-167. DOI: 10.1016/j.jad.2011.07.009

[13] Wagner GJ, Ghosh-Dastidar B, Robinson E, Ngo VK, Glick P, Mukasa B, et al. Effects of depression alleviation on ART adherence and HIV clinic attendance in Uganda, and the mediating roles of self-efficacy and motivation. AIDS and Behavior. 2017;**21**(6):1655-1664. DOI: 10.1007/s10461-016-1500-0

[14] Marinho M, Marques J, Bragança M, et al. Psychosis among HIV-infected patients –a serious and complex association. European Psychiatry.

2016;**33**(Supplement):S221. DOI: 10.1016/j.eurpsy.2016.01.542

[15] National Collaborating Center for Determinants of Health. 2022. Available from: https://www.nccdh.ca/glossary/entry/vulnerable-populations

[16] Nakimuli-Mpungu E, Wamala K, Okello J, Ndyanabangi S, Kanters S, Mojtabai R, et al. Process evaluation of a randomized controlled trial of group support psychotherapy for depression treatment among people with HIV/AIDS in northern Uganda. Community Mental Health Journal. 2017;**53**(8):991-1004. DOI: 10.1007/s10597-017-0129-4

[17] Nakimuli-Mpungu E, Wamala K, Okello J, Alderman S, Odokonyero R, Musisi S, et al. Group support psychotherapy for depression treatment in people with HIV/AIDS in Northern Uganda: A single-centre randomized controlled trial. The Lancet HIV. 2015;**2**(5):190-199

[18] Kessler RC, Chiu WT, Demler O, Merikangas KR, Walters EE. Prevalence, severity, and comorbidity of 12-month DSM-IV disorders in the national comorbidity survey replication. Archives of General Psychiatry. 2005;**62**(6): 617-627. DOI: 10.1001/archpsyc.62.6.617

[19] Brandt C, Zvolensky MJ, Woods SP, Gonzalez A, Safren SA, O'Cleirigh CM. Anxiety symptoms and disorders among adults living with HIV and AIDS: A critical review and integrative synthesis of the empirical literature. Clinical Psychology Review. 2017;**51**:164-184. DOI: 10.1016/j.cpr.2016.11.005

[20] Bolton P, Bass J, Betancourt T, Speelman L, Onyango G, Clougherty K, et al. Interventions for depression symptoms among adolescent survivors of war and displacement in northern Uganda: A randomized controlled trial. Journal of the American Medical Association. 2007;**298**(5):519-527

[21] Bass J, Neugebaur R, Clougherty KF, et al. Group interpersonal psychotherapy for depression in rural Uganda: A 6-month outcome. British Journal of Psychiatry. 2006;**188**:567-573

[22] Senyonyi RM, Underwood LA, Suarez E, Musisi S, et al. Cognitive behavioral therapy group intervention for HIV transmission risk behaviour in perinattally infected adolescents. Health. 2012;**4**(12):1334-1345

[23] David D, Davidson JRT. Treatment of anxiety and stress-related disorders. In: Schatzberg AF, Nemeroff CB, editors. Textbook of Psychopharmacology. 5th ed. Virginia: APA Publishing Arlington; 2017. pp. 1195-1239

[24] Tran BX, Ho R, Ho C, Latkin CA, Phan HT, Ha GH, et al. Depression among patients with HIV/AIDS: Research development and effective interventions ($GAP_{RESEARCH}$). International Journal of Environmental Research and Public Health. 2019;**16**(10):1772. DOI: 10.3390/Ijerph16101772

[25] Institute of Health Metrics and Evaluation. Global Health Data Exchange (GHDx). 2019. Available from: http://ghdx.healthdata.org/gbd-results-tool?params=gbd-api-2019-permalink/d780dffbe8a381b25e1416884959e88b

[26] Musisi S, Kinyanda E. The emotional and behavioral disorders in HIV-sero-positive adolescents in urban Uganda. East African Medical Journal. 2009;**86**(1):16-24

[27] Akena D, Musisi S, Kinyanda E. Clinical features of depression in HIV-positive patients in Uganda. African Journal of Psychiatry. 2010;**13**(1):2010

[28] Wagner G, Ngo V, Musisi S, Akena D, et al. INtegration of DEPression Treatment into HIV care in Uganda (INDEPTH-Uganda). Study Protocol For A Randomised Clinical Trial. 2014;**15**(1):248

[29] Wagner GJ, Ghosh-Dastidar B, Slaughter M, Akena D, Nakasujja N, Okello E, et al. Changes in condom use during the First Year of HIV treatment in Uganda and its relationship to depression. Annals of Behavioral Medicine. 2014;**48**(2):175-183

[30] Ngo VK, Wagner GJ, Nakasujja N, Musisi S, et al. Effectiveness of antidepressants and predictors of treatment response for depressed HIV-positive patients in Uganda. International Journal of STDs & AIDS. 2014;**26**(14):998-1006. DOI: 10.1177/0956462414564606

[31] Bobo WV, Shelton RC. Treatment of Depression. In: Schatzberg AF, Nemeroff CB, editors. Textbook of Psychopharmacology. 5th ed. Arlington, Virginia: APA Publishing; 2017. pp. 1151-1175

[32] Bobo WV, Shelton RC. Treatment of depression. In: Schatzberg AF, Nemeroff CB, editors. Textbook of Psychopharmacology. 5th ed. Arlington, Virginia: APA Publishing; 2017. pp. 1151-1175

[33] Nosik M, Lavrov V, Svitich O, Nosik M, et al. HIV Infection and Related Mental Disorders. Brain Sciences. 2021;**11**(2):248. DOI: 10.3390/brainsci11020248

[34] Nakimuli-Mpungu E, Musisi S, Katabira E, et al. Primary mania vs HIV-related secondary mania in Uganda. The American Journal of Psychiatry. 2006;**163**:8

[35] Nakimuli-Mpungu E, Musisi S, Kiwuuwa S, et al. Early onset versus late onset HIV-related secondary mania in Uganda. Psychosomatics Journal. 2008;**49**:530-534

[36] Keck PE, McElroy SL. Treatment of bipolar disorder. In: Schatzberg AF, Nemeroff CB, editors. Textbook of Psychopharmacology. 5th ed. Arlington, Virginia: APA Publishing; 2017. pp. 1177-1194

[37] Harris MJ, Jeste DV, Gleghorn A, Sewell DD. New onset psychosis in HIV-infected patients. The Journal of Clinical Psychiatry. 1991;**52**(9):369-376

[38] Sikira H, Murga SS, Muhić M, Kulenović AD and Priebe S: Common patient experiences across three resource-oriented interventions for severe mental illness: a qualitative study in low-resource settings. BMC Psychiatry. 2022;**22**:408. DOI: 10.1186/s12888-022-04055-2

[39] Sacktor N, Wong M, Nakasujja MS, et al. Risk factors for HIV-dementia in sub-Saharan Africa. Journal of Neurovirology. 2004;**10**(S3):83

[40] Signh D. What is in name? AIDS dementia complex, AIDS dementia complex, HIV associated dementia, HIV associated neurocognitive disorder or HIV encephalopathy. African Journal of Psychiatry. 2012;**15**(3):172-175

[41] Antinori A, Arendt G, Becker JT, et al. Updated research nosology of HIV-associated neurocognitive disorder. Neurology. 2007;**69**(18):1789-1799

[42] Sacktor N, Nakasujja N, Musisi S, Wong M, et al. The international HIV dementia scale : A new rapid screening test for dementia. AIDS. 2005;**19**:1367-1374

[43] HIV Mental Treatment Issues Fact Sheet. American psychiatric association:

practice guidelines for the treatment of patients with delirium. American Journal of Psychiatry. 1999;**156**(May Suppl):1-20

[44] Remien RH, Stirratt MJ, Nguyen N, Robbins RN, Pala AN, Mellins CA, et al. Mental health and HIV/AIDS: The need for an integrated response. AIDS. 2019;**33**(9):1411-1420. DOI: 10.1097/QAD.0000000000002227

Section 5

Stigma and Society

Chapter 10

Implications of Social Stigma on the Health Outcomes of Marginalised Groups

Jacqueline Carol Matthews-Mthembu and Gadija Khan

Abstract

Research Focus: Stigma is a longstanding issue for South Africa as it is influenced by a history of typification. Social marginalisation is influenced by a myriad of socially structured norms and those who experience stigma, are often faced with social devaluation within their society. In addition, experiences of discrimination may lead to internalised stigma that may lower the self-esteem and agency as well as negatively affect the well-being of many. *Methods:* This chapter uses current literature to propose that stigma, remain a public health concern. *Recommendations:* The findings suggest recommendations that are likely to enhance programme and policy interventions aimed to decrease stigma. Overview Stigma has been a longstanding issue for South Africa as it is influenced by a history of typification. Social marginalisation is influenced by a myriad of socially structured norms and those who experience stigma, are often faced with social devaluation within their society. This policy brief proposes that stigma, and in particular its association with certain marginalised groups, remain a public health concern. It further discusses possible recommendations that are likely to enhance both programme and policy interventions aimed to decrease stigma or at the least, make individuals aware of their complicity in reproducing and maintaining social stigmatisation.

Keywords: social stigma, marginalisation, internalised stigma, mental health, sexual orientation and gender identity, HIV

1. Introduction

The sociologist Erving Goffman [1], provided a widely used definition of stigma which asserts that stigma is a means through which an individual's image is tainted because of a certain characteristic or identity. More recent, definitions suggests that stigma is a concept that is socially constructed and situational; it is shaped by the culture and history of a society and may not transcend time and space [1, 2]. "Rather, the stigmas that prevail about a certain group are located in essentialist stereotypes that have been patterned over time" [3]. Stigmatisation therefore gives root to generalised stereotypes (or ideas) about a person or group which in turn may lead to blatant discriminatory and prejudiced attitudes toward that person or group [4]. There are different types of stigma such as public (externalised or experienced stigma) as well as self-stigma i.e. internalised stigma [5].

South Africa's Apartheid history is entrenched in essentialized ideas about its people, with racism at its core. So much so, that it seems like typifying each other in terms of race, gender and sexuality is a normative measure of the 'worth' of an individual. These ideas are socially constructed and ingrained in the fabric of society and has become the yardstick in health-related situations, including attitudes toward people living with HIV and those with mental disorders. As such, social stigma is shown to have a devastating effect on society [4]. Nevertheless, our country, with its progressive Constitution, has made immeasurable strides in the attempt to curb stigma, but much is still to be done to improve the level of tolerance toward those we "other".

Stigma is a major social determinant of health, it is a cross-sectoral phenomenon, which penetrates at various levels of the health care system including interpersonal, organisational and structural levels [6, 7]. Literature documents a variety of social, physical and physiological consequences of stigma such as isolation and rejection, blatant discrimination and ridicule and violence [3, 5, 8, 9]. Stigma has also been found to have direct and indirect effects on health seeking behaviours and health outcomes. As such, there has been calls for increased attention and urgency toward reducing stigma against marginalised groups, considering its implications on health and wellbeing [6, 10, 11]. This brief broadly focus on the public health implications of stigma for three marginalised groups namely: people with mental disorders, people whose sexual orientation and gender identity (SOGI) is different from their assigned sex at birth and people living with HIV (PLHIV).

2. Mental health disorders

There is sufficient evidence to demonstrate the health system defects in terms of mental health users, stigma and negative traumatic experiences (ill-treatment) at health facilities or by health care providers [12]. The health policy framework integrates chronic conditions including mental health care into primary health care (PHC), which in itself, serves as a way to destigmatize people with mental disorders. However, although the PHC 101 guideline, train health care providers on the diagnoses and treatment of people with mental conditions, it fails to address stigma and discrimination attached to these conditions. This shows implications for access and utilisation of mental health services (e.g. delayed health seeking and non-adherence) as well as the quality of life and well-being of those diagnosed with mental disorders [5, 6].

In regard to interventions to reduce mental disorder-related stigma within society, evidence suggest that family focused interventions, specifically, that of psycho-education on the causes, symptoms and how to care for someone with a mental disorder, is imperative. This is particularly important given the shift toward deinstitutionalisation, which renders the involvement of family members and reintegration into society crucial steps toward improving the health outcomes of people with mental disorders [5].

3. Sexual orientation and gender identities (SOGI)

Sexual orientation and gender identities or SOGI-related stigma is highly prevalent in South Africa and is often grounds upon which LGBTIQ+ people experience various degrees of abuse at the hand of those who hold heteronormative ideals. In the same vein, although progressive legislation legally protect the rights of LGBTIQ+ people to health services, it has also been restricted by heteronormative gatekeepers at local health facility level [11]. Furthermore, there is evidence to suggest that the public health care system is non-responsive to the diverse health needs of LGBTIQ+ people [9, 11]. The LGBTIQ+ population is often grouped together, yet they are very diverse groups. For example, the National Strategic Plan for HIV, TB and STIs (2007–2011) acknowledges that stigma reduction for the LGBTIQ+ population make them less vulnerable to HIV while the 2017–2022 plan encourages the scaling up of programmes geared toward zero stigma. However, greater programmatic and legislative commitment is focused on those who identify as gay and men who have sex with men (MSM) [9, 11, 13]. Reportedly, the development of policy that reflect the diversity within LGBTIQ+ and the necessary guidelines needed to offer specialised health care to sub-populations, is still underway. In the interim, there are important lessons to be learned from private healthcare and NGOs/civils society organisations where the majority of LGBTIQ+ users prefer to access services as opposed to public health facilities. The advocacy and activism emanating from LGBTIQ+ civil society organisations emphasises a rights based approach to (health) care to ensure equity and access to appropriate health services – this should be at the core or health provider training country-wide.

4. HIV

There have been breakthroughs in HIV prevention, treatment programme implementation and human rights realisation, which makes "an AIDS free generation" possible. However, the uptake, adaptation, and successful use of these innovations are hindered by ever-persistent HIV-related stigma [14]. To date, only two studies surveyed stigma experienced by PLHIV. Using the Stigma Index, 799 PLHIV were surveyed in the O. R. Tambo district of the Eastern Cape, in 2012. This was followed by the 2014 survey of over 10,000 PLHIV, across 18 districts (2 per province) in South Africa. Both surveys showed continued significant levels of HIV-related externalised (where stigma or unfair treatment is experienced) and internalised stigma (where stigma, discrimination or negative treatment by others is anticipated or expected) reported by PLHIV [15, 16]. The 2017 national population-based household HIV survey showed mainly positive attitudes toward PLHIV [17], which may be reflective of the improved HIV knowledge in the same survey and even the possible awareness of political correctness around reporting stigma. However, HIV-related stigma still persist and those who experience internalised stigma remain silenced due to fear of stigma. In an effort to mitigate stigma, treatment initiation and disclosure is delayed which nullifies positive prevention efforts.

5. Intersectionality of stigma

Stigma is often experienced on a continuum where race, HIV status, mental health and SOGI intersects [6, 7]. Experiences of stigma, whether real or imagined may influence an individual's health seeking behaviour, which may result in a diminished quality of life. Thus, while we progress toward effective treatment and management of HIV, a greater understanding of mental illness and a more inclusive society in terms of SOGI, social and structural dynamics and determinants of health including stigma are just as important when aiming to improve health outcomes [6].

The multi-layered nature of stigma makes the design and implementation of stigma-reduction interventions more challenging. Addressing stigma on multiple levels is complex and may require greater resources, and be more burdensome to implement successfully amongst all target groups [7]. The greatest impacts in addressing stigma and discrimination have been observed when national responses employ a range of approaches that are monitored, evaluated and re-designed where necessary [6, 14].

6. Recommendations

In reflecting on the current influence of social stigma on the health of South Africans, the country has institutionalised policies for the reduction of stigma for people with mental health conditions as well as those living with HIV, while we are still in the process of developing progressive policies and laws around health care that promotes all SOGI. In view of continued social stigma, we propose the following recommendations for policy development as well as programmatic implementation.

Policy development level:

- Promote the full inclusion and participation of stigmatised groups in the development of programmes, agenda setting and policy formation. This would empower groups and serve as a social accountability mechanism where public health and social systems are held accountable for the commitments made. We suggest that there is concerted efforts to build capacities of different actors in the health care system (providers, patients, civil society organisations) that would create an enabling environment for advocacy and for user groups. This would include legitimising the role patient and user representative groups in decision-making and policy development spaces.

- We recommend that the ministry of health prioritise LGBTIQ+ inclusive health policy development and implementation, and that these processes be spear-headed by the LGBTIQ+ community.

Implementation level:

- Civil society organisations have been at the forefront of advocacy and activism for many marginalised groups. They have been found to mobilise and empower communities and hold government accountable for the infringements of users' rights. We therefore, recommend that civil society organisations be prioritised as implementing partners, receiving support from the ministry to provide appropriate service that marginalised groups find acceptable and accessible.

- The need to improve health provider characteristics (attitudes, beliefs, skills and competencies) to reduce stigma at point of care and facility level. We suggest behavioural and psycho-educational health provider training that goes beyond diagnosis and treatment, to address issues of stigma, fears and attitudes of providers in regard to stigmatised populations. Health professional students should receive more substantive sensitization training during their undergraduate programmes. Continuous in-service training are imperative as well as monitoring the efficacy of the trainings overtime, to determine whether it improves the experiences of users at facilities, as well as the attitudes and culture of facilities.

- Develop an institutional culture of zero tolerance for stigmatisation where providers hold each other accountable and where the statements made in public against stigma must be reflected in action and not be refuted by qualifications and contradictory statements.

- There needs to be greater efforts to obtain feedback about the perceptions, needs and preferences of the health care system for marginalised groups, to create more equitable access to services and improve the inclusivity of services. Within facilities, it is imperative to provide enabling environments for users from marginalised groups to provide feedback regarding their expectations, views and experiences (experiences of care and satisfaction of services) of the health care system without being victimised. More importantly, such feedback should be used to make health care services less stigmatising and more responsive.

Author details

Jacqueline Carol Matthews-Mthembu[1*] and Gadija Khan[2]

1 eMterprise Consultancy, Pretoria, South Africa

2 University of the Western Cape, Cape Town, South Africa

*Address all correspondence to: jacquemthembu@gmail.com

References

[1] Goffman E. Embarrassment and Social Organization. 1963

[2] Hatzenbuehler ML, Phelan JO, Link BG. Stigma as a fundamental cause of population health inequalities. American Journal of Public Health. 2013;**103**(5):813-821

[3] Mthembu JC. Negotiating masculinities: Studying risk behaviours associated with performances of 'coloured' masculinities. 2015

[4] Frost DM. Social stigma and its consequences for the socially stigmatized. Social and Personality Psychology Compass. 2011;**5**(11):824-839. DOI: 10.1111/j.1751-9004.2011.00394.x

[5] Egbe CO, Brooke-Sumner C, Kathree T, Selohilwe O, Thornicroft G, Petersen I. Psychiatric stigma and discrimination in South Africa: Perspectives from key stakeholders. BMC Psychiatry. 2014;**14**(1):1-14. DOI: 10.1186/1471-244X-14-191

[6] Kane JC, Elafros MA, Murray SM, Mitchell EMH, Augustinavicius JL, Causevic S, et al. A scoping review of health-related stigma outcomes for high-burden diseases in low- and middle-income countries. BMC Medicine. 2019;**17**(1):17. DOI: 10.1186/s12916-019-1250-8

[7] Rao D, Elshafei A, Nguyen M, Hatzenbuehler ML, Frey S, Go VF. A systematic review of multi-level stigma interventions: State of the science and future directions. BMC Medicine. 2019;**17**(1):1-11. DOI: 10.1186/s12916-018-1244-y

[8] Manago B. Understanding the Social Norms, Attitudes, Beliefs, and Behaviors Towards Mental Illness in the United States. Proceedings of the National Academy of Sciences; Indiana University. 2015 (September)

[9] Rispel LC, Metcalf CA. Breaking the silence: South African HIV policies and the needs of men who have sex with men. Reproductive Health Matters. 2009;**17**(33):133-142. DOI: 10.1016/S0968-8080(09)33442-4

[10] Egbe CO, Brooke-Sumner C, Kathree T, Selohilwe O, Thornicroft G, Petersen I. Psychiatric stigma and discrimination in South Africa: perspectives from key stakeholders. BMC Psychiatry. 2014;**14**(1):1-14

[11] Luvuno ZP, Mchunu G, Ngidi H, Ncama B, Mashamba-Thompson T. Evidence of interventions for improving healthcare access for lesbian, gay, bisexual and transgender people in South Africa: A scoping review. African Journal of Primary Health Care & Family Medicine. 2019;**11**(1):1-10

[12] Knaak S, Mantler E, Szeto A. Mental illness-related stigma in healthcare: Barriers to access and care and evidence-based solutions. Healthcare Management Forum. Mar 2017;**30**(2):111-116. DOI: 10.1177/0840470416679413. Epub 2017 Feb 16. PMID: 28929889; PMCID: PMC5347358

[13] Cloete A, Sanger N, Simbayi LC. Are HIV positive women who have sex with women (WSW) an unrecognized and neglected HIV risk group in South Africa? Journal of AIDS and HIV Research. 2011;**3**(1):1-5

[14] Paul Pronyk B, Lutz B. Policy and Programme Responses for Addressing the Structural Determinants of HIV AIDS Support and Technical Assistance

Resources Project Recommended Citation. 2013 (June). Available from: http://strive.lshtm.ac.uk/

[15] Simbayi L, Zuma K, Cloete A, Jooste S, Zimela S, Blose S, et al. The people: Living with HIV stigma index: South Africa. 2014: Summary Report; 2015

[16] Boyle MP. Enacted stigma and felt stigma experienced by adults who stutter. Journal of Communication Disorders. 2018;**73**:50-61

[17] Simbayi L, Zuma K, Zungu N, Moyo S, Marinda E, Jooste S, et al. South african national HIV prevalence, incidence, behaviour and communication survey 2017. Towards Achieving the UNAIDS 90-90-90 Targets. 2019

Section 6

Human Rights and Health Rights

Chapter 11

The Global Impact of HIV/AIDS on the Realisation of Health Rights

Nirmala Pillay

Abstract

The chapter critically examines the extent to which the HIV/AIDS litigation advanced the prevention, control and treatment of HIV/AIDS and the realisation of health rights. The justiciability of socio-economic (SC) rights underpins the discussion on health rights but questions about justiciability still leaves unanswered the enforceability of measures against duty bearers to achieve health equity so that vulnerable communities, bearing the greatest burden of HIV/AIDS, are targeted. Advancing health rights through the courts highlights the limitations of law as a human rights tool in holding duty bearers accountable.[1] Ultimately, the full realisation of health rights to achieve health equity may require rights-based approaches to be embedded across public and private health service delivery, research, national strategies, and plans.

Keywords: health rights, law, justiciability, HRBA

1. Introduction

Irrespective of the advances made in science in the form of therapies and drugs, the public health challenge posed by deadly infectious diseases is targeting those who are most susceptible with appropriate strategies to prevent, control and treat the disease. This chapter critically examines the challenges HIV/AIDS posed for the most vulnerable communities and the impact of HIV/AIDS litigation on advancing the health rights of those most affected. HIV/AIDS produced an impressive amount of litigation especially in the late 1990s and early 2000s. Several landmark judgements materially advanced the health rights of the litigants with far reaching implications for people living with HIV (PLHIV). This success contributed to a general view that the justiciability of health rights, a key socio-economic (SC) right was being advanced by the courts and this will make a material difference to states' taking their obligations seriously and holding states accountable. If the human rights legal framework were strengthened so that SC rights achieved the same standing as civil and political (CP) rights, enjoying the same levels of justiciability, then equal health for all will be easier to achieve. The argument presupposes a central role for the courts. This chapter examines health rights in the context of international human rights law (IHRL), the

[1] Courting Rights: Case Studies in Litigating the Human Rights of People Living with HIV. Published jointly by the Canadian HIV/AIDS Legal Network and the Joint UN Programme on HIV/AIDS, UNAIDS/06.01E, March 2006. p. 8.

extent of the gains made by HIV/AIDs litigation for the judicialization of the right and the implications of this for addressing the health inequalities that underpin HIV/AIDS. The chapter is divided into three parts. The first part discusses the global response to HIV/AIDS and the challenge HIV/AIDS poses to public health efforts; the second with the realisation of health rights through HIV/AIDS litigation, and the third discusses broader human rights-based approaches (HRBA) to HIV/AIDS that focus on the underlying determinants of health to address health inequities.

2. Global response to HIV/AIDS

Since the beginning of the epidemic 84.2 million people were infected with the HIV virus and about 40.1 million people died from AIDs.[2] As startling as these figures are the yearly tally of people infected with HIV has dramatically fallen in part because of the development of antiretroviral treatment (HAART) and pre-exposure prophylaxis (PrEP).[3] These therapies are vital to attempts by public health authorities to bring HIV and AIDS under control. The drugs prevent people at risk from contracting HIV and dramatically reduces morbidity from AIDS of those infected with HIV. At the end of 2021 75% of PLHIV were accessing anti-retroviral drugs, up from 25% in 2010. There were 1.3 million pregnant women with HIV in 2021 of which an estimated 81% received anti-retroviral drugs to prevent mother-to-child transmission. Between 2010 and 2021, the number of children living with globally HIV decreased from 2.5 million to 1.7 million.[4] Yet, this impressive success was also the result of concerted efforts by PLHIV to access treatment. The figures also obscure the persistence of the underlying conditions that lead to high rates of HIV/AIDS and continue to inhibit access to treatment or prevent the rise of new infections. In 2021 there were still 38.4 million PLHIV and 650 000 deaths. Alarmingly, 1.5 million new infections were recorded in 2021 alone.[5] Although HIV remains a problem in both first world and developing countries, it is the latter, especially Africa, that bears the biggest burden of the disease accounting for two thirds of PLHIV worldwide.[6] Early in the pandemic it became apparent that the poorest and most unequal societies bore the brunt of HIV/AIDs infection. The inequitable distribution of health care that was "available, accessible or of good quality"[7] affected mostly people afflicted by poverty, illiteracy, and discrimination and lead directly to high rates of infection, predominantly among women, and high rates generally.

In the first five years of the HIV/AIDS pandemic, governments across the world, the public and employers, motivated by ignorance and the fact that the disease seemed endemic to "risk groups" tried to prevent transmission with measures such as mandatory testing, isolation, detention, and quarantine. This meant that infected people suffered "the double jeopardy of disease and discrimination" [1]. Stigmatising individuals and groups did not have the desired effect of slowing down transmission because infected people avoided treatment. This affected the ability of public

---

[2] WHO The Global Health Observatory, who.int/data/glo/data/themes/hiv-aids

[3] PrEP is the "provision of antiviral medication to uninfected persons that reduces transmission by 99% among men who have sex with men (MSM)".

[4] Global HIV and AIDS statistics-Fact Sheet – UNAIDS.

[5] Global HIV and AIDS statistics-Fact Sheet – UNAIDS.

[6] Global HIV and AIDS statistics-Fact Sheet – UNAIDS.

[7] WHO Human Rights and Health wto.int.

authorities to bring the disease under greater control regardless of the availability of sophisticated therapies [2]. HIV/AIDs advocacy groups and activists, including those with HIV, changed attitudes to the disease, locally and internationally, by drawing attention to the human rights dimension of the pandemic [2]. Allan Brandt observed that "AIDS activists...served as collaborators and colleagues rather than constituents and subjects, changing the trajectory of research and treatment" [1]. Inequitable access to treatment had relegated some communities to the margins of prevention and control strategies. Better approaches to tackling the disease were needed that would pinpoint the most vulnerable communities. In other words, approaches that would address both the underlying determinants of health that cause greater susceptibility among some groups and access to therapies.

The work of advocacy groups and a new approach that paid attention to the human rights of PLHIV, adopted by the first director of the (WHO) Global Program on AIDS, Jonathan Mann, linked human rights directly to prevention and control strategies to bring the pandemic under control. If people with HIV/AIDS were marginalised and their human rights denied, this would drive the disease underground where it would be impossible to manage and would spread. Mann argued that to treat the infected would protect society. Thus, epidemiological, and clinical approaches to HIV/AIDS became inextricably intertwined with the protection of human rights [1]. HIV/AIDS brought together health and human rights in a way that was not obvious before. According to Michael Kirkby the "linkage between human rights and effective HIV prevention and care is "more than a moral imperative ...it [is] an epidemiological necessity."[8] It accelerated the development of global health initiatives as the scale of the disease and its impact on the world, especially in developing countries, necessitated co-ordinated medical, financial and policy responses. The approach taken by the UN, from the 1990s, onward was to try and embed human rights in strategies for tackling HIV/AIDS. A co-ordinated international effort was undertaken through a series of measures: In 1996 the Joint United Nations Program on HIV/AIDS (UNAIDS) was created bringing together the world's public health officials, community leaders and politicians [5, p. 2210]. Five years later, in 2001, the UN General Assembly made its Declaration of Commitment on HIV/AIDS which they renewed in 2011. This led to the creation of the Global Fund to Fight AIDS, Tuberculosis, and Malaria targeted at providing financial support to the prevention, control and treatment of HIV/AIDs in developing countries. The USA, under President George W. Bush also made a major funding intervention in 2003 with the President's Emergency Plan for AIDS Relief (PEPFAR) as lifesaving drugs were too expensive to scale up for national roll outs in middle-and low-income countries [6].

3. Human rights norms and public health

Human rights are protected in international law in the Universal Declaration of Human Rights (UDHR), two legally binding international covenants: the International Convention of Civil and Political Rights (ICCPR) and the International Convention of Economic, Social and Cultural Rights (ICESCR), and numerous regional treaties. While CP

and SC rights are treated as qualitatively different, they are fundamental to public health in different ways. Public health authorities have some powers to restrict the

[8] [3] quoted in [4].

fundamental rights of people when circumstances warrant it. They are empowered by national and international law to take measures to prevent, control and treat infectious and contagious diseases such as HIV/AIDS. Within democracies at least, the limits of those powers are also set out to avoid any unnecessary restrictions on the rights of individuals in the pursuit of the laudable goal of protecting the nation's health. The ICCPR ensures that only reasonable restrictions and derogations from rights are acceptable if circumstances demand them.[9] The criteria for the limitation or restriction of rights under the ICCPR by public health authorities is set out in the Siracusa Principles.[10] For example, public health emergencies may provide grounds for limiting certain rights when the rationale for the restriction is the protection of the nation's health. It is legitimate, under IHRL to institute quarantine restrictions that breach the right to freedom of movement of people infected with serious communicable diseases such as Ebola fever, dengue fever, SARS, syphilis, typhoid or tuberculosis, provided they meet the criteria for restrictions [7]. These criteria are standards of legality, evidence-based necessity, proportionality, and gradualism; are of limited duration and subject to review.[11]

The ICESCR also includes a limitation clause (Article 4) intended to protect the rights of individuals. In General Comment No. 14 on the right to health the Committee highlighted PLHIV to explain the limitation. "...a state party which, for example, restricts the movement of, or incarcerates, persons with transmissible diseases such as HIV/AIDS...on grounds such as national security or the preservation of public order... must do so in accordance with the law, international human rights standards, in the interest of legitimate aims pursued, and "strictly necessary for the promotion of the general welfare in a democratic society".[12] Despite these limited restrictions to fundamental rights, the rights of PLHIV were frequently breached. They challenged the breaches of their civil liberties, fundamental freedoms, and rights in various jurisdictions.[13] However, challenging discrimination against PLHIV for their HIV status in employment or club membership or breaches of privacy and confidentiality, at an individual level, does not promote the health rights of HIV sufferers nor does it help deliver the requisite treatment, or bring the disease under control. This requires that the health rights of PLHIV are respected, protected and fulfilled.[14]

[9] Absolute rights in the ICCPR, such as the prohibition against torture, slavery, and genocide may not be restricted under any circumstances and bind all states even those who have not signed up to the treaties.

[10] Siracusa Principles on the Limitation and Derogation Provisions ion the international covenant on Civil and Political Rights. American Association for the International Commission of Jurists icj.org

[11] [8]. See also para 29 General Comment No. 14. In line with Article 5.1, such limitations must be proportional, i.e. the least restrictive alternative must be adopted where several types of limitations are available. Even where such limitations are ...permitted, they should be of limited duration and subject to review.

[12] CESCR General Comment on the Right to the Highest Attainable Standard of Health, (2000), General Comment No. 14, U.N. Doc. E/C. 12/2000/4. 2 para 30.

[13] See for example: *Canada (Attorney General) v Thwaites,* [1994] 3 FC 38 (Federal Court of Canada – Trail Division, 1994); *XX v. Gun Club Corporation et al.*, Constitutional Court, Judgement No. SU-256/96 (1996); *A,C & Others v Union of India & Others,* High Court of Judicature at Bombay [Mumbai], Writ Petition No. 1322 of 1999; *JRB et al v. Ministry of Defence,* Case No. 14000, Supreme Court of Justice of Venezuela (Political-Administrative Bench) (1998); *Hoffmann v South African Airways*, Constitutional Court of South Africa, Case CCT 17/00 (2000); 2001 (1) SA 1 (CC); 2000 (11) BCLR 1235 (CC); *Diau v. Botswana Building Society* (BBS), Case No IC 50/2003, Industrial Court of Botswana (2003).

[14] CESCR General Comment on the Right to the Highest Attainable Standard of Health, (2000), General Comment No. 14, U.N. Doc. E/C. 12/2000/4.

4. Health rights and states obligations in international law

It is the responsibility of the state to implement the rights of both Covenants. Yet, despite signing up to targets to reduce HIV such as the MDGs and the commitment to eradicate HIV in 2030 and the SDGs,[15] governments responded with limited urgency to adopt strategies to address the health rights of HIV sufferers who were mainly among the poorest. In the early 1990s the rate of litigation by PLHIV soared. The cases involved mainly access to treatment, especially to antiretroviral treatments (ART) and were based on the right to health guarantees of national constitutions and right to health provisions in international law. The resulting jurisprudence produced the optimistic assessment that the justiciability of health rights was being accelerated through HIV litigation. The HIV/AIDS highlighted what a constitutionally enforceable health right could mean for the lives and dignity of people but a closer look at the right to health as an international legal norm and HIV case law is instructive with respect to revealing the scope and limitations of the litigation for the realisation of the right to health in all its aspects.

The right to health was first described in 1946 by the WHO constitution as "a state of complete physical, mental and social well-being, and not merely the absence of disease or infirmity" [9]. This definition is broad, all-encompassing, and not possible to operationalise.[16] Article 12 of the ICESCR, that opened for signature in 1966, defines the right to health more precisely. "The state parties to the present covenant recognise the right of everyone to the enjoyment of the highest attainable standard of physical and mental health."[17] The steps states need to take to achieve the full realisation of the right are spelt out. The following are directly relevant to PLHIV:

1. The provision for the reduction of the stillbirth rate and of infant mortality and the healthy development of the child;

2. The prevention, treatment and control of epidemic, endemic, occupational, and other diseases

3. The creation of conditions that would assure to all medical services and medical attention in the event of sickness.[18]

Unfortunately, the formulation is weak as State parties are only required to "recognise" the right to health. Furthermore, Article 2 stipulates that state parties will undertake to the "maximum of available resources" to achieve progressively the full realization of the rights in the covenant".[19] The formulation is not an urgent imperative for states to address the underlying determinants and reasons for poor health

[15] There are 10 Sustainable Development Goals (SDGs) for ending AIDS that refer mainly to the underlying conditions that determine health. The third SDG is to end AIDS by 2030 unaids.org; the Millennium Development Goals has two HIV targets – to ensure access to treatment by those in need by 2010 and to reverse the spread of AIDS by 2015.un.org

[16] See [10].

[17] International Covenant on Economic, Social and Cultural Rights. Adopted 16 December 1966 GA Res 2200A(XXI). Ohchr.org

[18] UN Article 12 International Covenant on Economic, Social and Cultural Rights, (Dec 1966) G.A.Res 2200 (XXI) Art 12, U.N. Doc. A/6316.

[19] Article 2, International Covenant on Economic, Social and Cultural Rights. Adopted 16 December 1966 GA Res 2200A(XXI). Ohchr.org

outcomes. The 1978 Declaration of Alma-Ata on Primary Health Care came closer to treating health as a social goal involving not only the health sector but other social and economic sectors as well.[20] The declaration emphasised correctly that health rights involved the creation of health systems that "ensure effective and equitable distribution of resources for maintaining health" [11, p. 4]. Imposing obligations on states was being developed in international law, however, it remained unclear what obligations the right to health as a legal norm imposed on states and in what ways states were accountable to move the right from concept to implementation.[21]

In the 1990s the HIV/AIDS pandemic produced a spate of health litigation globally that forced courts in several jurisdictions to implement constitutional and international law provisions on health rights. The cases were connected to PLHIV being denied the new life-saving antiretroviral therapy [12]. "The uniqueness of HIV/AIDS as a threat to public health on a global scale, the availability of life-saving ART drugs, and inclusion of SC rights in constitutions in various countries either as directly justiciable or directive principles, created the perfect environment for the rise of right to health litigation. One researcher found that 110 national constitutions make reference to a right to health care [13]. For example, South Africa (SA) and Brazil included the right to health, in their constitution as directly justiciable;[22] and the UDHR and the ICESCR are entrenched in the constitution of Argentina.[23]

In several significant judgements in various jurisdictions courts ruled in favour of the applicants basing their rulings on violations of fundamental rights and the positive obligations of the state that flow from health rights. In several instances the courts creatively interpreted the constitutional rights of individuals even when there was no directly applicable right in the national law. In the *Alonso Munoz Ceballon* case, the Columbian Constitutional Court,[24] in a first judgement of its kind in Latin America, held that the Institute of Social Security could not withhold treatment for HIV/AIDS that the applicant had been receiving. The court based its ruling on the Columbian constitution that required the state to take positive steps to promote the conditions necessary for health equality especially for groups in need or those who are marginalised. In a ruling on the right to free access to health care services and freedom from discrimination based on HIV/AIDS status, the court could not rely on the non-discrimination provisions of Columbian law as the national law does not prohibit discrimination based on disability. The court relied instead on the equality provision which entitled the applicant to equal access to health care-benefits and held that withdrawing treatment would have been discriminatory. Similar conclusions were reached by the Costa Rican courts in the *Luis Guillermo Murrillo Rodriguez et al* and *William Garcia Alvarez* cases. [25] The applicants argued that their constitutional right to life was being violated if they were denied access to ART. The Costa Rican court reversed a previous decision that refused to order the Costa Rican Social Security Fund to supply medication because of the costs involved and ruled in favour of the applicants.

[20] Declaration of Alma Ata 1978. WHO and the United Nations Children's Fund. Unicef.org

[21] Article 16 International Covenant on Economic, Social and Cultural Rights. Adopted 16 December 1966 GA Res 2200A(XXI). Ohchr.org

[22] 13 successful lawsuits in Latin America until 2000.

[23] Article 75.22. [14, p. 26]. See also [15].

[24] *Alonso Munoz Ceballon v Instituto de Seguros Sociales constitutional a Court of Columbia*, Judgement No. T-484-92 (1992).

[25] *Luis Guillermo Murrillo Rodriguez et al* v Caja Costarricence de Seguro Social, Constitutional Chamber of the Supreme Court of Justice, Decision No. 6096-97 (1997); *William Garcia Alvarez v Caja Costarricense de Seguro Social*, Constitutional Chamber of the Supreme Court of Justice, Decision No 5934-97 (1997).

The judgement noted that the cost of the medication had come down and that HIV was the main cause of death in Costa Rica. The court went further and ordered the Fund to develop a plan to provide ART coverage to all PLHIV in need of the treatment.[26]

The case is interesting for the factors the court considered in its ruling. The court took into account the cost and efficacy of the available therapies; the impact of treatment on the health and lives of PLHIV and the fact that HIV was a major cause of death in Costa Rica. The court ordered the government to take positive steps to roll out a national plan for PLHIV.

In the Venezuelan *Cruz del Valle Bermudez et al case*[27] the applicants demanded HIV treatment and treatment for opportunistic infections basing their case on their rights to life and equality, health, liberty and security, freedom from discrimination and access to benefits of science and technology that were protected in the Venezuelan law. The way in which the court arrived at its conclusions is similar in many respects to the Columbian court. It rejected the inequality and discrimination claims on the basis that people with HIV were not in a worse position as people with other conditions. However, the court accepted the applicants' right to health and right to life arguments regarding both as positive rights. The state has a duty to ensure that plaintiffs health rights are protected, especially when the plaintiff lacks sufficient means. Rejecting the government's arguments that supplying ART to everyone who needs it would be very expensive, the court's wide-ranging order required the Ministry to develop policies, provide information and undertake research for PLHIV.

In addition to these national court decisions there was an important regional ruling by the Inter American Commission on health rights in the *Jorge Odir Miranda Cortez et al case.*[28] This ruling was significant in raising the political profile of PLHIV. Several HIV sufferers with no access to ART petitioned the Supreme Court of El Salvador for relief. Frustrated with the the tardiness of the court in dealing with the issue the petitioners took their case to the inter-American Commission asking first for an interim order (*amparo*) compelling the Government of El Salvador to provide PLHIV with the necessary therapies and then for a ruling on the full merits of the case. The petitioners claimed discrimination based on their HIV status and a breach of their right to life saving therapies. The Commission ordered the El Salvador government to supply the treatment and medication, including the nutrition necessary for their immunity. However, before the Commission could rule on the merits of the case the national court of El Salvador ordered the Social Security Institute to provide the necessary ART. This was the first case before any regional court on access to medication for HIV. The impact of a ruling from an international human rights court prompted the EL Salvador court to make a decision and the law in El Salvador changed as well so that PLHIV would have a right to health care that included surgical and phycological treatment and measures to slow down the progression of the infection.[29] The ruling had far reaching effects on the judgements of the national courts in Latin America and health activism for HIV in the region.[30]

---

[26] UN AIDS. Courting Rights. Case Studies in Litigating the Human Rights of People living with HIV.

[27] *Cruz del Valle Bermudez et al Ministry of Health and Social Action,* Supreme Court of Venezuela (Political-Administrative Chamber), Decision No. 916, Court File No. 15789 (1999).

[28] *Jorge Odir Miranda Cortez et al. v. El Salvador,* Inter-American Commission on Human Rights, Report No. 29/01, Case 12.249 (2001).

[29] Law on the Prevention and Control of the Infection caused by the Human Immunodeficiency Virus (Decree No 588, 24 October 2001), Article 5(a).

[30] See *AV & CM v. Ministerio de Salud de la Nacion,* Federal Civil & commercial Court (No. 7), 26 April 2002 where people living with HIV sought ART from the Ministry of Health.

These cases, including the Commission's ruling showed that the courts were willing, not only to uphold the rights of individuals but to force government departments to address the plight of PLHIV who were not the litigants. The courts treated the cases as class actions or collective rights holding governments accountable for not paying attention to groups of people for whom basic lifesaving drugs were inaccessible. According to Cabrera and Ayala "it is fair to state that HIV/AIDS-related litigation played a key role in shaping the right to health litigation at the global scale" [14, p. 27]. They are also right to point out that health rights litigation was a response to states' neglect of or inability to "adequately address the health needs of its people..." [14, p. 26].

In 2000, the CESCR published important clarifications on the right to health and states' responsibilities for realising health rights in General Comment No. 14. The case law on health rights discussed predates the Comment and clarified the approach the courts would take to the adjudication of health rights and the types of orders they were willing to make. The Comment 'codifies' this by requiring that states take deliberate, concrete and targeted measures, through legislative and other means to implement rights and tied this to benchmarks and reporting mechanisms.[31] Importantly, for litigation purposes, the committee included the following formulation: "While the Covenant provides for progressive realisation and acknowledges the constraints due to the limits of available resources, it also imposes on state parties various obligations which are of *immediate effect*."[32] The Comment emphasised that the state has immediate legal "obligations in relation to the right to health, such as the guarantee that the right will be exercised without discrimination of any kind (Article 2.2)."[33] Additionally, the Comment clarified the implications of General Comment No. 3, that related to state obligations to implement the "core minimum" of SC rights, for health rights. The core obligations to fulfil health rights include, at a minimum: (a) the right of access to health facilities, goods and services on a non-discriminatory basis, especially for vulnerable or marginalised people; (b) access to the minimum essential food; (c) basic shelter, sanitation and potable water; (d) essential drugs; (e) equitable distribution of health facilities; (f) a national public health strategy and plan of action, including indicators and benchmarks... that prioritise marginalised groups. In its lengthy explanation of the meaning of non-discrimination as it relates to health, the committee stated that "even in times of severe resource constraints, the vulnerable members of society must be protected by the adoption of relatively low-cost targeted programmes."[34] The right to health means no discrimination in the provision of health services, equality of access to health care and health services, and even obligations to provide health insurance and health care facilities for those without sufficient means. To achieve these outcomes states had to focus on the underlying determinants of health such as "non-discrimination, health information, participation," and inhibiting cultural and social norms, such as gender inequality [11, p. 3]. The Comment tried to ensure that states were accountable and appropriately monitored in realising rights [16]. It distinguished

[31] CESCR General Comment on the Right to the Highest Attainable Standard of Health, (2000), General Comment No. 14, 30, U.N. Doc. E/C. 12/2000/4. See also General Comment on the Nature of States Parties Obligations, (1990) General comment No. 3 at 9, 130, U.N. Doc. E/1991/23.

[32] CESCR General Comment on the Right to the Highest Attainable Standard of Health, (2000), General Comment No. 14, U.N. Doc. E/C. 12/2000/4. 2 para 30.

[33] CESCR General Comment on the Right to the Highest Attainable Standard of Health, (2000), General Comment No. 14, U.N. Doc. E/C. 12/2000/4. 2 para 30.

[34] CESCR General Comment on the Right to the Highest Attainable Standard of Health, (2000), General Comment No. 14, U.N. Doc. E/C. 12/2000/4. para 18.

between steps states can take to realise some aspects of health rights immediately and positive actions using "maximum available resources" to progressively realise national public health strategies that address the health concerns of the whole population.[35]

The development of state obligations in General Comment No. 14 is consistent with the court's approach in two significant right to health cases from South Africa (SA), one of the worst afflicted countries with HIV/AIDS. Whether PLHIV manage to achieve access to ART is as much dependant on government responsibility to ensure that the least worse off get can also access the necessary treatment and affordability of national programmes for the supply of ART. This issue was the basis for a significant ruling on accessing ART in SA, The SA government amended its Medicines Act to make medicines more affordable. Several pharmaceutical companies challenged these amendments[36] seeking a declaration that the changes were unconstitutional as it affected their property rights and were against WTO[37] rules. Treatment Action Campaign (TAC), a national activist group, whose aim was to ensure access to treatment for PLHIV, were granted standing to join the defence as *amicus curiae* (friend of the court) to defend the constitutional rights of PLHIV "that were being undermined by the failure to implement the legislation's measures to reduce the price of medicines."[38] TACs argument revolved around parallel importation of affordable drugs, cheaper generic substitution, and fair pricing. They claimed that the human right to access to health was not as important as the property rights of the petitioners, especially if patients were being abused. They made representation that ART and medicines that treat and prevent opportunistic infections should be made affordable and that government had a positive duty to take steps to ensure the accessibility of health, especially for the poor and marginalised. Additionally, TAC organised protests nationally and internationally and defiance campaigns against the pharmaceutical companies for price-gouging.[39] The activism of TAC outside the court generated, an enormous amount of negative publicity which combined with the legal arguments produced a number of important successes directly relevant to health rights for PLHIV. The US President recognised the right of African countries to "enact legislation that seeks to improve access to medicines" although American interests (companies) are involved; the pharmaceutical companies bowed to pressure, dropped their objections to the amendments and withdrew the lawsuit agreeing to pay court costs[40]; and Pfizer donated Diflucan for the treatment of AIDS related opportunistic infections for use in the SA public health system. Despite the fact that the pharmaceutical companies withdrew their case before a ruling could be made, the courts had been

---

[35] CESCR, 2000 General Comment 14: The right to the highest attainable standard of health (Article 12 of the International Covenant on Economic, Social and Cultural Rights). Committee on Economic, Social and Cultural Rights (CESCR): Geneva, para 43.

[36] *Pharmaceutical Manufacturers' Association and 41 Others v. President of South Africa and 9 Others,* High Court of South Africa, Transvaal Provincial Division, Case No. 4183/98 (2001).

[37] WTO Agreement on Trade-Related Aspects of the Intellectual Property Rights. https://www.wto.org/english/docs_e/legal_e/27-trips_01_e.htm

[38] UNAIDS courting Rights Case Studies in Litigating the Human Rights of People Living with HIV. UNAIDS/06.01E p. 68.

[39] See also a 2003 case Hazel Tau 7 Others v GlaxoSmithKline and Boehringer Ingelheim, Competition Commission of South Africa (2003).

[40] Treatment Action Campaign homepage: http://www.tac.org.za/about.htm 14 Ibid. May 2002 | The International Guidelines on HIV-AIDS and Human Rights, 14.

used as an instrument of corrective and distributive justice.[41] Mark Heywood claimed that that the victory emboldens "people in developing countries and around the world to stand up for medicines that are affordable" [17, p. 45].

TAC followed up on this victory with one of the most analysed cases on health rights and HIV/AIDs. In *Minister of Health and Others v Treatment Action Campaign and Others (No 2)* [42] the SA government appealed a successful legal challenge to their limited use of the ART drug, nevirapine, in the public sector and the absence of a national programme of action to prevent mother-to-child transmission of HIV.[43] TAC relied on several constitutionally protected rights, namely, the "right to access health-care services, including reproductive health care (Section 27) and children's' right to basic health care services (Section 28).[44] They claimed that mothers and children were denied access to medication available free to patients in the private sector and a few public sector pilot programmes. TAC argued that the limited provision was unfair and breached the right of access to public health care services and the right of children to be afforded special protection.[45] Also, they contended that the government is constitutionally obliged "to plan and implement an effective, comprehensive and progressive programme for the prevention of mother-to-child transmission of HIV throughout the country."[46] The breach of this right meant that disease transmission and death rates would be disproportionate among the poor resulting is greater health inequity.

In addition to considering the legal disputes particular to this case, the Constitutional Court considered several points of law about the nature of SC rights important for an assessment of how far the judiciary is prepared to go in enforcing SC rights and by extension health rights: (a) do SC rights give rise to individual rights and claims, (b) the difference between individual entitlements and government obligations to meet "core minimum" SC rights. The case makes no reference to IHRL but is based on Section 27(1)[47] of the SA Bill of Rights that incorporates a positive right to health with similar in wording in parts to Article 12 ICESCR.

The government did not contest the justiciability of ESC rights since this was constitutionally protected and there was established precedent. Their defence was based on the doctrine of the separation of powers.[48] Courts have a different role in a democracy from the legislature and the executive, and it is the executive that is tasked with formulating health policies. Courts should show due deference to this and take care not to make an order that would have the effect of requiring the executive to

---

[41] Treatment Action Campaign homepage: http://www.tac.org.za/about.htm 14 Ibid. May 2002 | The International Guidelines on HIV-AIDS and Human Rights, 14.

[42] Minister of Health and Others v Treatment Action Campaign and Others (No 2) (CCt8/02) [2002] ZAACC 15; 2002 (5) SA 721; 2002 (10) BCLR (5 July 2002).

[43] Minister of Health and Others v Treatment Action Campaign and Others (No 2) (CCt8/02) [2002] ZAACC 15; 2002 (5) SA 721; 2002 (10) BCLR (5 July 2002).

[44] Para 22.14. They also argued that the government violated a binding 8 (I) constitutional provision requiring the state to "protect, promote and fulfil the rights in the Bill of Rights" and was in breach of its international human rights treaty obligations.

[45] Sections 27 and 28 of the SA Constitution.

[46] Minister of Health and Others v Treatment Action Campaign and Others (No 2) (CCt8/02) [2002] ZAACC 15; 2002 (5) SA 721; 2002 (10) BCLR (5 July 2002) para 4.

[47] The right to have access to (a) health care services, including reproductive health care; and (2) The state must take reasonable legislative and other measures, within *its available resources*, to achieve the *progressive realisation* of each of these rights".

[48] *Grootboom etc.*

pursue a particular policy.[49] This would undermine the notion of the separation of powers. The government further argued that "courts are ill-suited to adjudicate upon issues where court orders could have multiple social and economic consequences for the community."[50]

Rejecting the idea that Section 27(1) gave rise to "a self-standing, independent positive, enforceable right," the court held that the right to health is about the scope of positive rights and, in this case, "access to services that the state is obliged to provide."[51] The SA government had fallen short of its constitutional obligations to provide access to health care services for HIV-positive mothers and their new-born babies.[52] The court ruled that since a whole class of persons were excluded, this was a denial of rights. Even though the court did not rely on international law, the reasoning reflects the non-discrimination, "core minimum" provisions of SC rights that are immediately justiciable and not subject to "progressive implementation". The court also ruled that the government had failed in its responsibilities by not setting out a "timeframe for a national programme to prevent mother child transmission of HIV."[53] The judgement recognised that the state balances health rights with other SC rights such as education, land, housing, health care, food, water and social security, but the state must also take "reasonable legislative and other measures *within its available resources* to achieve the *progressive realisation* of each of them."[54] Therefore, legislation and policies need to be reasonable and "programmes must be reasonably implemented" to comply with the State's obligations.[55] The ruling confirmed that states will be held accountable for not setting out benchmarks and indicators with "timeframes" for positive rights. The ruling marked a watershed for the adjudication of health rights in SA and globally. For many commentators the ruling also exemplified a "transformative" constitution that could achieve concrete results for PLHIV [18]. According to Cooper, the justiciability of SC combined with the urgency of the HIV/AIDs crisis "placed the right to health at the centre of promoting social justice and framed litigation as a mode of social transformation in South Africa" [19].[56]

While the HIV case law should not be underestimated, it is also important not to overestimate its achievements. The extent to which HIV litigation expanded the

---

[49] *Minister of Health and Others v Treatment Action Campaign and Others* (No 2) (CCt8/02) [2002] ZAACC 15; 2002 (5) SA 721; 2002 (10) BCLR (5 July 2002).

[50] *Minister of Health and Others v Treatment Action Campaign and Others* (No 2) (CCt8/02) [2002] ZAACC 15; 2002 (5) SA 721; 2002 (10) BCLR (5 July 2002).

[51] See Sections 26(2) and 27(2) of the SA constitution.

[52] *Minister of Health and Others v Treatment Action Campaign and Others* (No 2) (CCt8/02) [2002] ZAACC 15; 2002 (5) SA 721; 2002 (10) BCLR (5 July 2002) para 4.

[53] Minister of Health and Others v Treatment Action Campaign and Others (No 2) (CCt8/02) [2002] ZAACC 15; 2002 (5) SA 721; 2002 (10) BCLR (5 July 2002) para 3.

[54] Minister of Health and Others v Treatment Action Campaign and Others (No 2) (CCt8/02) [2002] ZAACC 15; 2002 (5) SA 721; 2002 (10) BCLR (5 July 2002) para 4.

[55] Minister of Health and Others v Treatment Action Campaign and Others (No 2) (CCt8/02) [2002] ZAACC 15; 2002 (5) SA 721; 2002 (10) BCLR (5 July 2002) para 4.

[56] [14, p. 27], [19]. See also Brand a "[T]ransformative constitutionalism emphasises attaining SC justice by having a pro-poor (or anti-poverty) orientation that focuses on addressing inequalities. [20]. The imperative for the court when interpreting the law, is to deploy constitutionally entrenched human rights to transform the lives of all SAs. [21]. Former Chief Justice Langa went even further in stating that "that at the heart of transformative constitutionalism is the objective to create a truly equal society and 'to heal the wounds of the past and guide us to a better future.' (Langa 2006: 352 quoted in [21]).

right to health is related to the question of the suitability of the law and the efficacy of courts in addressing all the components of health rights. The right to health has both justiciable and non-justiciable elements and the role of the court is to both adjudicate on breaches of rights where the violation is clear and hold governments accountable for duties that only the executive can undertake. The latter role involves monitoring States for accountability for treaty obligations that do not form part of the non-justiciable "core minimum." The general assumption is that since rights are legal entitlements the more effective the adjudication of health rights becomes through the courts, and the more the differences between CP and SC rights are reduced, the better the health outcomes for those suffering the biggest burden of disease. The differences between CP and SC rights are not as great as once presumed and there is a significant body of literature on this question, but the pressing issue is how far the courts are able to protect the right to health in all its aspects. In other words, how effective is the law as a human rights tool.

The cases before the courts were clearly defined and generally involved access to medication. There was a clear causal link between having access to ART and life. In the *Jorge Odir Miranda Cortez* case 10 of the original 36 petitioners died even before a judgement could be rendered. The urgency of the issues before the courts and the resulting impact on the lives and health of large numbers of people, if the cases were unsuccessful, would have been apparent to any judiciary. HIV case law in Latin America and SA was important for the impact the rulings had on the lives of PLHIV, especially in developing countries and for those who could not afford ART; and for developing the legal framework of the right to health. It showed:

a. that the courts were willing to act where governments had failed;

b. where the right to health was entrenched in national constitutions, and where SC rights were directly justiciable, the courts applied it to protect the constitutional rights of people;

c. that in many cases the courts were creative in their application of the rights provisions in the national law reading the law in the light of international law (which was usually cited). For example, in cases prohibiting discrimination against people for their HIV status;

d. that courts were willing to make wide ranging orders covering not only the petitioners before the court but classes of people who were denied access to ART;

e. regional courts were willing to order governments to comply with the right to health provisions in regional treaties when petitioned

The litigation on HIV/AIDs demonstrated the justiciability of health rights but it is important to consider how effective the courts were and how far the jurisprudence went in protecting the health rights of PLHIV and in helping to bring down new infections. The reasoning of the courts in the cases discussed are interesting as they often applied a combination of rights provisions in their reasoning. For example, interpreting the right to life positively, relying on anti-discrimination provisions and in one instant on the right to S&T, to grant the petitioners relief. Additionally, the rulings of the court were largely engaged with "core minimum" justiciable sections of General Comment No. 14 such as the non-discrimination clauses, equal access to medication and health services[57] and prioritising of the rights of children.[58] These rights are immediately justiciable and not "progressively realised."[59] Yet, successful litigation often did not produce the necessary relief for the applicants. Delivery of accessible treatment, properly financed, did not follow court orders and the law failed to solve the access to medication issue. Ultimately, it is the executive that must devise the policies to implement rights. In Argentina, for example, successful court cases that imposed a positive duty on governments to supply PLHIV with ART had disappointing results and in SA it was a long time before the country achieved a successful rollout of ART that also included a plan to stop mother-to-child transmission. As Heywood pointed out in the TAC case, it was still up to the SA government to demonstrate commitment by making good on the ruling and on their constitutional obligations to ensure that any new act will be effective in making treatment accessible [22]. The rollout of nevirapine was patchy with some SA provinces significantly increasing access and others failing to do so children continued to be infected. Governments were not always able or willing to commit resources or address systemic problems in the health care sector. Too often litigants had to follow up legal action with more legal action to compel states to comply with previous orders.

The implementation of SC rights, with serious implications for PLHIV, cannot be left up to governments without international accountability mechanisms through the UN and local accountability through the courts. The Universal Periodic Review and other UN monitoring systems require governments to report on progress made on the implementation of SC rights, including the right to health. When governments still fail to implement at least the core minimum of the right, the courts can intervene. But discrete intervention of the courts only in instances when individuals and groups are successful in getting their cases heard make for uneven attempts to provide relief to marginalised communities suffering the highest burden of the disease. The courts should be the last resort in forcing governments to act and cannot be the only means of ensuring attention to human rights within the public health system.

The development of a legally binding right to health in national constitutions made it easier for courts to hold governments accountable for the justiciable elements of the right but they are careful in their interventions. The HIV cases reveal that the courts acted in a supervisory capacity, within their administrative law remit, and held the executive accountable for omissions in their constitutional duties. The role of the courts is to evaluate whether the measures the government takes to meet its constitutional obligations are reasonable. This approach restricts the judiciary to its proper role in a democracy and prevents the judiciary from intruding on the role of the executive. "In this way the judicial, legislative and executive functions achieve appropriate constitutional balance."[60] However, accountability is a central plank of rights discourse, litigation does not seem effective in holding governments' accountable for addressing the underlying determinants of health. The HIV case law highlighted the

---

[57] CESCR, General Comment No. 3: The Nature of State Parties Obligations (Art. 2. Para 1, of the Covenant. E/1991/23.

[58] [20, p. 124]. The exception is in the case of children, where the court has recognised in the Grootboom (right to housing) and TAC (right to healthcare) cases amongst others that the state has a special duty to protect and uphold the rights of children, especially in circumstances where parents are unable to fulfil their obligations towards their children.".

[59] General Comment No. 14.

[60] *Minister of Health and Others v Treatment Action Campaign and Others* (No 2) (CCt8/02) [2002] ZAACC 15; 2002 (5) SA 721; 2002 (10) BCLR (5 July 2002) .

extent to which the burden of disease fell on the poorest and most vulnerable as most PLHIV are the victims of chronic health inequities.

The main themes of this debate are well rehearsed and revolve around the appropriate spheres of the judiciary, legislature, and the executive; and the appropriateness of the courts to make orders that have major budgetary implications. Restricting the role of the courts is reasonable if the full scope of health rights, that includes unaccounted for environmental and social factors, that have an impact on health, is considered. There are, therefore, built in limitations to the role of the judiciary in the expansion of health rights and there are good reasons not to expect an ever-expanding role for the courts to implement SC rights. A former UK High Court justice, Lord Sumption, highlighted an added danger of an overreaching judiciary in his Reith lectures. He posed the question, "How far is it legitimate for democracies to create a body of law that is independent of democratic choice and protected against abrogation and amendment by a democratic legislature" [17].[61]

Sumption's question is not about the justiciability of SC v CP rights, or the proper function of the courts, but the proper limits of human rights law [17, p. 47]. He acknowledges that the law plays an important role in holding the executive accountable and can even act as a corrective, but he raises a concern about the creation of an "empire of law" where an expanded idea of the rule of law means that courts can claim a "wider supervisory authority over other organs of the state" [17, p. 47]. Law derives its legitimacy from elected law makers, the legislators, while elected government, the executive, determine policy and set budgets. Hence, is litigation "really the right way to resolve differences of opinion about what are really questions of policy". According to Sumption "the judicial resolution of policy issues would undermine the single biggest advantage of the political process, which is to accommodate the divergent interests and opinions of citizens" [17, p. 45]. Sumption is not in favour of the law taking over the role of the executive as the law is part of a "larger system of public decision making" namely politics. The mediating role of politics to produce policies which the broadest possible range of people can live with. This is why politics, not law is the more powerful engine of national compromise and effective mediators between the state and the electorate" [17, p. 29]. While law is black and white the concept of representation mediates the variety of clashing opinions in policy making through compromises.

Sumption, in his consideration of the relationship of the United Kingdom courts with the Human Rights Act 1998 (HRA'98) that incorporated the regional human rights treaty the European Convention of Human Rights (ECHR) into the law of the UK, claims that the Convention "ties the United Kingdom to a dynamic system of law whose development is the task of a court standing entirely outside its own political institutions." He concedes that HRA 98 (which only protects CP rights) successfully "protects the interests of vulnerable groups, with no natural body of support among the electorate or the press. It has forced more humane and inclusive values on ministers and officials. It has obliged decision makers to listen to the objections of people whose interests are adversely affected and to provide a coherent and objective justification for their decisions. These are major concessions to the power of human rights law but Sumption's claim that these "concessions were capable of being provided by domestic law without recourse to international treaty" is problematic. It is precisely

[61] [16, p. 47]. This is an interesting question in the UK context since, unlike SA, the UK does not have a constitution that protects positive rights. The human rights act incorporates the ECHR, and the UK is a signatory to the European Social Charter of positive rights. The UK regularly reports to the European Committee of Social Rights on progress made on implementing positive rights.

because the political system excluded PLHIV a group with no support "among the electorate or press" that PLHIV took their grievances to court in countries where SC rights were constitutionally protected. However, Sumption's larger point is that the law, by overreaching, can either fail to deliver relief or force the issue on behalf of the excluded and become the enemy of democracy.

If the role of the courts is to ensure that governments give effect to their international human rights treaty obligations and constitutional obligations the courts can make careful interventions on issues of equality of access. These are not individual entitlements, but policy matters and the courts can require the government and relevant departments to apply their minds to equitable policies without taking over the role of government. This leaves open the issue of who sets priorities when policy choices are a competition between education, health, housing, clean water and adequate nutrition. Addressing the HIV crisis was a priority as the death rate would have soared. This is where courts have little moral or constitutional unease on the separation of powers issues. States always had a responsibility to prevent infectious diseases and provide primary health care, however, this was difficult to conceptualise as rights or translate into rights language until the UDHR and especially the ICESCR which lists rights and duties of government. It is true that the judiciary cannot be relied upon to enforce health rights as this means taking steps to reduce health inequities, but they do have a role in holding the government accountable, for failing to comply with their constitutional and treaty obligations. This is a limited role of which the courts are quite conscious, as evidenced in a major ruling by the SA court on housing.

The *Grootboom*[62] case provided the court with an opportunity to make a determination on the justiciability of SC rights, Yacoob J, held that the constitution included positive rights requiring the state to provide access to housing, healthcare, sufficient food and water, and social security to those in need and unable to support themselves. However, "[T]he obligation does not require the State to do more than its available resources permit."[63] Moreover, the insertion of the words "progressive realisation shows that it was contemplated that the right would not be realised immediately." The constitutional qualifications to positive rights restrict the scope of the courts' decisions. However, as the constitution does oblige the state to give effect to these rights it is an obligation that courts in appropriate circumstances can enforce.[64]

It would appear from an analysis of the HIV case law that rights litigated before court were within the court's capacity to order the state to "respect and protect" but not to "fulfil." Courts are likely to be circumspect in interpreting the right to health in a way that leads to making orders the state can't meet. The role of the courts is significant but limited in advancing the right to health. While current HIV data shows that the situation has dramatically improved with the rollout of ART, and the part the courts played in ensuring access to the drug by upholding the rights of excluded groups, the disease remains a challenge with new infections being reported every year. Global data for malaria, TB and HIV/AIDS showed a clear link between poverty, discrimination, marginalisation and poor access to treatment with direct implications for rates of infection and death. Higher rates of HIV infection are continuing to occur

---

62 *Government of the Republic of South Africa and Others v Grootboom and Others,* (CCT11/00)[2000]ZACC 19;2001 (1) SA 46; 2000 (11) BCLR 1169 (4 October 2000).

63 *Government of the Republic of South Africa and Others v Grootboom and Others,* (CCT11/00)[2000]ZACC 19;2001 (1) SA 46; 2000 (11) BCLR 1169 (4 October 2000) para 45.

64 *Government of the Republic of South Africa and Others v Grootboom and Others,* (CCT11/00)[2000]ZACC 19;2001 (1) SA 46; 2000 (11) BCLR 1169 (4 October 2000) para 45.

mainly among young women. For health rights to become a reality for PLHIV the focus needed to be on the underlying determinants of health.

5. Implementing health rights: the human rights-based approaches (HRBA) and health inequities

The progressive realisation of health should be part of the ongoing work of public health authorities as mandated by international human rights treaty obligations. Key to the realisation of health rights is getting to grips with the underlying determinants of health that predispose people to disease and early death pernicious. Poverty, disease, illiteracy, and ignorance can so impair a person's ability to imagine and realise life plans that their lives fail, in important ways, to be realised [23]. Stephen Marks observed that "the essence of the right to health is access to the conditions necessary for the realisation of healthy lives" [11, p. 11] and it is the "duty of the State to ensure those conditions, whether through a regular market or through government services" [11, p. 11]. The denial of, or poor quality education or health care directly affects human agency and human dignity meaning that the enjoyment of CP rights are also impaired if SC rights are not fulfilled [23]. This is what is meant by the indivisibility of rights. Systemic health inequalities is outside the remit of judicial review to remedy. For governments to make progress in the implementation of health rights so that the distribution of health is more equitable in society, the state and society need to shoulder the responsibility.

In his attempt to bring HIV under control, treat PLHIV and protect the health of the whole society, Jonathan Mann developed an approach to public health that was rights-based. The pandemic highlighted the 'social dimension' of the disease that inhibited control and treatment strategies. Mann's plan was to offer a "coherent, comprehensive and practical framework for analysis and action on the societal root causes of vulnerability" to HIV/AIDS [24]. Embedding human rights in the structure and development of public health policy making reorientates public health to focus on the whole society. The conventional approach to dealing with the social determinants of health have significant limitations that a HRBA tries to complement.

The conventional approach to addressing health inequalities is to "focus on universally targeted health interventions designed to benefit as many people as possible" [25]. The public health approach to control the spread of highly contagious and deadly infections is a universal intervention based on achieving the maximum benefit for the greatest number of people. It involves messaging, regulations, statistical analysis, supervision. This approach successfully mobilises the nation, but it fails to have an impact those communities where the infection and death rates are the highest. J. Scott's analysis of the extent of the failure of development programmes of many 20th century schemes concluded that ... [P]revious public health research on efforts to control TB, malaria and HIV/AIDs that investigated why some communities failed to take the required action irrespective of the resources deployed, discovered unidentified factors that prevented people from acting on rational information [26]. These may be "social and cultural practices," attitudes and beliefs embedded in communities that "affect 'trust' in government programmes and external messaging" [27] The conventional approach neglected to address these embedded attitudes and beliefs and conspicuously failed to close gaps and disparities in health outcomes within the society with some communities experiencing far worse health outcomes than others. The lack of success was because the programmes lacked "sufficient engagement with communities" [27] Closing gaps requires interventions that work better in particular communities than interventions aimed at benefitting the population at large.

A HRBA to health crucially incorporates an understanding of the "individual characteristics of the population groups concerned" [28] It would pinpoint communities most at risk of HIV and identify the politics, religion, traditional practices, social and institutional norms and gender issues that act as barriers to health and prevent public health authorities from controlling and treating HIV/AIDs, not only for the targeted group but for society. The model "treats people not as passive recipients of goods and services but as "participants and key actors in decisions that that affect their wellbeing" [29] HRBA centralises the concept of agency – of individuals (as rights claimants) and of communities – to take decisions for their own health and capacity to make rational health choices. Therefore, a HRBA includes an investigation into barriers to the health of individuals and communities amenable to remedial interventions.

When good quality health services are inaccessible to the most susceptible to disease, health inequalities could be structural or the result of poor policy making. Even access to anti-retroviral treatment, as the HIV case law showed, required overcoming political and economic resistance.[65] Gruskin and Tarantola argue that the point of health rights activism, is to hold governments accountable by establishing what amount of government action or inaction contributes to existing violations, "looking at how a government deals or does not deal with identified problems and recommending solutions" [31, p. 449].

HRBA requires an enabling legal and conceptual framework for advancing health rights that is normatively based on international human rights standards [32, 33]. The aim of HRBA is to tackle the effects of human rights breaches on disease prevention and treatment and to ensure that governments fulfill their constitutional and human rights treaty obligations with respect to implementing the right to health [31, p. 449]. The components of HRBA are: (a) the social determinants of health that takes into account the "family, the community, civil society, local and national authorities;" and (b) the legal framework to determine individual, collective, and institutional claims, duties and accountabilities for health.

The main purpose of HRBA is to address inequities. A HRBA demands reasons for high correlations between social inequalities and health outcomes to determine whether perceived health inequalities are health inequities [29]. If an analysis of the underlying determinants of health exposes gaps in the social, political, cultural, historical, and institutional determinants of health, it is crucial to determine if the disparities are "preventable, avoidable or justifiable" [34]. A HRBA offers a "framework for accountability" on inequities in health outcomes by identifying the human rights at issue; determining who owes duties and has obligations at the community and national level; whose health rights needs safeguarding and promotion and whether the inequities are the result of human rights breaches [29]. The United Nations (UN) outlined the pillars of HRBA to development—universality, indivisibility, interdependence and interrelatedness, non-discrimination and equality, participation and inclusion, accountability and the rule of law that need to be "operationalised in the policy, programmes, projects and other health related interventions with a view to enhancing effectiveness" [35] An example of this is the approach of the Indian National AIDS control Organisation (NACO) that was created to control AIDS. Phase three "involved implementing targeted interventions and preventive measures for high-risk populations, and expanding treatment, medical and support services nationwide" [2].

[65] [30]. Quoted in [24].

By 2000, HRBA had already produced some notable successes for PLHIV. The pharmaceutical industry lowered the price of anti-retroviral drugs in low-income countries to less than 10% of their cost [31, p. 451]. They responded to the right of "access to treatment" [31, p. 451]. However, the fact that there were still massive inequalities in the distribution of the drugs with low-income countries suffering the severest shortages showed a lack of international co-operation and resources and that could have benefitted the poorest. Other systematic reviews of HRBA in the context of to HIV/AIDS noted "promising evidence of the impact of human rights programmes on key and vulnerable populations most at risk of HIV" [36] A reduced incidence of HIV could be attributed to a range of HRBA targeted interventions that resulted in "decreased HIV risk behaviours to increased HIV testing to reduced incidence" [36] In a more recent review of 29 studies of HRBA programmes between 2015 and 2019 analysing "influence of context,... conflicting rights and added value" of HRBAs, "... positive changes were reported at individual and programme level" [37] The studies highlight the fact that HRBA targeted the legal, social, political, and economic environments "needed to reach and engage in care, key and vulnerable populations most at risk of HIV infection" [36] The studies measured the outcomes of HRBA initiatives such as the reduction of infections or deaths. Since HRBA centralises participation and agency the implication is that the success of the approach is also a measure of the involvement of people in the understanding and claiming of their rights.

HRBA provides *intrinsic, instrumental, and institutional* rationales for adoption in policies and strategies aimed at the treatment of infectious diseases. The *intrinsic* rationale is that it is the right thing to do, morally and legally and in the interests of justice. Embedding universal human rights values of freedom, equality, and solidarity into policies that affect mainly the poorest prioritises the social determinants of health including cultural norms, traditional practices, and discriminatory practices which might explain the causes of poor health decisions and outcomes. HRBA moves health inequities into the realm of policy and law. The *instrumental rationale* is better and more sustainable health outcomes because HRBA focuses on groups bearing a disproportionate burden of poor health outcomes. It emphasizes and enables participation of the community in bespoke policies addressing the communities' health challenges in the interests of long-term sustainability. The flexible framework addresses many and varied health challenges because the "situation assessment, analysis, design, implementation, monitoring" and evaluation of interventions and policies is informed by international rights.[66] The *Institutional rationale* anchors policy development and implementation in a state's international law reporting obligations underscoring the government's responsibility, as primary duty bearers, to ensure that health rights are "respected, protected and fulfilled" including the fair distribution of health rights [29]. A RBA includes accountability mechanisms for duty-bearers to meet their obligations and fulfil their duties leading to better UPR reporting.[67] A rights-based approach complements the traditional/conventional approach to public health by building into health strategies and plans key HRBA indicators that ensure health rights are being progressively realised. The value of HRBA is that it builds in "systemizing attention" on core indicators that centralise equity and rights in the larger goal of preventing and treating diseases namely: [1] HRBA:

[66] The Human Rights Based Approach to Programming. Practical Implementation Manual and Training Materials. NY. United Nations Population Fund [38] p. 81.

[67] The Human Rights Based Approach to Programming. Practical Implementation Manual and Training Materials. NY. United Nations Population Fund [38] p. 81.

DOI: http://dx.doi.org/10.5772/intechopen.109382

1. Ensures that policy options to prevent and treat infection do not treat people as a means to an end;

2. Prioritises agency by recognising that prevention depends on people volunteering for testing and treatment. People affected by disease have a "crucial role in the discovery and advocacy of new modes of treatment and prevention and their equitable access;" [1]

3. Examines the laws and policies under which programmes take place as policy options could either encourage or discourage people from accessing treatment and hghlights gaps in the enabling legal and policy framework that have an impact on health inequities.

4. Uncovers the buried social, cultural and economic inequities that lead to health inequities. Interventions are designed to take into account the identified barriers to participation and the human rights of the most at-risk people so that adequate and appropriate medical care can be appropriately targeted to also stop disease transmission to the rest of the population

5. Ensures that health information is evidence-based? It is impossible to address inequities in health if data collection is not disaggregated to provide evidence needed to tackle complex health challenges. " …disaggregating data beyond traditional markers could detect discrimination" on the basis of ethnicity, poverty, and status revealing "underlying determinants of overall poor health status" [7]

6. Integrates core human rights principles such as participation, non-discrimination and transparency into laws and policies designed to target infectious diseases;

7. Builds accountability into policy and programme responses;

8. Focusing on the key elements of the right to health—availability, accessibility; acceptability and quality when defining standards for provision of services" [31, p. 451].

These elements of HRBA help policy makers ensure that benchmarks and targets are set to guarantee that health rights are realised progressively. It also ensures transparency and accountability for "what decisions are made and their ultimate outcomes" [31, p. 451] HRBA informs the work of International and national NGOs, governments, and individuals by basing the development of strategies and programmes for service delivery on legal standards [31, p. 451]. This helps target new treatments and medical services to the worst hit communities. A health rights framework prevents the neglect of areas of health that could be overlooked and examines the impact of different policies on different communities. It ensures consultation and proper participation making health policies more effective for target populations and puts in place "effective monitoring and accountability arrangements" [16].

6. Conclusions

The failure of governments to address serious health issues in a timely manner and to narrow inequities in health has increased the demand for the involvement of the law and the courts.

In the end no single intervention curtailed the spread of HIV/AIDs or provided the requisite treatment. Prevention, control and treatment programmes combined with aggressive HIV litigation, brought together biomedical interventions, behavioural changes (such as adherence to condom use, prevention of behaviours associated with an increased risk of infection) in better nationally mandated plans that successfully reduced the incidence of HIV infection and achieved better control of the epidemic [5, p. 2215].

HIV litigation, especially in developing countries, tested the ability of the courts to support the poorest and most susceptible communities in accessing anti-retroviral drugs and holding governments accountable for the health of the population. A combination of legal challenges and well organised activism and advocacy based on breaches of fundamental rights, non-discrimination and states' obligations for health rights achieved a sustainable reduction in HIV incidence.

HIV litigation involved mainly free or affordable access to medication. The litigation tested the states obligations to supply lifesaving medication to the poorest and most afflicted through social security programmes. The cases also tested the regulatory framework of the state to ensure affordability of medication. This meant ensuring that the pricing policy of private pharmaceutical companies did not disproportionality impact the indigent where the preponderance of the HIV cases existed. These cases were a significant intervention in the pandemic and ensured that the tardiness and poor responses from governments that characterised the early phases of the HIV/AIDs outbreak, shifted to a more interventionist approach when it became clear that poverty and inequality were "the primary determinants of the success or failure of attempts at curtailing new HIV infections" [4].

The case law on HIV shows that significant sections of health rights are justiciable since they required immediate implementation and do not have to wait to be "progressively realised." The litigation addressed circumscribed groups of people who were denied access to medication and who would have perished if no relief were granted. Although, some of the court orders were far reaching with the courts being prepared to make orders that involved government spend and extending relief to all poor people with HIV, from the perspective of cost-effectiveness, focussing on populations at highest risk for transmission form HIV/AIDs would have been a better and more effective public health approach to the disease in the first place [5, p. 2215].

However, the review of the case law also showed the limits of the courts in advancing health rights. First, it was easier for courts to rule on health when SC rights were included in the national constitution [39]. Second, the courts can only rule when petitioned which means their interventions are sporadic. This does not constitute systematic monitoring of states' responsibility to implement rights. Third, the courts' rulings were restricted to what became the "core minimum" SC rights of General Comment No. 3. Many of the immediate obligations of states identified in General Comment No. 14 had already been made explicit by the courts in the HIV case law. Hence, the extent to which the law is useful in advancing health rights was also clarified by the case law. The cases did not present the courts with the prospect of "adjudicating complex policies with significant budgetary implications" that would involve the courts in redressing systemic health inequity [14, p. 26]. This is a difficult area to litigate and strengthening litigation or the role of the court to implement SC/health rights may involve an undemocratic expansion of the courts role.

The issues in the HIV case law highlight the original debate between the implementation of the ICCPR and the ICESCR treaties and the argument that that the treaties represent qualitatively different rights. It is more difficult for the courts to hold governments accountable for breaches of SC rights. The implementation of SC rights, in this case health rights, remains the primary responsibility of the legislature and executive with the courts holding duty bearers accountable for not taking steps to "progressively realise" all aspects of the rights. While the AIDS epidemic provided the foundation for a revolution in SC rights that upended traditional approaches to human rights enforcement and the proper focus of the courts, it highlighted the fact that health rights can only be partially protected in the courts. To ensure that health related interventions are "responsive, equitable and of good quality" [16] early and routine consideration of the HRBA indicators should be embedded in all government health initiatives dealing with infectious diseases. The monitoring and accountability for health rights ultimately lies NGOs, citizens, researchers, and public health officers. The interest groups are better than courts in monitoring governments for their "action or inaction that contributes to existing violations, looking at how a government deals or does not deal with identified problems, and recommending solutions" [31, p. 451].

Therefore, health rights and the underlying determinants of health have to be the included in policy making, national plans and programmes. According to Paul Hunt, the first UN Special rapporteur on the right to the highest attainable standard of health "...too often, human rights are seen only as standards contained in treaties and declarations. However, human rights have concrete contributions to make in guiding policy formulation and implementation, and constructively addressing major global challenges. A human rights-based approach educates duty bearers about their obligations and how to meet them, and empowers people to claim their rights, which would otherwise remain far away."[68]

[68] Office of the United Nations High Commissioner for Human Rights, Scenario and talking points for High Commissioner on Human Rights event to launch the technical guidance on the application of a human rights based approach to the implementation of policies (September 2012). Available at http:llwww.ohchr.org/EN/NewsEvents/Pages/DisplayNews.aspx-?NewsJD=12559&LangJD=;

Author details

Nirmala Pillay
Leeds Law School, Leeds Beckett University, Leeds, United Kingdom

*Address all correspondence to: n.pillay@leedsbeckett.ac.uk

References

[1] Brandt AM. How AIDS invented global health. New England Journal of Medicine. 2013;**368**:2149-2152. DOI: 10.1056/NEJMp1305297

[2] Mehta A, Quinn TC. Addressing future epidemics: Historical human rights lessons from the AIDS pandemic. Pathogens and Immunity. 2016;**1**(1):2, 3, 5. Available from: www.PAIJOURNAL.COM

[3] Kirkby M. "Obituary: Dr Jonathan Mann," HIV/AIDS Legal Link [quarterly newsletter published by the Australian Federation of AIDS Councils]. 1998;**9**(4)

[4] Heywood M, Altman D. CONFRONTING AIDS: Human rights, law and social transformation. Health and Human Rights. 2000;**5**(1):150

[5] Poit P, Quinn T. Response to the global AIDs pandemic—A global health problem. The New England Journal of Medicine. 2013;**368**:2210-2218. DOI: 10.1056/NEJMra1201533

[6] Lange JMS et al. The discovery and development of antiretroviral agents. Antiviral Therapy. 2014;**19**(Suppl. 3):5-14

[7] WHO. 25 Questions and Answers on Health and Human Rights. Health and Human Rights Publication Series, No. 1. July 2002. p. 17. Available from: http://www.who.int/hhr/NEW37871OMSOK.pdf

[8] Todrys KW, Howe E, Amon JJ. Failing Siracusa: Governments' responsibility to find the least restrictive options to tuberculosis control. Public Health Action. 2013;**3**(1):7-10

[9] Constitution of the World Health Organisation. 1946. In: World Health Organisation. Basic Documents. 45th ed. Geneva: WHO; 2005

[10] Bok S. "WHO Definition of Health, Rethinking the," in International Encyclopedia of Public Health. Vol. 6 (ed. Heggenhougen and Quah). San Diego: Academic Press; 590-597

[11] Marks SP. The emergence and scope of the human right to health in Jose' M. Zuniga et al. Advancing the Human Right to Health (OUP, 2013). p. 3, 4, 17

[12] Yamin AE. A power, suffering and courts: Reflections on promoting health rights through judicialization. In: Yamin A, Gloppen S, editors. Can Courts Bring More Justice to Health? Cambridge, MA: Harvard University Press; 2011. pp. 333-372

[13] Kinney E, Clarke B. Provisions for health and health care in the constitutions of the countries of the world. Cornell International Law Journal. 2004;**37**(2)

[14] Cabrera OA, Ayala AS. Advancing the right to health through litigation. In: The Emergence and Scope of the Human Right to Health in Jose' M. Zuniga et al, Advancing the Human Right to Health (OUP, 2013). p. 26, 27

[15] Bergallo P. Courts and social change: Lessons in the struggle to universalise access to HIV/AIDS treatment in Argentina. Texas Law Review. June 2011;**89**(7)

[16] Hunt P. Forward in Jose' M. Zuniga et al, Advancing the Human Right to Health. OUP, 2013. p. vi

[17] Sumption J. Trails of the State Law and Decline of Politics. London: Profile Books Ltd; 2019. p. 29, 44, 45, 47

[18] Klare K. Legal culture and transformative constitutionalism. South African Journal of Human Rights. 1998;**14**(1):146-188

[19] Cooper C. South Africa: Health rights litigation: Cautious constitutionalism. In: Yamin AE, Gloppen S, (Eds). Litigating Health Rights. Can Courts Bring More Justice to Health? Cambridge, MA: Harvard University Press; 2011. pp. 190-229

[20] Brand J. Courts, socio-economic rights and transformative politics. PhD Thesis, Stellenbosch University quoted. In: Bohler N, Pienaar G, Davids YD (2018). Realising socioeconomic rights: A reconceptualised constitutional dialogue in Poverty and Inequality. Academia.edu. 2009. p. 123

[21] Pienaar G. Realising socioeconomic rights: A reconceptualised constitutional dialogue State of the Nation—HSRC 2018. p. 123

[22] International Council of AIDS Service Organisations. The International Guidelines on HIV/AIDS and Human Rights. How are they being used and applied? May 2002

[23] Gauri V. Social rights and economics: Claims to health care and education in developing countries. World Development. 2004;**32**(3):465-477

[24] Sarelin AL. Human rights-based approaches to development cooperation, HIV/AIDS and food security. Human Rights Quarterly. 2007:29(2):460-488, 464

[25] Harris J, Croot L, Thompson J, Springett J. How stakeholder participation can contribute to systematic reviews of complex interventions. Journal of Epidemiology and Community Health. 2016;**70**:207-214

[26] Scott J. Seeing Like a State: How Certain Schemes to Improve the Human Condition Have Failed. New Haven: Yale University Press; 1988

[27] Chopra M, Ford N. Scaling up health promotion interventions in the era of HIV/AIDS: Challenges for a rights-based approach. Health Promotion International. 2005;**20**(4):386. Available from: https://academic.oup.com/heapro/article/20/4/383/2182087

[28] WHO. "25 Questions and Answers on Health and Human Rights", Health and Human Rights Publication Series. July 2002;**1**:17. Available from: http://www.who.int/hhr/NEW37871OMSOK.pdf

[29] Yamin AE. Will we take suffering seriously? Reflections on what applying a human rights framework to health means and why we should care. Health and Human Rights. 2008;**10**(1):49

[30] Jones PS. On a never-ending waiting list: Toward equitable access to anti retroviral treatment? Experiences from Zambia. Health and Human Rights. 2005;**8**:77, 79, 136

[31] Gruskin S, Mills EJ, Tarantola D. History, principles and practice of health and human rights. Lancet. 2007;**370**:449. Available from: www.thelancet

[32] OHCHR. Frequently Asked Questions on a Human Rights-Based Approach to Development Cooperation. NY and Geneva: UN; 2006. p. 15

[33] The United Nations Population Fund. The Human Rights Based Approach to Programming. Practical Implementation Manual and Training Materials. NY: United Nations Population Fund; 2015. p. 93

[34] Chang W-C. The meaning and goals of equity in health. Journal of

Epidemiology and Community Health. 2002;**56**:488-491

[35] Hunt P, Yamin AE, Bustreo F. Making the case: What is the evidence of impact of applying human rights-based approaches to health? Health and Human Rights Journal. 2015;**17**(2):1

[36] Strangl A et al. A systematic review of selected human rights programs to improve HIV-related outcomes from 2003-2015: What do we know? BMC Infectious Diseases. 2019;**19**(209):12

[37] Noh J-E. Review of human rights-based approaches to development: Empirical evidence from developing countries. The International Journal of Human Rights. 2022;**26**(5):883-901

[38] UN Population Fund. 2015

[39] Rasanathan K et al. Realising human rights-based approaches for action on the social determinants of health. Health and Human Rights. 2010;**12**(2):49-59